Image-Based Computer-Assisted Radiation Therapy

Hidetaka Arimura
Editor

Image-Based Computer-Assisted Radiation Therapy

Springer

Editor
Hidetaka Arimura
Department of Health Sciences
Kyushu University
Fukuoka, Japan

ISBN 978-981-10-2943-1 ISBN 978-981-10-2945-5 (eBook)
DOI 10.1007/978-981-10-2945-5

Library of Congress Control Number: 2017931395

Printed on acid-free paper

This Springer imprint is published by Springer Nature
The registered company is Springer Nature Singapore Pte Ltd.
The registered company address is: 152 Beach Road, #21-01/04 Gateway East, Singapore 189721, Singapore

Foreword

Cancer incidence and death rates started to decline after 1990 in the USA, largely because of improvements in the ability to detect cancer at early stages and in more accurate disease staging, which in turn were facilitated by advances in imaging and the advent of a multidisciplinary approach to caring for patients with cancer.

At this time, early-stage cancer or small metastatic lesions can be treated by stereotactic ablative radiotherapy to the lung, liver, adrenal glands, or other organs. Some brain metastases can be also eliminated by stereotactic radiosurgery.

However, eliminating small lesions with high-dose irradiation requires that irradiation be exquisitely precise, such as that used in stereotactic radiosurgery. An important component of that precision, in terms of both killing the tumor and avoiding damage to surrounding normal tissues, is the use of imaging that combines visualization of anatomic detail (such as computed tomography [CT] or magnetic resonance imaging [MRI]) with visualization of tumor metabolism (such as positron emission tomography [PET]).

Once tumors became too large to be ablated by radiation or removed by surgery, current practice involves combining chemotherapy with radiation therapy. Chemotherapy is well known to act as a radiation sensitizer, enhancing the ability of both modalities to kill cancer cells. However, most traditional chemotherapy regimens are quite toxic to normal tissues. Improving the therapeutic ratio under these conditions will require improving the ability to kill cancer cells while reducing the toxic effects of therapy on surrounding normal cells. Before the advent of sophisticated imaging techniques for cancer diagnosis, such as CT, PET, or MRI, very large radiation treatment fields were needed to encompass areas thought to be harboring metastases or microscopic extensions of the tumor.

Now, even though we can delineate tumor extension and metastasis much more precisely with imaging, we still need histologic confirmation of small nodal metastases by means of biopsy by interventional radiologists or endoscopists.

The next step after diagnosis and staging is radiation treatment simulation, which also requires sophisticated imaging techniques such as CT, PET, or MRI depending on the site of the tumor. Sometimes, we use contrast solution for simulating treatment of gastrointestinal tumors. Another important aspect of treatment simulations is to control or account for tumors that move, such as lesions of the lung, gastrointestinal tract, or other anatomic sites. Respiration-induced motion is often accounted for with 4-dimensional CT.

Another important application of imaging is in confirming that each radiation fraction has been directed toward the appropriate target or targets. Daily imaging is used for this purpose, to account for irregularities in patient positioning or other uncertainties involved in the delivery of radiation. This is even more important for hypofractionated treatments (involving smaller numbers of larger-dose fractions), such as stereotactic radiosurgery or stereotactic ablative radiation therapy. More prolonged courses of radiation should involve verification with cone-beam CT and adjustments made or treatments replanned depending on the response of the tumor to the treatment. This is especially important for small cell lung cancer or other very radiosensitive (or chemosensitive) tumors that tend to respond to treatment quickly.

Finally, imaging is crucial for evaluating tumor response. Regardless of whether the outcome is local tumor control or ablation of distant metastasis, further improvements in treatment strategies require that we accurately—and quickly—identify tumor recurrence. If tumors recur in the middle of the radiation treatment field, then higher-dose radiation may be needed. If tumors recur at the margin, then methods for controlling tumor motion such as fiducial markers and/or larger margins would be required.

If tumors appear at distant sites before local recurrence, then more effective systemic treatments are needed. Such therapies may be based on molecular targets, tumor histopathologic characteristics, and the ability of the patient to tolerate the proposed treatment, which ideally comes from close communication with medical oncologists. Although the ability to image molecular targets is still in the development stage, the ability to visualize hypoxia or other aspects of the tumor microenvironment would be valuable as well. The use of PET, particularly uptake of the tracer by tumor or normal tissues, is being explored for its potential to predict failure sites so that the radiation dose or type of systemic treatment can be modified early in the course of the treatment. Although this topic is currently the subject of intense study, information that is gathered prospectively rather than after the fact will be crucial.

I highly recommend this book not only for radiation oncologists and radiologists but also for radiology technologists, medical physicists, medical dosimetrists, and engineers as well as for medical oncologists and surgeons, all of whom make important contributions to the multidisciplinary approach to caring for patients with cancer.

Ritsuko Komaki, MD, FACR, FASTRO

Professor,
Gloria Lupton Tennison
Distinguished Professorship
in Lung Cancer Research,
Department of Radiation Oncology
The University of Texas
MD Anderson Cancer Center
Houston, TX

Preface

X-rays were discovered by Wilhelm Conrad Röntgen in 1895, leading to the initial investigations of the ionizing effect of radiation. The effects were considered beneficial for curing malignant tumors. The applications of radiation to curing cancer around this time are relevant to the birth of radiation therapy and medical physics. In early times, medical physics appeared to be a field that combined only medicine and physics. However, current medical physics is a multidisciplinary field, which requires a wide range of knowledge, including medicine, biology, physics, chemistry, mathematics, and engineering, as shown in Fig. 1. The field of medical physics is therefore dependent on the other fields. We feel proud as medical physics researchers that outcomes from the medical physics field such as computed tomography, magnetic resonance imaging, and medical linear accelerators are so useful in clinical practice. Medical physics researchers play a bridging role between cancer patients and diagnosis or radiation therapy by discovering and investigating novel medical physics technologies that have been helpful for the detection, differentiation, and treatment of cancer. Since the editor believes that we need a wide range of knowledge (imaging, computer science, and mathematics, as well as physics and medicine) in order to perform medical physics researches, the policy in the editor's laboratory is "Diverse knowledge in various fields is better than a lot of knowledge in a specific narrow field. Multifaceted knowledge is best." (with apologies to Blaise Pascal) In spite of the fact that we need a wide range of knowledge to do medical physics researches, the academic field is still very small. That is why the editor has been attracted by this niche field, which requires the wisdom to apply diversified knowledge to problems in diagnosis and radiation therapy.

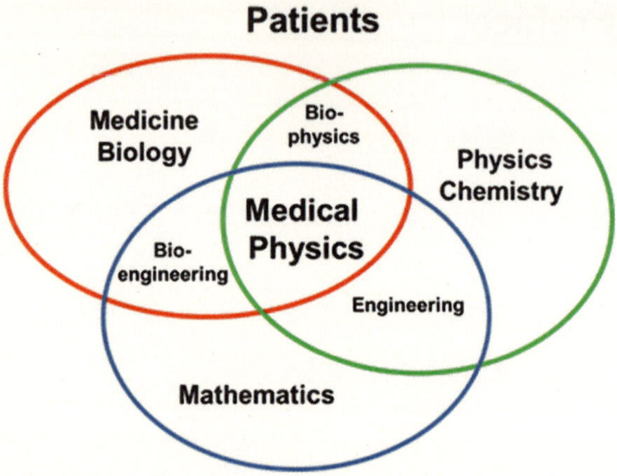

Fig. 1 Relationship between medical physics and other academic fields. Actually, there are a number of other fields, which are not shown in this figure

All the authors in this book believe that the readers will enjoy learning diverse knowledge from a wide range of fields, which they might not be familiar with, but could inspire them to do something new and unique.

Fukuoka, Japan Hidetaka Arimura

Contents

Chapter 1
Introduction

Hidetaka Arimura

Radiation therapy can ideally maintain organ functions and reduce the physical burden of patients compared with surgery, particularly elderly patients. Consequently, radiation therapy has attracted rising attention, and this modality is considerably important for developed countries that have been rapidly moving toward an aging society, such as Japan, China, Korea, European Union countries, and the United States of America. In Japan, the percentage of elderly people of 65 years old and over was estimated to be around 26.5 % in 2011 (MIC 2015). Radiation therapy can be greatly beneficial for many patients, especially elderly patients, whose quality of life could be improved.

The primary aim of radiation therapy is to deliver as a high dose as possible to a cancerous tumor, while causing as little damage as possible to normal tissues and organs at risk (OAR), in order to reduce adverse effects (Dawson and Sharpe 2006; Evans 2008). The OAR are critical organs whose radiation sensitivity may significantly influence radiation treatment planning (RTP) and/or the prescribed dose (ICRU 1999). In order to achieve the primary aim of radiation therapy, high-precision radiation therapy approaches have been developed, such as stereotactic body radiation therapy (SBRT), intensity-modulated radiation therapy (IMRT), adaptive radiotherapy (ART), real-time tumor-tracking radiotherapy (RTRT), and image-guided radiation therapy (IGRT). In recent years, these advanced approaches have led to outstanding outcomes with respect to the precision of radiation delivery. As a result, high-precision radiation therapy has been reported to provide clinical results that were comparable to surgery for some cancers (Onishi et al. 2011). In these radiation therapies, novel methods of multidimensional image analysis are used, including multimodalities, image transformation, region segmentation, pattern recognition, radiomics, and so on. These methods play considerable roles in

H. Arimura (✉)
Division of Medical Quantum Science, Department of Health Sciences, Faculty of Medical Sciences, Kyushu University, 3-1-1 Maidashi, Higashi-ku, Fukuoka 812-8582, Japan
e-mail: arimurah@med.kyushu-u.ac.jp

H. Arimura (ed.), *Image-Based Computer-Assisted Radiation Therapy*,
DOI 10.1007/978-981-10-2945-5_1

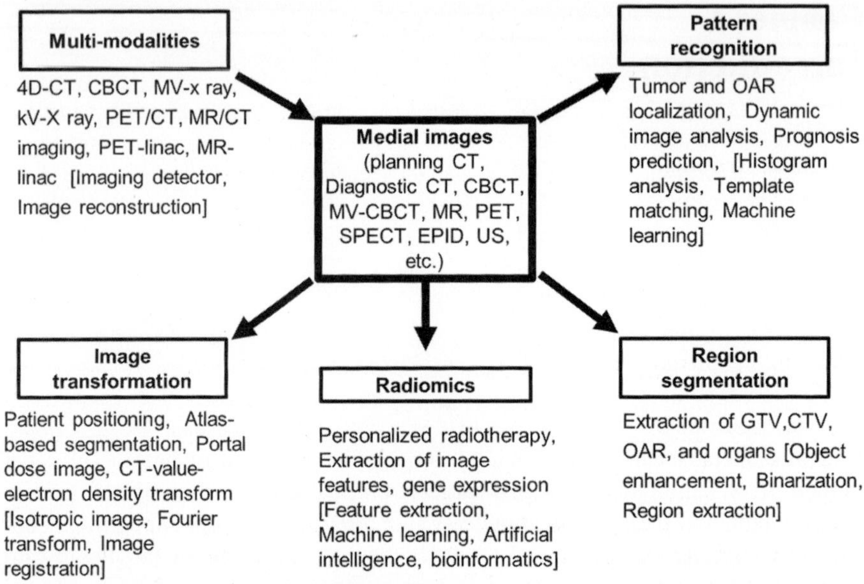

Fig. 1.1 "Harmonic" collaborations of radiation therapy with multidimensional image analysis

improving the accuracy of radiation therapy and assisting radiation oncology professionals such as radiation oncologists, radiation technologists, and medical physicists in their decision-making. Figure. 1.1 illustrates the "harmonic" collaboration of radiation therapy with multidimensional image analysis.

This book is dedicated to image-based computer-assisted radiation therapy, which requires diverse knowledge from many different fields such as imaging technology, image processing, radiation physics, radiation measurement, image registration, pattern recognition, machine learning, and radiomics. The radiation therapy procedure consists of five steps: diagnosis, treatment planning, patient setup, radiation treatment, and follow-up. The five steps of radiation therapy are shown with several approaches relevant to image-based computer-assisted radiation therapy below:

1. Diagnosing a cancer patient (computer-aided diagnosis, CAD)
2. Design of treatment plans (computer-assisted radiation treatment planning, CARTP)
3. Patient positioning (image-guided patient positioning, IGPP)
4. Performing the radiation treatment (intelligent radiation treatment systems)
5. Follow-up (computerized prediction of treatment outcomes)

The first step is to diagnose a cancer patient. Radiation oncologists should determine the treatment policies, e.g., curative treatment or palliative treatment, based on reports from radiologists. CAD systems such as automated detection and differentiation of lung cancer (Chap. 2, Suzuki) or breast cancer (Chap. 3,

Nakayama) may be helpful for the diagnosis and decision-making of treatment policies. Pathological CAD will be a significant tool for diagnostic pathology such as cancer detection, grade differentiation, and the decision of treatment approaches (Chap. 4, Yamaguchi). Recently, "radiomics" has emerged as an innovative area, which can be applied to personized medicine based on image features (phenotypes) extracted from several types of medical images (Lambin et al. 2012, Aerts et al. 2014). The radiomics has been studied to be applied to customizing radiation treatment approaches for individual patients (Chap. 14, El Naqa).

The second step is to construct the treatment plans. Radiation oncologists should estimate the regions of gross tumor volume (GTV), clinical target volume (CTV), and the OAR, and then treatment planners should design the optimum plan by changing the planning parameters so that the dose distributions for the tumor and OAR can be maximized and minimized, respectively. The GTV is defined by the gross demonstrable extent and location of a malignant growth (ICRU 1999). In current clinical practices, the GTV regions are manually delineated by radiation oncologists using treatment planning computed tomography (CT). The subjective manual contouring of tumor regions is tedious and time-consuming, and the reproducibility is relatively low, which could cause intra- and inter-variability of tumor regions (van de Steene et al. 2002; El Naqa et al. 2007; Nakamura et al. 2008). Therefore, automated frameworks for segmentation of GTVs have been developed to overcome these problems (Chap. 5, Arimura). Furthermore, computational approaches for determination of the CTV-to-PTV margins have been studied (Chap. 5, Arimura).

The determination of treatment parameters (e.g., beam arrangements in SBRT and IMRT) is a very demanding task for both inexperienced and experienced treatment planners. This may result in intra- and inter-planner variabilities of treatment plans. Computer-assisted radiation treatment planning can reduce intra- and interobserver variability of target delineations (observer noise) and the subsequent intra- and interobserver variability of the treatment plans. Actually, computer-assisted planning systems for SBRT could help treatment planners by utilizing past similar cases that are stored in treatment planning databases with knowledge and skills of treatment planners (Chap. 6, Magome). The IMRT planning approaches assist planners to automatically optimize dose distributions around the PTVs except setting of initial parameters, but it is still on trial-and-error basis (Chap. 8, Haryanto). Treatment procedures for particle beam therapy are similar to those for the photon beam therapy, but beam range (penetration depth) should be taken into account carefully in the particle beam therapy due to different physical characteristics (Chap. 7, Mori).

The third step is the patient positioning. In this step, the radiation technologist should manually position the patient as accurately as possible on the treatment couch. Correcting patient setup errors is then performed using image registration techniques. The image registration involves registering a moving image with a reference image with respect to a common object between the two images. Digitally reconstructed radiograph (DRR) images and planning CT images are generally used as the reference images to aid the patient positioning. Electronic portal imaging device (EPID) and cone-beam CT (CBCT) images are employed as the moving images at the treatment time. Past studies have revealed that these techniques are effective in reducing setup errors (Ploquin et al. 2008; Wang et al. 2009). Several techniques with the X-ray-based patient positioning have been utilized based on digitally reconstructed radiograph, cone-beam computed tomography reconstruction, and patient registration (Chap. 9, Haga). Recently, a number of optical imaging-based approaches have been researched and developed for estimation of the intra-fractional patient motion without ionizing radiation (Kang et al. 2012; Schaerer et al. 2012) (Chap. 10, Soufi).

The fourth step is to perform the radiation treatment (treatment execution). An X-ray or charged particle beam is delivered to the planning target volume (PTV) in the patient according to the treatment plan. However, it is difficult to deliver the radiation to moving tumors such as lung or liver cancers. Pattern recognition techniques, e.g., the detection of tumors and fiducial markers (e.g., gold markers), are needed to minimizing the internal margin in these cases. For example, the RTRT system employs pattern recognition techniques in order to track surrogate tumors (actually gold markers) and switch the X-ray beam on and off (Shirato et al. 2000). The real-time tumor tracking can reduce the internal margin for the PTV, which could result in sparing the healthy tissues near the tumor (Chap. 11, Ishikawa). Furthermore, the visualization approaches of dose distributions during the treatment time have been investigated to ensure the treatment quality in SBRT (Chap. 12, Nakamoto). In the proton treatment room, a beam ON-LINE PET system was constructed for dose-volume delivery-guided proton therapy by visualization of activity distribution in proton irradiation (Chap. 13, Nishio).

Finally, the fifth step is the follow-up. In this step, the radiation oncologist evaluates the treatment outcomes using multimodality imaging devices. Pattern recognition techniques have also been applied during the follow-up to predict the radiation therapy outcomes and normal tissue complications (Su et al. 2005; Kakar et al. 2009; El Naqa et al. 2009; Jayasurya et al. 2010; Atsumi et al. 2012) (Chap. 14, El Naqa).

The main requirements in radiation therapy from a medical physics point of view are (1) high conformity and homogeneity of the dose distributions to the tumor regions and (2) accurate tumor localization and patient positioning. To achieve these requirements, radiation therapy researchers have dedicated their efforts to the development of novel technologies such as conformal radiotherapy (Takahashi 1965), IMRT (Brahme 1988), RTRT (Shirato et al. 2000), and IGRT (Dawson and Sharpe 2006; Evans 2008).

The five steps of radiation therapy are covered in this book by the following chapters, each including content from dedicated authors as shown below:

1. Diagnosis of cancer patients

   - Computer-aided detection of lung cancer (Chap. 2, Kenji Suzuki)
   - Computer-aided detection and differentiation of breast cancer on mammograms (Chap. 3, Ryohei Nakayama)
   - Computer-aided differentiation for pathology images (Chap. 4, Masahiro Yamaguchi)

2. Construction of treatment plans
    - Computer-assisted target volume determination (Chap. 5, Hidetaka Arimura)
    - Computer-assisted treatment planning approaches for SBRT (Chap. 6, Taiki Magome)
    - Computer-assisted treatment planning approaches for carbon-ion beam therapy (Chap. 7, Shinichiro Mori)
    - Computer-assisted treatment planning approaches for IMRT (Chap. 8, Freddy Haryanto)
3. Patient positioning
    - X-ray image-based positioning (Chap. 9, Akihiro Haga)
    - Surface-imaging-based patient positioning in radiation therapy (Chap. 10, Mazen Soufi)
4. Performing of radiation treatments
    - Tumor tracking approaches (Chap. 11, Masayori Ishikawa)
    - Visualization of dose distributions for photon beam radiation therapy during treatment delivery (Chap. 12, Takahiro Nakamoto)
    - Visualization of dose distributions for proton (Chap. 13, Teiji Nishio)
5. Follow-up: Prediction of treatment outcomes
    - Computerized prediction of treatment outcomes and radiomics analysis (Chap. 14, Issam El Naqa)

Epoch-making innovations caused by a new type of researchers encourage paradigm shifts to higher levels. They always make leaps or quantum jumps in science. I believe that all the authors are this type of researchers. They have collaborated in this book to open a new field of medical physics.

References

Aerts HJ, Velazquez ER, Leijenaar RT, Parmar C, Grossmann P, Carvalho S, Bussink J, Monshouwer R, Haibe-Kains B, Rietveld D, Hoebers F, Rietbergen MM, Leemans CR, Dekker A, Quackenbush J, Gillies RJ, Lambin P (2014) Decoding tumour phenotype by noninvasive imaging using a quantitative radiomics approach. Nat Commun 5:4006. doi:10.1038/ncomms5006

Atsumi K, Shioyama Y, Arimura H et al (2012) Esophageal stenosis associated with tumor regression in radiation therapy for esophageal cancer: frequency and prediction. Int J Radiat Oncol Biol Phys 82(5):1973–1980

Brahme A (1988) Optimization of stationary and moving beam radiation therapy techniques. Radiother Oncol 12(2):129–140

Dawson LA, Sharpe MB (2006) Image-guided radiotherapy: rationale, benefits, and limitations. Lancet Oncol 7(10):848–858

El Naqa I, Yang D, Apte A et al (2007) Concurrent multimodality image segmentation by active contours for radiotherapy treatment planning. Med Phys 34(2):4738–4749

El Naqa I, Bradley JD, Lindsay PE et al (2009) Predicting radiotherapy outcomes using statistical learning techniques. Phys Med Biol 54(18):S9–S30

Evans PM (2008) Anatomical imaging for radiotherapy. Phys Med Biol 53(12):R151–R191

International Commission on Radiation Units & Measurements (ICRU) (1999) Prescribing, Recording and Reporting Photon Beam Therapy, (Supplement to ICRU Report 50) ICRU Report, vol 62. Bethesda, ICRU

Jayasurya K, Fung G, Yu S et al (2010) Comparison of Bayesian network and support vector machine models for two-year survival prediction in lung cancer patients treated with radiotherapy. Med Phys 37(4):1401–1407

Kakar M, Seierstad T, Røe K et al (2009) Artificial neural networks for prediction of response to chemoradiation in HT29 xenografts. Int J Radiat Oncol Biol Phys 75(2):506–511

Kang HJ, Grelewicz Z, Wiersma RD (2012) Development of an automated region of interest selection method for 3D surface monitoring of head motion. Med Phys 39(6):3270–3282

Lambin P, Rios-Velazquez E, Leijenaar R, Carvalho S, van Stiphout RG, Granton P, Zegers CM, Gillies R, Boellard R, Dekker A, Aerts HJ (2012) Radiomics: extracting more information from medical images using advanced feature analysis. Eur J Cancer 48(4):441–446

Ministry of Internal Affairs and Communications (MIC) (2015) http://www.stat.go.jp/data/jinsui/pdf/201512.pdf

Nakamura K, Shioyama Y, Tokumaru S et al (2008) Variation of clinical target volume definition among Japanese radiation oncologist in external beam radiotherapy for prostate cancer. Jpn J Clin Oncol 38(4):275–280

Onishi H, Shirato H, Nagata Y et al (2011) Stereotactic body radiotherapy (SBRT) for operable stage I non-small-cell lung cancer: can SBRT be comparable to surgery? Int J Radiat Oncol Biol Phys 81:1352–1358

Ploquin N, Rangel A, Dunscombe P (2008) Phantom evaluation of a commercially available three modality image guided radiation therapy system. Med Phys 35(12):5303–5311

Schaerer J, Fassi A, Riboldi M et al (2012) Multi-dimensional respiratory motion tracking from markerless optical surface imaging based on deformable mesh registration. Phys Med Biol 57:357–373

Shirato H, Shimizu S, Kitamura K et al (2000) Four-dimensional treatment planning and fluoroscopic real-time tumor tracking radiotherapy for moving tumor. Int J Radiat Oncol Biol Phys 48:435–442

Su M, Miften M, Whiddon C et al (2005) An artificial neural network for predicting the incidence of radiation pneumonitis. Med Phys 32(2):318–325

Takahashi S (1965) Conformation radiotherapy rotation techniques as applied to radiography and radiotherapy of cancer. Acta Radiol Suppl 242:1–142

van de Steene J, Linthout N, de Mey J, Vinh-Hung V, Claassens C, Noppen M, Bel A, Storme G (2002) Definition of gross tumor volume in lung cancer: inter-observer variability. Radiother Oncol 62:37–49

Wang Z, Nelson JW, Yoo S et al (2009) Refinement of treatment setup and target localization accuracy using three-dimensional cone-beam computed tomography for stereotactic body radiotherapy. Int J Radiat Oncol Biol Phys 73(2):571–577

Part I
Computerized Diagnosis for Cancer

Chapter 2
Computer-Aided Detection of Lung Cancer

Kenji Suzuki

Abstract As medical imaging technologies advance, a large number of medical images are produced which physicians/radiologists must interpret. Consequently, computer aids are becoming indispensable in physicians' decision-making based on medical images. Computer-aided diagnosis (CAD) has been investigated and becomes an active research area in medical imaging. CAD is defined as detection and/or diagnosis made by a radiologist/physician who takes into account the computer output as a "second opinion." In CAD research, detection of lung cancer in thoracic imaging constitutes a major research area, because lung cancer is the leading cause of cancer death worldwide, including the United States, Japan, and other countries. In this chapter, CAD for the detection of lung cancer in thoracic computed tomography (CT) is overviewed with emphasis on machine learning that plays an essential role in CAD systems. Massive training artificial neural network (MTANN) technology is one of the most promising machine learning techniques in image analysis. The MTANNs have substantially improved the sensitivity and specificity of CAD systems in detection and diagnosis of lung cancer. MTANN CAD systems offer high performance in detection and diagnosis of lung cancer in CT. Thus, MTANN CAD systems would be useful for improving the diagnostic performance of radiologists/physicians in early detection of lung cancer.

Keywords Computer-aided detection • Computer-aided diagnosis • Screening • Lung nodule • Thoracic CT • Classifier • Pixel-based machine learning • Machine learning in medical imaging • Patch-based machine learning • Image-based artificial neural network • Massive training artificial neural network

K. Suzuki, Ph.D. (✉)
Medical Imaging Research Center & Department of Electrical and Computer Engineering, Illinois Institute of Technology, 3440 South Dearborn Street, Chicago, IL 60616, USA
e-mail: ksuzuki@iit.edu

H. Arimura (ed.), *Image-Based Computer-Assisted Radiation Therapy*,
DOI 10.1007/978-981-10-2945-5_2

2.1 Introduction

2.1.1 CAD Field

Medical imaging has been indispensable in modern medicine since the discovery of x-rays by Wilhelm C. Röntgen in 1895. Medical imaging provides helpful information on medical conditions of patients and clues to causes of their diseases and symptoms. Medical imaging has unique advantages in the localization of lesions, diseases, and/or causes of symptoms over other examinations such as blood tests. As imaging technologies have been advancing, a large number of medical images are produced which physicians/radiologists have to read and interpret. Thus, computer aids have been strongly demanded by physicians and radiologists, and they are becoming indispensable in physicians' decision-making based on medical images. Consequently, computer-aided detection and diagnosis (CAD) (Giger and Suzuki 2007; Doi 2005; Doi 2007; Giger et al. 2008) have been an active research area in medical imaging. CAD is defined as detection and/or diagnosis made by a radiologist/physician who takes into account the computer output as a "second opinion" (Doi 2005). CAD is often categorized into two major groups: computer-aided detection (CADe) and computer-aided diagnosis (CADx). CADe focuses on a detection task, i.e., detection (or localization) of lesions in medical images. CADx focuses on a diagnosis (characterization) task, e.g., classification among different lesion types and distinction between malignant and benign lesions.

The history of CAD started in 1955. A radiologist, Lee Lusted, mentioned the potential use of digital computers (people at that time called ordinary computers today as digital computers, as there were analog computers.) for large-scale data problems in medicine in (Lusted 1955) in 1955. Notably, it was only 9 years after the first general-purpose computer, ENIAC, was introduced in 1946. Becker et al. developed an automated measurement of the cardiothoracic ratio in chest radiographs in 1964 (Becker et al. 1964; Meyers et al. 1964). In 1967, the first study on CADe of abnormalities in mammograms was published by Winsberg et al. (1967). In 1973, Toriwaki et al. (1973) reported the first study on CADe of a focal abnormality in chest radiographs, and Roellinger et al. (1973) reported the first study on CADe of a heart abnormality in chest radiographs. In the mid-1980s, investigators in the Kurt Rossmann Laboratories in the Department of Radiology at the University of Chicago began studies on the development and evaluation of CAD. Chan et al. (1987), Fujita et al. (1987), Giger et al. (1988), and Katsuragawa et al. (1988) published a series of papers on CADe of microcalcifications in mammography, CAD for vessel size measurement in angiography, CADe of lung nodules in chest radiography, and CADe of interstitial lung disease in chest radiography, respectively. In 1988, a venture company, R2 Technology (acquired by Hologic), which obtained licenses for CAD technologies from the University of Chicago, received approval for the first commercial CAD system for mammography from the US Food and Drug Administration (FDA).

2.1.2 *Overview of CADe for Lung Cancer Detection*

Lung cancer continues to rank as the leading cause of cancer death in the United States and in other countries such as Japan. Some evidence suggests that early detection of lung cancer may allow more timely therapeutic intervention and thus a more favorable prognosis for the patient. Because CT is more sensitive than chest radiography in the detection of small nodules (i.e., potential lung cancer) and of lung carcinoma at an early stage (Kaneko et al. 1996; Sone et al. 1998; Henschke et al. 1999; Miettinen and Henschke 2001), lung cancer screening programs were conducted in the United States (Swensen et al. 2003; Henschke et al. 2004), Japan (Kaneko et al. 1996; Sone et al. 1998), and other countries with low-dose helical CT as the screening modality. Helical CT, however, generates a large number of images that must be read by radiologists. This may lead to "information overload" for the radiologists. Furthermore, radiologists may miss some cancers during interpretation of CT images. Therefore, a CAD scheme for the detection of lung nodules in low-dose CT images has been investigated as a useful tool for lung cancer screening.

Many investigators have developed a number of methods for the automated detection of lung nodules on CT scans (Suzuki 2012b). In 1994, Giger et al. (1994) developed a CADe scheme for the detection of lung nodules in CT based on the comparison of geometric features. They applied their CADe scheme to a database of thick-slice diagnostic CT scans of eight patients with 47 nodules. They achieved a sensitivity of 94 % with 1.25 false positives (FPs) per case. In 1999, Armato et al. (1999, 2001) extended the method to include 3D feature analysis, a rule-based scheme, and linear discriminant analysis (LDA) for classification. They tested their CADe scheme with a database of thick-slice diagnostic CT scans of 43 patients with 171 nodules. They achieved a sensitivity of 70 % with 42.2 FPs per case in a leave-one-out cross-validation test. Gurcan et al. (2002) employed a similar approach, i.e., a rule-based scheme based on 2D and 3D features, followed by LDA for classification. They achieved a sensitivity of 84 % with 74.4 FPs per case for a database of thick-slice (mostly 5 mm) diagnostic CT scans of 34 patients with 63 nodules in a leave-one-out test. Lee et al. (2001) employed a simpler approach which is a rule-based scheme based on 13 features for classification. They achieved a sensitivity of 72 % with 30.6 FPs per case for a database of thick-slice (10 mm) diagnostic CT scans of 20 patients with 98 nodules.

Suzuki et al. (2003a) developed a pixel-based machine learning technique called a massive training artificial neural network (MTANN) for reduction of a single source of FPs and a multiple MTANN scheme for reduction of multiple sources of FPs that had not been removed by feature-based LDA. They achieved a sensitivity of 80.3 % with 4.8 FPs per case for a database of thick-slice (10 mm) screening low-dose CT (LDCT) scans of 63 patients with 71 nodules with solid, part-solid, and nonsolid patterns, including 66 cancers in a validation test. This MTANN approach did not require a large number of training cases: the MTANN was able to be trained with ten positive and ten negative cases (Suzuki and Doi 2005), whereas feature-based classifiers generally require 400–800 training cases (Chan et al. 1999; Sahiner et al. 2008). Arimura et al. (2004) employed a rule-based scheme followed by LDA or by an MTANN (Suzuki et al. 2003a) for classification. They tested their scheme with a database of 106 thick-slice (10 mm) screening LDCT scans of 73 patients with 109 cancers that had solid, part-solid, and nonsolid patterns, and they achieved a sensitivity of 83 % with 5.8 FPs per case in a validation test (or a leave-one-patient-out test for LDA). Farag et al. (2005) developed a template modeling approach that uses level sets for classification. They achieved a sensitivity of 93.3 % with an FP rate of 3.4 % for a database of thin-slice (2.5 mm) screening LDCT scans of 16 patients with 119 nodules and 34 normal patients. Ge et al. (2005) incorporated 3D gradient field descriptors and ellipsoid features in LDA for classification. They employed Wilks' lambda stepwise feature selection for selecting features before the LDA classification. They achieved a sensitivity of 80 % with 14.7 FPs per case for a database of 82 thin-slice (1.0–2.5 mm) CT scans of 56 patients with 116 solid nodules in a leave-one-patient-out test. Matsumoto et al. (2006) employed LDA with eight features for classification. They achieved a sensitivity of 90 % with 64.1 FPs per case for a database of thick-slice (5 or 7 mm) diagnostic CT scans of five patients (four of which used contrast media) with 50 nodules in a leave-one-out test.

Yuan et al. (2006) tested a commercially available CADe system (ImageChecker CT, LN-1000, by R2 Technology, Sunnyvale, CA; acquired by Hologic). They achieved a sensitivity of 73 % with 3.2 FPs per case for a database of thin-slice (1.25 mm) CT scans of 150 patients with 628 nodules in an independent test. Pu et al. (2008) developed a scoring method based on the similarity distance of medial axis-like shapes for classification. They achieved a sensitivity of 81.5 % with 6.5 FPs per case for a database of thin-slice (2.5 mm) screening CT scans of 52 patients with 184 nodules, including 16 nonsolid nodules. Retico et al. (2008) used a voxel-based neural approach (i.e., a class of the MTANN approach) with pixel values in a subvolume as input for classification. They obtained sensitivities of 80–85 % with 10–13 FPs per case for a database of thin-slice (1 mm) screening CT scans of 39 patients with 102 nodules. Ye et al. (2009) used a rule-based scheme followed by a weighted SVM for classification. They achieved a sensitivity of 90.2 % with 8.2 FPs per case for a database of thin-slice (1 mm) screening CT scans of 54 patients with 118 nodules including 17 nonsolid nodules in an independent test. Golosio et al. (2009) used a fixed-topology ANN for classification, and they evaluated their CADe scheme with a publicly available database from the Lung Image Database Consortium (LIDC) (Armato et al. 2004). They achieved a sensitivity of 79 % with 4 FPs per case for a database of thin-slice (1.5–3.0 mm) CT scans of 83 patients with 148 nodules that one radiologist detected from an LIDC database in an independent test.

Murphy et al. (2009) used a k-nearest neighbor classifier with features selected from 135 features for classification. They achieved a sensitivity of 80 with 4.2 FPs per case for a large database of thin-slice screening CT scans of 813 patients with 1525 nodules in an independent test. Tan et al. (2011) developed a feature-selective classifier based on a genetic algorithm and ANNs for classification. They achieved a sensitivity of 87.5 % with 4 FPs per case for a database of thin-slice CT scans of 125 patients with 80 nodules that four radiologists agreed from the LIDC database in an independent test. Messay et al. (2010) developed a sequential forward selection process for selecting the optimum features for LDA and quadratic discriminant analysis (QDA). They obtained a sensitivity of 83 % with 3 FPs per case for a database of thin-slice CT scans of 84 patients with 143 nodules from the LIDC database in a sevenfold cross-validation test. Riccardi et al. (2011) used a heuristic approach based on geometric features, followed by an SVM for classification. They achieved a sensitivity of 71 % with 6.5 FPs per case for a database of thin-slice CT scans of 154 patients with 117 nodules that four radiologists agreed on from the LIDC database in a twofold cross-validation test.

Thus, various approaches have been proposed for CADe schemes for lung nodules in CT. Sensitivities for detection of lung nodules in CT range from 70 to 95 %, with FPs from a few to 70 per case. Major sources of FPs are various-sized lung vessels. Major sources of false negatives are ground-glass nodules, nodules attached to vessels, and nodules attached to the lung wall (i.e., juxtapleural nodules). Ground-glass nodules are difficult to detect, because they are subtle, of low-contrast, and have ill-defined boundaries. The MTANN approach was able to enhance and thus detect ground-glass nodules (Suzuki et al. 2003a). The cause of false negatives due to vessel-attached nodules and juxtapleural nodules is mis-segmentation and thus inaccurate feature calculation. Because the MTANN approach does not require segmentation or feature calculation, it was able to detect such nodules (Suzuki et al. 2003a).

2.1.3 Overview of CADx for Lung Cancer Diagnosis

Although CT has been shown to be sensitive to the detection of lung nodules, it may be difficult for radiologists to distinguish between benign and malignant nodules on LDCT images. In a screening program with LDCT in New York, 88 % (206/233) of suspicious lesions were found to be benign on follow-up examinations (Henschke et al. 1999). In a screening program in Japan, only 83 (10 %) among 819 scans with suspicious lesions were diagnosed to be cancer cases (Li et al. 2002). According to findings at the Mayo Clinic, 2792 (98.6 %) of 2832 nodules detected by a multidetector CT were benign, and 40 (1.4 %) nodules were malignant (Swensen et al. 2003). Thus, a large number of benign nodules were found with CT; follow-up examinations such as high-resolution CT (HRCT) and/or biopsy were performed on these patients. Therefore, CADx schemes for distinction between benign and malignant nodules in LDCT would be useful for reducing the number of "unnecessary" follow-up examinations.

A number of researchers developed CADx schemes for distinguishing malignant nodules from benign nodules automatically and/or determining the likelihood of malignancy for the detected nodules. The performance of the schemes was generally evaluated by using receiver operating characteristic (ROC) analysis (Metz

1986), because this task is a two-class classification. The area under the ROC curve (AUC) (Hanley and Mcneil 1983) was often used as a performance index.

In 1999, McNitt-Gray et al. (1999) developed a classification scheme based on LDA for distinction between malignant and benign nodules in HRCT. They achieved a correct classification rate of 90.3 % for a database of 17 malignant and 14 benign nodules. Matsuki et al. (2002) used an ANN with subjective features determined by radiologists for classification between 99 malignant and 56 benign nodules in HRCT and achieved an AUC value of 0.951. Aoyama et al. (2002) used LDA for distinction between malignant and benign nodules in thick-slice (10 mm) screening LDCT. They achieved an AUC value of 0.846 for a database of 73 patients with 76 primary cancers and 342 patients with 413 benign nodules. Mori et al. (2005) developed a classification scheme for distinction between malignant and benign nodules in contrast-enhanced (CE) CT by using LDA with three features (i.e., attenuation, shape index, and curvedness value). They used a database of thin-slice (2 mm) CE-CT scans of 35 malignant and 27 benign nodules for testing their CADx scheme. They achieved AUC values of 0.91 and 1.0 with non-CE-CT and CE-CT, respectively, in a leave-one-out test.

Shah et al. (2005) employed different classifiers such as logistic regression and QDA with features selected from a group of 31 by using stepwise feature selection based on the Akaike information criterion. Their scheme with logistic regression achieved an AUC value of 0.92 in the distinction between 19 malignant and 16 benign nodules in thin-slice CE-CT. Suzuki et al. (2005a) developed a pixel-based machine-learning technique called a multiple MTANN scheme for the classification task. They achieved an AUC value of 0.88 for thick-slice screening LDCT scans of 73 patients with 76 primary cancers and 342 patients with 413 benign nodules. Iwano et al. (2008) achieved a sensitivity of 76.9 % and a specificity of 80 % with their scheme based on LDA with two features in their evaluation of HRCT images of 52 malignant and 55 benign nodules. Way et al. (2009) incorporated nodule surface features into their classification based on LDA or an SVM, and they achieved an AUC value of 0.857 in the classification of 124 malignant and 132 benign nodules in 152 patients. Chen et al. (Chen et al. 2010) employed an ANN ensemble to classify 19 malignant and 13 benign nodules, and they achieved an AUC value of 0.915. Lee et al. (2010) developed a two-step supervised learning scheme combining a genetic algorithm with a random subspace method, and they achieved an AUC value of 0.889 in the classification between 62 malignant and 63 benign nodules.

Thus, various approaches to CADx schemes have been proposed. The database size varied in different studies; CT scans in the databases included screening LDCT, standard diagnostic CT, and HRCT. This chapter does not review CADx due to the limitation of the space, but focuses on CADe.

2.2 Generic Architectures of CADe Schemes

2.2.1 Generic Architecture

A flowchart for a generic CADe scheme of lesions in medical images is shown in Fig. 2.1. A CADe scheme generally consists of seven major steps: (1) segmentation of the organ(s) of interest, (2) enhancement of lesions, (3) detection of lesion candidates from the segmented organ, (4) segmentation of the detected lesion candidates, (5) feature analysis of the segmented lesion candidates, (6) classification of the lesion candidates by using a classifier with features, and (7) reduction of false-positive (FP) detections. Segmentation of the organ(s) of interest is the first necessary step that aims to make the rest of the steps focus on the organ(s). The development of the detection of lesion candidates generally aims to obtain a high sensitivity level, because we cannot recover a sensitivity loss in this step in the later steps. In the next step, the detected lesion candidates are segmented, and connected-component labeling (He et al. 2009; Suzuki et al. 2003b) is performed for the identification of each segmented candidate as an individual isolated object. Pattern features such as gray-level-based features, texture features, and morphologic features are extracted from the segmented candidates. Feature selection (Xu and Suzuki 2014) is generally performed to select a subset of "effective" features from an entire set of features to remove redundant or unnecessary features. Finally,

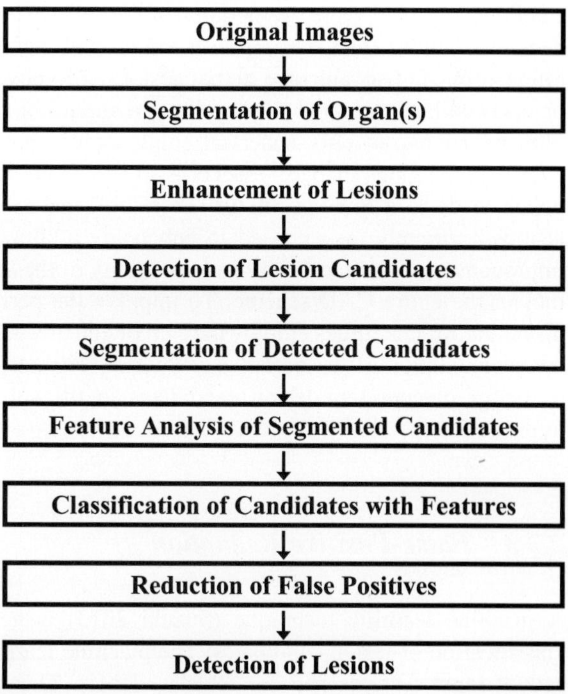

Fig. 2.1 Flowchart for a generic CADe scheme for detection of lesions in medical images

the detected lesion candidates are classified into lesions or non-lesions by using a classifier with the extracted features. The development of the classification step aims to remove as many non-lesions (i.e., FPs) as possible, while minimizing the removal of lesions (i.e., true-positive detections).

2.2.2 Enhancement of Lesions in CADe

Among the steps in CADe schemes, thresholding-based methods such as multiple thresholding (Xu et al. 1997; Aoyama et al. 2002; Bae et al. 2002; Giger et al. 1988) are often used for detection of lesion candidates in CT. With such methods, the specificity can generally be low, because normal structures of gray levels similar to those of lesions could be detected erroneously as lesions. To obtain a high specificity as well as sensitivity, some researchers employ a filter for enhancement of lesions before the lesion candidate detection step. Such a filter aims at enhancement of lesions and sometimes the suppression of noise. The filter enhances objects similar to a model employed in the filter. For example, a blob enhancement filter based on the Hessian matrix enhances sphere-like objects (Frangi et al. 1999). A difference image technique employs a filter designed for the enhancement of nodules and the suppression of noise in chest radiographs (Xu et al. 1997).

Actual lesions, however, are not simple enough to be modeled accurately by a simple equation in many cases. For example, a lung nodule is generally modeled as a solid sphere, but there are nodules of various shapes and with internal inhomogeneities such as spiculated opacity and ground-glass opacity. Thus, conventional filters often fail to enhance actual lesions. Moreover, such filters enhance any objects similar to a model employed in the filter. For example, a blob enhancement filter enhances not only spherical solid nodules but also any spherical parts of objects in the lungs such as vessel crossing, vessel branching, and a part of a vessel, which leads to a low specificity. Therefore, methods which can enhance actual lesions accurately (as opposed to enhancing a simple model) are demanded for improvement of the sensitivity and specificity of the lesion candidate detection and thus of the entire CAD scheme. To improve the performance of CADe schemes, investigators sometimes employ the step of enhancement of lesions after the step of the segmentation of the organ(s) of interest. This step aims to improve the sensitivity for detection of lesion candidates in the subsequent step. It often helps improve the specificity as well.

2.2.3 False-Positive Reduction

A machine learning technique (Suzuki 2013) is generally used in the step of classification of lesion candidates. The machine learning technique is trained with sets of input features and correct class labels. This class of machine learning is referred to as feature-based machine learning or simply as a classifier. The task of the machine learning here is to determine "optimal" boundaries for separating classes in the multidimensional feature space which is formed by the input features (Duda et al. 2001). Feature-based machine-learning algorithms include linear discriminant analysis (LDA) (Fukunaga 1990), quadratic discriminant analysis (QDA) (Fukunaga 1990), multilayer perceptron (one of the most popular artificial neural network (ANN) models) (Rumelhart et al. 1986), support vector machines (SVMs) (Vapnik 1995), and random forests. The structure of an ANN may be designed by using an automated design method such as sensitivity analysis (Suzuki et al. 2001; Suzuki 2004).

Investigators often employ an additional step of the reduction of FPs at the end in a CADe scheme. The FP reduction step aims to improve the specificity of the CADe scheme. Reduction of FPs is very important, because a large number of FPs could adversely affect the clinical application of CADe. A large number of FPs are likely to confound the radiologist's task of image interpretation and thus lower his/her efficiency. In addition, radiologists may lose their confidence in CADe as a useful tool.

Recently, as available computational power has increased dramatically, pixel-/patch-based machine learning (Suzuki 2012a) emerged in medical image processing/analysis which uses pixel values in images directly, instead of features calculated from segmented regions, as input information; thus, feature calculation or segmentation is not required. Pixel-/patch-based machine learning has been used in the classification of the detected lesion candidates in CADe and CADx schemes (Suzuki et al. 2003a, 2005a, b, 2006b, 2008b, 2010a; Arimura et al. 2004).

2.3 Supervised "Lesion Enhancement" MTANN Filter

We believe that enhancing actual lesions requires some form of "learning from examples"; thus, machine learning plays an essential role in this task. To enhance actual lesions accurately, we developed a supervised filter based on a machine-learning technique called a massive training artificial neural network (MTANN) (Suzuki et al. 2003a) filter in a CADe scheme for the detection of lung nodules in CT. By extension of "neural filters" (Suzuki et al. 2002a, b) and "neural edge enhancers" (Suzuki et al. 2003c, 2004b), which are ANN-based (Rumelhart et al. 1986) supervised nonlinear image-processing techniques, MTANNs (Suzuki et al. 2003a) have been developed for accommodating the task of distinguishing a specific opacity from other opacities in medical images. MTANNs have been applied for the reduction of false positives (FPs) in CADe of lung nodules in low-dose CT (Arimura et al. 2004; Suzuki et al. 2003a) and chest radiography (Suzuki et al. 2005b), for distinction between benign and malignant lung nodules in CT (Suzuki et al. 2005a), for enhancement of lung nodules in CT (Suzuki 2009), for suppression of ribs in chest radiographs (Suzuki et al. 2004a, 2006a; Chen et al.

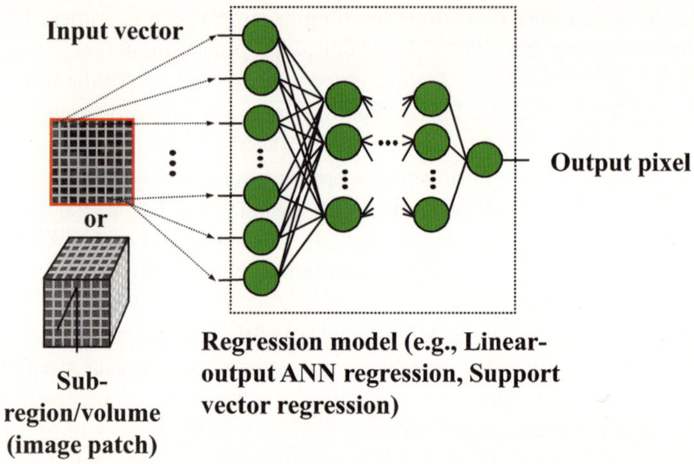

Fig. 2.2 Architecture of an MTANN consisting of a linear-output ANN regression model with multiple layers, with subregion/volume input and single-pixel output

2016; Chen and Suzuki 2013, 2014), and for reduction of FPs in computerized detection of nodules in CT colonography (Suzuki et al. 2006b, 2008b, 2010a, b).

2.3.1 Architecture of an MTANN Filter

The architecture of an MTANN supervised filter is shown in Fig. 2.2. An MTANN filter consists of a supervised regression model such as a linear-output ANN regression model (Suzuki et al. 2003c) which is a regression-type ANN capable of operating on pixel data directly. The MTANN filter is trained with input CT images and the corresponding "teaching" images that contain a map for the "likelihood of being lesions." The pixel values of the input images are linearly scaled such that –1000 Hounsfield units (HUs) correspond to 0 and 1000 HUs correspond to 1. The input to the MTANN filter consists of pixel values in a subregion/volume (image patch), V_S, extracted from an input image. The output of the MTANN filter is a continuous scalar value, which is associated with the center pixel in the subregion/volume (image patch) and is represented by

$$O(x, y, z) = NN\left(\vec{I}_{x,y,z}\right), \tag{2.1}$$

where

$$\vec{I}_{x,y,z} = \{I(x-i, y-j, z-k)|i, j, k \in V_S\} \tag{2.2}$$

is the input vector to the MTANN; x, y, and z are the coordinate indices; $NN(\cdot)$ is the output of a supervised regression model (e.g., linear-output ANN regression model); i, j, and k are the coordinate indices in V_s; and $I(x,y,z)$ is the normalized voxel value of the input isotropic volume. The linear-output ANN regression employs a linear function,$f_L(u) = a \cdot u + 0.5$, instead of a sigmoid function, $f_S(u) = 1/\{1 + \exp(-u)\}$, as the activation function of the output layer unit because the characteristics and performance of an ANN are improved significantly with a linear function when applied to the continuous mapping of values in image processing (Suzuki et al. 2003c). Note that the activation function in the hidden layers is still a sigmoid function. For processing of the entire image, the scanning of an input CT image with the MTANN is performed pixel by pixel, as illustrated in Fig. 2.3b.

2.3.2 *Training of an MTANN Filter*

For the enhancement of lesions and suppression of non-lesions in CT images, the teaching image $T(x,y,z)$ contains a map of the "likelihood of being lesions," as illustrated in Fig. 2.3a. To create the teaching image, we first segment lesions manually for obtaining a binary image with 1 being lesion pixels and 0 being non-lesion pixels. Then, Gaussian smoothing is applied to the binary image for smoothing down the edges of the segmented lesions, because the likelihood of being lesions should gradually be smaller as the distance from the boundary of the lesion decreases.

The MTANN filter involves training with a large number of pairs of subregions/volumes (image patches) and pixels/voxels. For enrichment of the training samples, a training image, V_T, extracted from the input CT image is divided pixel by pixel into a large number of subregions/volumes (image patches). Note that close subregions/volumes overlap each other. Single pixels are extracted from the corresponding teaching image as teaching values. The MTANN filter is massively trained by use of each of a large number of input subregions/volumes (image patches) together with each of the corresponding teaching single pixels/voxels, hence the term "massive training ANN." The error to be minimized by training of the MTANN filter is given by

$$E = \frac{1}{P}\sum_{c}\sum_{x,y,z\in V_T} \{T_c(x,y,z) - O_c(x,y,z)\}^2, \qquad (2.3)$$

where c is a training case number and P is the number of total training voxels in V_T. The MTANN filter is trained by a linear-output backpropagation algorithm (Suzuki et al. 1995, 2003c) where the generalized delta rule (Rumelhart et al. 1986) is applied to the linear-output ANN architecture (Suzuki et al. 2003c), which was derived for the linear-output ANN model by using the same method used for deriving the original BP algorithm (Rumelhart et al. 1986) (see Refs. (Suzuki et al. 1995, 2003c,) for the details and the property of the linear-output BP

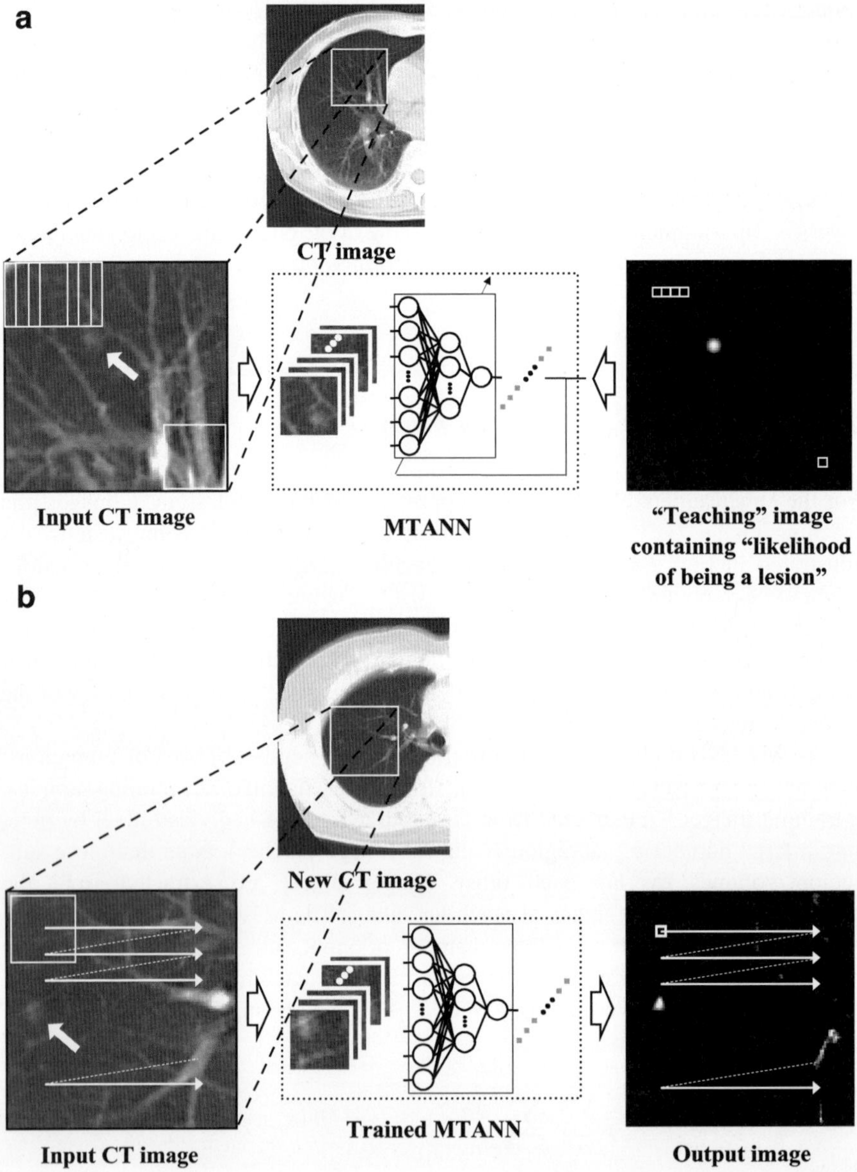

Fig. 2.3 Training and application of an MTANN filter for enhancement of lesions. (**a**) Training of an MTANN filter. (**b**) Application of the trained MTANN filter to a new CT image

algorithm). After training, the MTANN filter is expected to output the highest value when a lesion is located at the center of the subregion of the MTANN filter, a lower value as the distance from the subregion center increases, and zero when the input subregion contains a non-lesion.

In the computer vision field, a technology called deep learning (Lecun et al. 2015; Mnih et al. 2015) or deep convolutional neural networks (Krizhevsky et al. 2012) obtained enthusiastic attentions from the research communities and industries. The deep convolutional neural networks (Krizhevsky et al. 2012) were able to classify objects in images 20 % more correctly than did other existing classifiers that had been studied in the field in the past three decades. The MTANN approach is similar to deep convolutional neural networks, as both use image patches as input, but there are differences: (1) the output of the MTANN is images, whereas that of deep learning is class labels (e.g., cancer or non-cancer); (2) the MTANN can do image processing and pattern enhancement, but deep learning cannot; (3) the MTANN requires a very small number of training samples, but deep learning requires a million of samples; and (4) the MTANN has simpler architecture and training and thus easy to train.

2.3.3 Experiments

2.3.3.1 Database of Lung Nodules in CT

To test the performance of the MTANN filter, we applied it to our CT database consisting of 69 lung cancers in 69 patients (Li et al. 2002). The scans used for this study were acquired with a low-dose protocol of 120 kVp, 25 mA or 50 mA, 10 mm collimation, and 10 mm reconstruction interval at a helical pitch of two. The reconstructed CT images were 512 x 512 pixels in size with a section thickness of 10 mm. The 69 CT scans consisted of 2052 sections (slices). All cancers were confirmed either by biopsy or surgically. The locations of the cancers were determined by an expert chest radiologist.

2.3.3.2 Enhancement of Nodules in the Lungs in CT

To limit processing area to the lungs, we segmented the lung regions in a CT image by the use of thresholding based on Otsu's threshold value determination (Otsu 1979). Then, we applied a "rolling-ball" technique (Hanson 1992), which is a mathematical morphology operator, along the outlines of the extracted lung regions to include a nodule attached to the pleura in the segmented lung regions (Armato et al., 2001).

To enhance lung nodules in CT images, we trained an MTANN filter with 13 lung nodules in a training database which was different from the testing database and the corresponding "teaching" images that contained maps for the "likelihood of being nodules," as illustrated in Fig. 2.3a. To obtain the training regions, V_T, we applied a mathematical morphology opening operator to the lung nodules that were segmented manually (i.e., binary regions) such that the training regions sufficiently covered nodules and surrounding normal structures. The number of hidden units was selected to be 20 by use of a method for designing the structure of an ANN (Suzuki et al. 2001; Suzuki 2004). The method is a sensitivity-based pruning method, i.e., the sensitivity to the training error was calculated when a certain unit was removed experimentally, and the unit with the smallest training error was removed. Removing the redundant hidden units and retraining for recovering the potential loss due to the removal were performed alternately, resulting in a reduced structure where redundant units were removed. The size of the input subregion, R_S, was 9 by 9 pixels, which was determined experimentally in our previous studies, i.e., the highest performance was obtained with this size (Arimura et al. 2004; Suzuki and Doi 2005; Suzuki et al. 2003a); thus, the number of input units in the MTANN filter is 81. The slope of the linear function, a, was 0.01. With the parameters above, training of the MTANN filter was performed by 1,000,000 iterations. To test the performance, we applied the trained MTANN filter to the entire lungs. We applied thresholding to the output images of the trained MTANN filter to detect nodule candidates. We compared the results of nodule candidate detection with and without the MTANN filter.

2.3.3.3 A CAD Scheme Incorporating the MTANN Lesion Enhancement

A previously reported CAD scheme (Arimura et al. 2004) for detection of lung nodules in thoracic CT is shown in Fig. 2.4a. The CAD scheme employs a standard approach which consists of lung segmentation, difference image technique for enhancing nodules (Xu et al. 1997), multiple thresholding for detection of nodule candidates, segmentation of the detected nodule candidates, feature analysis of the segmented nodule candidates, rule-based scheme for reduction of FPs, and classification based on linear discriminant analysis (LDA) for the final FP reduction. The difference image technique uses two different filters: a matched filter is used for enhancing nodule-like objects in CT images, and a ring-average filter is used for suppressing nodule-like objects. We incorporated the MTANN lesion enhancement filter in our CAD scheme to improve the overall performance. A schematic diagram of our MTAN-based CAD scheme is shown in Fig. 2.4b. In the MTANN-based CAD scheme, nodule candidates are detected (localized) by the MTANN lesion enhancement filter followed by thresholding. The detected nodule candidates generally include true positives and mostly FPs.

2.3.4 *Results*

2.3.4.1 Enhancement of Nodules in the Lungs on CT Images

We applied the trained MTANN filter to original CT images. The results of enhancement of nodules in CT images by the trained MTANN filter (Suzuki et al.

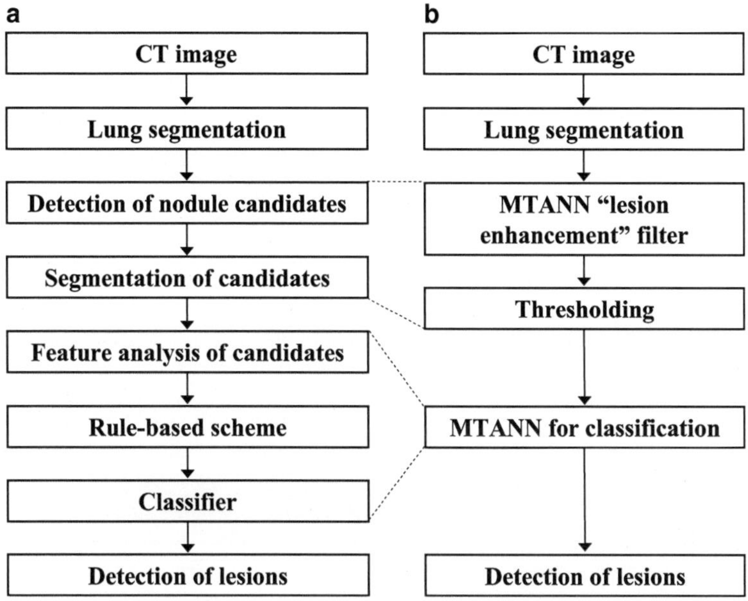

Fig. 2.4 Comparison of a standard CAD scheme with an MTANN-based CAD scheme. (**a**) Schematic diagram of a standard CAD scheme. (**b**) Schematic diagram of an MTANN-based CAD scheme

2008a) are shown in Fig. 2.5. The MTANN filter enhances nodules and suppresses most of the normal structures in CT images. Although some medium-sized vessels remain in the output image, the nodule with spiculation is enhanced well. We applied thresholding with a single threshold value (65 % of the maximum gray scale) to the output images of the trained MTANN filter. We compared the MTANN nodule enhancement filter with a sphere enhancement filter (Li et al. 2003) based on Hessian matrix (Frangi et al. 1999), as shown in Fig. 2.6. There are a smaller number of candidates in the MTANN-based images, whereas there are many nodule candidates in binary images obtained by using the sphere enhancement filter. The MTANN filter followed by thresholding identified 97 % (67/69) of cancers with 6.7 FPs per section, which is a substantial improvement over the performance (96 % sensitivity with 19.3 FPs/section) of our previously reported CAD scheme without MTANNs.

2.4 False-Positive Reduction with MTANNs

Reduction of FPs is very important, because a large number of FPs could adversely affect the clinical application of CADe. A large number of FPs are likely to confound the radiologist's task of image interpretation and thus lower his/her

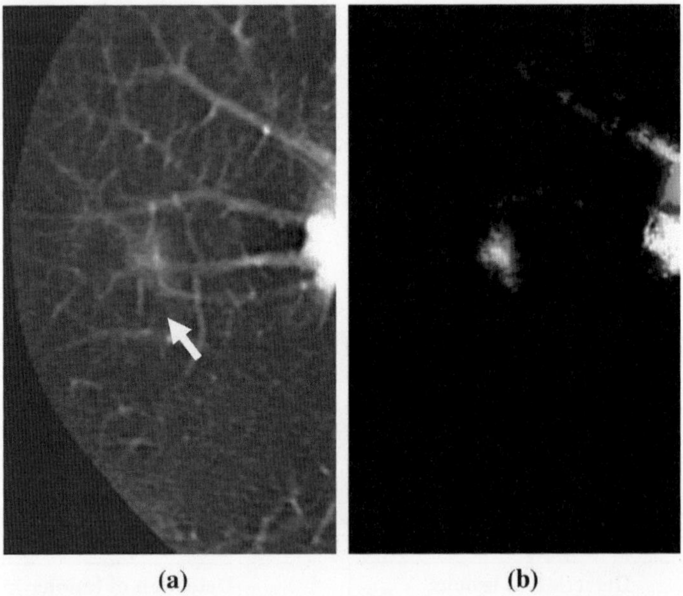

Fig. 2.5 Lesion enhancement by using a supervised MTANN lesion enhancement filter. (**a**) Original axial CT slice with a lung nodule (indicated by an *arrow*). (**b**) Output image of the trained MTANN nodule enhancement filter

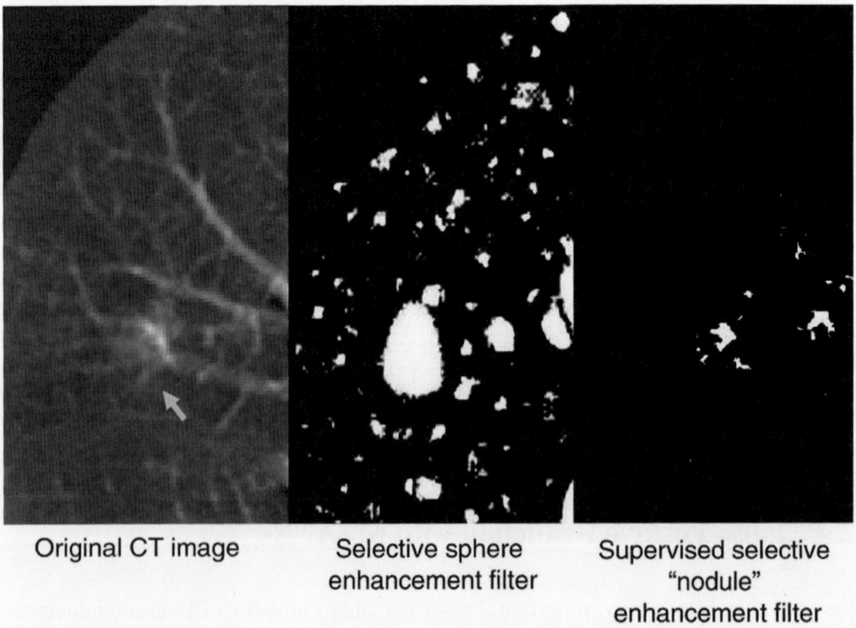

Fig. 2.6 Comparison of nodule enhancement by the conventional sphere enhancement filter based on the Hessian matrix and our supervised MTANN "nodule" enhancement filter

efficiency. In addition, radiologists may lose their confidence in CADe as a useful tool. Suzuki et al. developed an FP reduction technique based on MTANNs (Suzuki et al. 2003a) for reduction of FPs in a CADe scheme for lung nodules in CT. The MTANNs were trained to enhance lung nodules and suppress various types of FPs (i.e., non-nodules) such as lung vessels.

2.4.1 A. Database of Low-Dose CT Images

The database used in this study consisted of 101 noninfused, low-dose thoracic helical CT (LDCT) scans acquired from 71 different patients who participated voluntarily in a lung cancer screening program between 1996 and 1999 in Nagano, Japan.[3,18,7] The CT examinations were performed on a mobile CT scanner (CT-W950SR; Hitachi Medical, Tokyo, Japan). The scans used for this study were acquired with a low-dose protocol of 120 kVp, 25 mA (54 scans) or 50 mA (47 scans), 10 mm collimation, and 10 mm reconstruction interval at a helical pitch of two.[18] The pixel size was 0.586 mm for 83 scans and 0.684 mm for 18 scans. Each reconstructed CT section (slice) had an image matrix size of 512×512 pixels. We used 38 of 101 LDCT scans which were acquired from 31 patients as a training set for our CAD scheme. The 38 scans consisted of 1057 sections and contained 50 nodules, including 38 "missed" nodules that represented biopsy-confirmed lung cancers and were not reported or misreported during the initial clinical interpretation.7 The remaining 12 nodules in the scans were classified as "confirmed benign" ($n = 8$), "suspected benign" ($n = 3$), or "suspected malignant" ($n = 1$). The confirmed benign nodules were determined by biopsy or by follow-up over a period of 2 years. The suspected benign nodules were determined by follow-up less than 2 years. The suspected malignant nodule was determined on the basis of results of follow-up diagnostic CT studies; no biopsy results were available. We used 63 of 101 LDCT scans which were acquired from 63 patients as a test set. The 63 scans consisted of 1765 sections and contained 71 nodules, including 66 primary cancers that were determined by biopsy and five confirmed benign nodules that were determined by biopsy or by follow-up over a period of 2 years. The scans included 23 scans from the same 23 patients as those in the training set, which were acquired at a different time (the interval was about 1 year or 2 years). Thus, the training set consisted of 38 LDCT scans including 50 nodules, and the test set consisted of 63 LDCT scans including 71 confirmed nodules.

The nodule size was determined by an experienced chest radiologist and ranged from 4 to 27 mm. The mean diameter of the 50 nodules in the training set was 12.7 ± 6.1 mm, and that of the 71 nodules in the test set was 13.5 ± 4.7 mm. In the training set, 38 % of nodules were attached to the pleura, 22 % of nodules were attached to vessels, and 10 % of nodules were in the hilum. As to the test set, 30 % of nodules were attached to the pleura, 34 % of nodules were attached to vessels, and 7 % of nodules were in the hilum. Three radiologists determined the nodules in the training set as three categories such as pure ground-glass opacity (pure GGO; 40 % of nodules), mixed GGO (28 %), and solid nodule (32 %); the nodules in the test set were determined as pure GGO (24 %), mixed GGO (30 %), and solid nodule (46 %).

2.4.2 Scheme for Lung Nodule Detection in Low-Dose CT

Technical details of our current scheme have been published previously (Armato et al., 1999, Armato et al., 2001). With our current CAD scheme, the multiple gray-level thresholding technique initially identified 20 743 nodule candidates in 1057 sections of LDCT images in the training set. Forty-five of 50 nodules were correctly detected. Then a rule-based classifier followed by a series of two linear discriminant classifiers was applied for removal of some false positives, thus yielding a detection of 40 (80.0 %) of 50 nodules (from 22 patients) together with 1078 (1.02 per section) false positives. The sizes of the 10 false-negative nodules ranged from 5 mm to 25 mm, and the mean diameter was 13.2±6.1 mm. In this study, we used all 50 nodules, the locations of which were identified by the radiologist, and all 1078 false positives generated by our CAD scheme in the training set, for investigating the characteristics of the MTANN and training the MTANN. The use of radiologist-extracted true nodules with computer-generated false positives was intended to anticipate future improvements in the nodule detection sensitivity of our CAD scheme. When a nodule was present in more than one section, the section that included the largest nodule was used. When we applied our current CAD scheme to the test set, a sensitivity of 81.7 % (58 of 71 nodules) with 0.98 false positives per section (1726/1765) was achieved. We used the 58 true positives (nodules from 54 patients) and 1726 false positives (non-nodules) for testing the MTANN in a validation test.

2.4.3 MTANN for FP Reduction

2.4.3.1 Architecture

The architecture and training method of the MTANN for FP reduction are shown in Fig. 2.7. When the task is the distinction between nodules and non-nodules, the output would be interpreted as the "likelihood of being a nodule." In order to distinguish between nodules and various types of non-nodules, we extended the capability of the single MTANN and developed a multiple MTANN (multi-MTANN). The architecture of a mixture of expert MTANNs (multi-MTANN) is shown in Fig. 2.8. The multi-MTANN consists of plural MTANNs that are arranged in parallel. Each MTANN is trained by using a different type of non-nodule, but

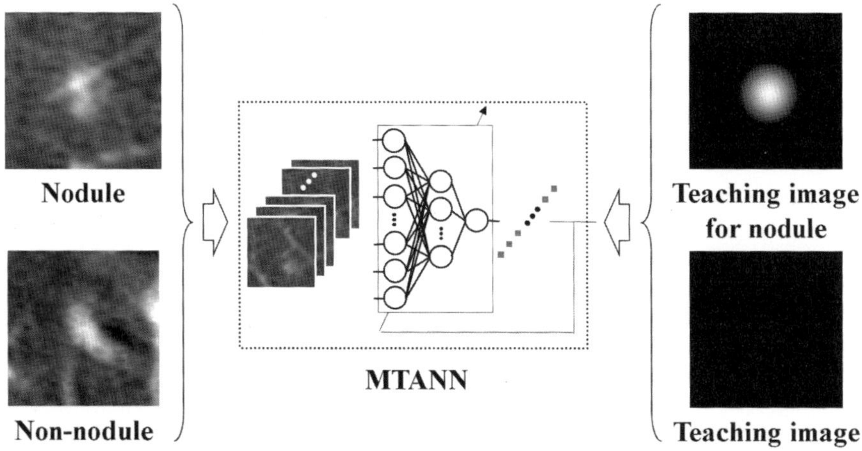

Fig. 2.7 Architecture and training of an MTANN for classification of candidates into a nodule or a non-nodule. A teaching image for a nodule contains a Gaussian distribution at the *center* of the image, whereas that for a non-nodule contains zero (i.e., it is completely *dark*)

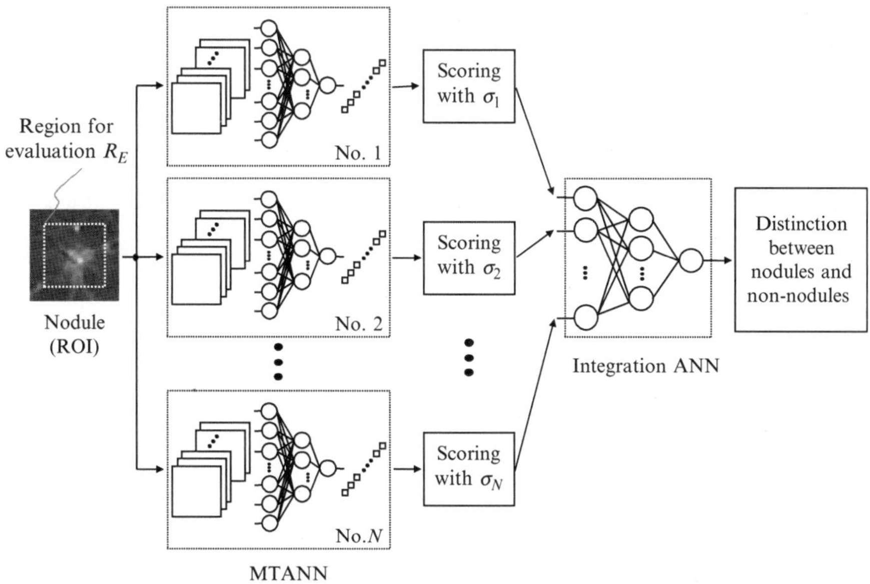

Fig. 2.8 Architecture of a mixture of expert MTANNs consisting of multiple MTANNs combined by the integration ANN

with the same nodules. Each MTANN acts as an expert for the distinction between nodules and a specific type of non-nodule, e.g., MTANN No. 1 is trained to distinguish nodules from false positives caused by medium-sized vessels; MTANN No. 2 is trained to distinguish nodules from soft-tissue-opacity false positives caused by the diaphragm; and so on. A scoring method is applied to the output of each MTANN, and then thresholding of the score from each MTANN is performed for distinction between nodules and the specific type of non-nodule. The output of each MTANN is then integrated by the integration ANN or the logical AND operation. If each MTANN can eliminate the specific type of non-nodule with which the MTANN is trained, then the multi-MTANN will be able to reduce a larger number of false positives than does a single MTANN.

2.4.3.2 Training of MTANN

For the enhancement of nodules and suppression of non-nodules in CT images, the teaching volume contains a 3D distribution of values that represent the "likelihood of being a nodule." We used a 3D Gaussian distribution with standard deviation σ_T, the peak of which is located at the center of the nodule, as a teaching volume for a nodule and a volume that contains all zeros for a non-nodule, represented by

$$T(x,y,z) = \begin{cases} \frac{1}{\sqrt{2\pi}\sigma_T}\exp\left\{-\frac{(x^2+y^2+z^2)}{2\sigma_T{}^2}\right\} & \text{if an actual nodule} \\ 0 & \text{otherwise} \end{cases}. \tag{2.4}$$

The MTANN involves training with a large number of subvolume-voxel pairs; we call it a massive-subvolumes training scheme. A training volume V_T extracted from the input CT volume is divided voxel by voxel into a large number of overlapping subvolumes (image patch). Single voxels are extracted from the corresponding teaching volume as teaching values. The 3D MTANN is massively trained by use of each of a large number of the input subvolumes together with each of the corresponding teaching single voxels. A training set of pairs of a subvolume and a teaching voxel is represented by

$$\left\{\vec{I}(x,y,z),T(x,y,z)|x,y,z\in V_T\right\} = \left\{\left(\vec{I}_1,T_1\right),\left(\vec{I}_2,T_2\right),\ldots,\left(\vec{I}_p,T_p\right),\ldots,\left(\vec{I}_{N_T},T_{N_T}\right)\right\}, \tag{2.5}$$

where V_T is a training volume, p is a voxel number in V_T, T_p is a teaching value in the teaching volume that corresponds to the center voxel in $\vec{I}_p$, and N_T is the number of voxels in V_T. In order to learn the relationship between the input image and the teacher image, the MTANN is trained with a set of input images and the teacher images by adjusting the weights between layers. The error to be minimized by training is defined in Eq. (2.3). After training, the MTANN is expected to output the highest value when a nodule is located at the center of the subvolume of the MTANN, a lower value as the distance from the subvolume center increases, and zero when the input subvolume contains a non-nodule.

2.4.3.3 Scoring of the MTANN Output for Testing

When an original image for the *s*th nodule candidate is entered into the *n*th trained MTANN for testing, the output image for the *s*th nodule candidate is obtained by scanning of the original image with the trained MTANN. The distinction between a nodule and a non-nodule is determined by use of a score defined from the output image of the *n*th trained MTANN, described as follows:

$$S = \sum_{x,y,z \in V_E} f_G(\sigma; x, y, z) \cdot O(x, y, z), \tag{2.6}$$

where

$$f_G(\sigma; x, y, z) = \frac{1}{\sqrt{2\pi}\sigma} \exp\left\{ -\frac{(x^2 + y^2 + z^2)}{2\sigma^2} \right\} \tag{2.7}$$

is a 3D Gaussian weighting function with standard deviation σ with its center corresponding to the center of the volume for evaluation, V_E; V_E is the volume for evaluation that is sufficient to cover a nodule or a non-nodule; and $O(x,y,z)$ is the output of the trained MTANN. The use of the 3D Gaussian weighting function allows us to combine the individual voxel-based responses (outputs) of a trained MTANN as a single score. The score obtained by the above equations represents the weighted sum of the estimates for the likelihood that the volume (nodule candidate) contains an actual nodule near the center, i.e., a higher score would indicate a nodule and a lower score would indicate a non-nodule. We use the same 3D Gaussian weighting function as is used in the nodule teaching volumes. Thresholding is performed on the scores to distinguish between nodules and non-nodules.

2.4.4 Results

2.4.4.1 MTANN Performance

An imaging expert selected ten representative non-nodules from each of the nine groups as the training samples for each MTANN; thus, the multi-MTANN employed nine MTANNs. The same ten nodules were used as training samples for all nine MTANNs. Therefore, ten nodules and 90 non-nodules were used for training the multi-MTANN. The single MTANN trained with medium-sized vessels (with relatively high contrast) was used as MTANN No.1. Non-nodules for the training of MTANN No. 1 to No. 5 ranged from medium-sized vessels to small (peripheral) vessels. Non-nodules for the training of MTANN No. 6 to No. 9 were large vessels in the hilum, relatively large vessels with some opacities, soft-tissue opacities caused by the partial volume effect between peripheral vessels and the diaphragm, and some abnormal opacities (focal interstitial opacities), respectively. Each MTANN was trained in the same way as a single MTANN.

The trained MTANN was applied to 1068 false-positive nodule candidates not used for training. The results for non-training cases are shown in Fig. 2.9. In the output image of the MTANN for nodules, the nodules are represented by light distributions near the center as expected, whereas the output images for false positives (non-nodules) are relatively dark, as shown in Fig. 2.10.

The scoring method was applied to the output images of the individually trained MTANNs. The free-response receiver operating characteristic (FROC) curve expresses a classification rate as a function of the number of false positives per section at a specific operating point. With the single MTANN (MTANN No.1), we can achieve a classification rate of 100 % (40/40) with 0.36 false positives per section, as shown in Fig. 2.11. With the single MTANN (MTANN No.1), the false-positive rate of our current scheme could be improved from 1.02 to 0.36 false positives per section, while maintaining the current sensitivity. Note that 38 out of 50 nodules used in this study were missed by radiologists. When the multi-MTANN employed nine MTANNs, 91 % (902/988) of false positives (non-nodules) were removed without eliminating any true positives, i.e., we can achieve a classification rate of 100 % (40/40) with 0.08 false positives per section.

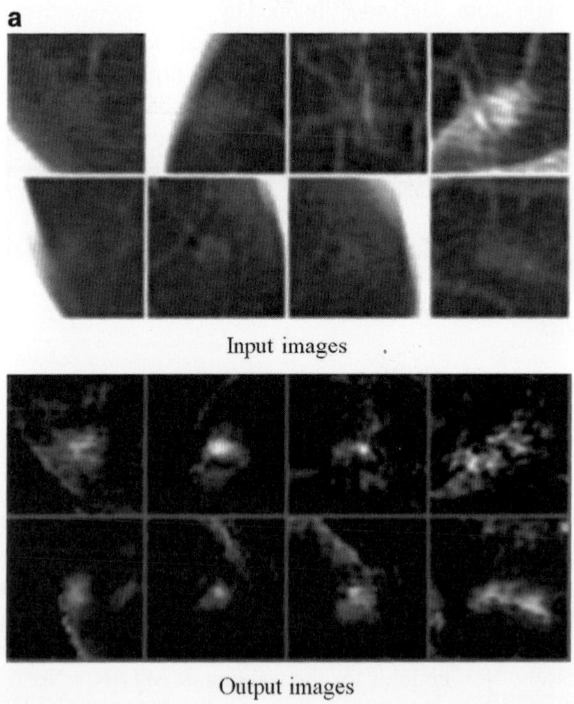

Fig. 2.9 Actual nodules (**a**) and the output images of the trained MTANN (**b**). Nodules are enhanced and represented by light distributions in the output images

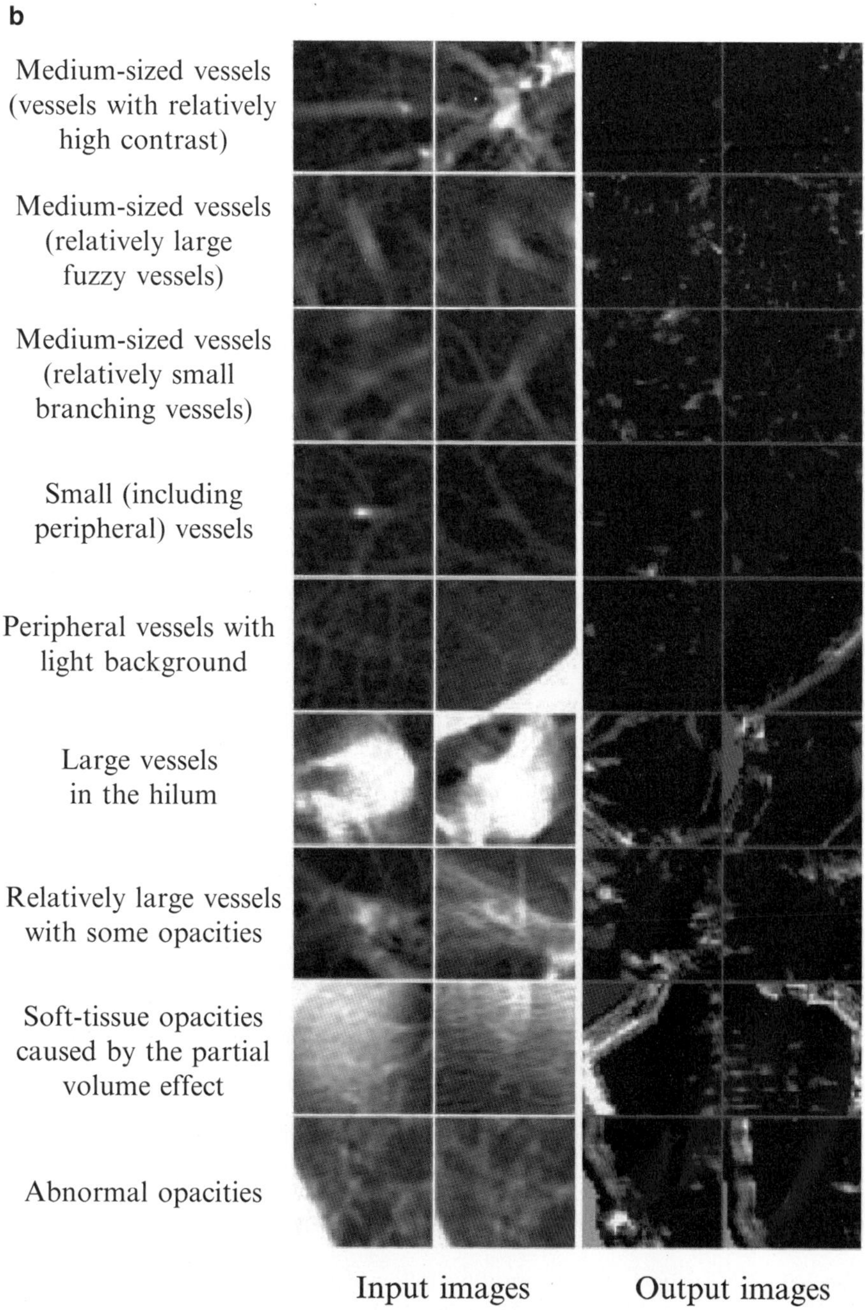

Fig. 2.9 (continued)

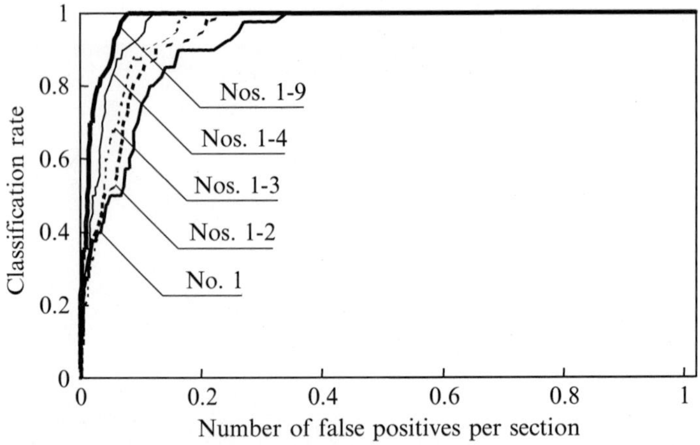

Fig. 2.10 FROC curves indicating the performance of multi-MTANNs with different numbers of MTANNs

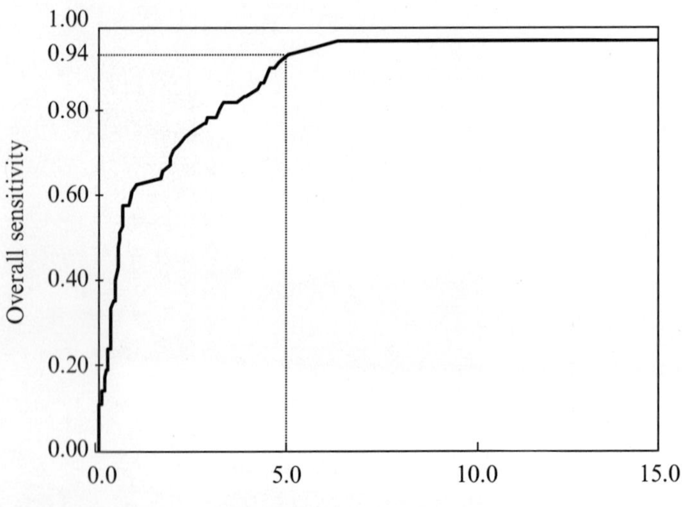

Fig. 2.11 FROC curve for the performance of the multi-MTANN for CAD for thin-slice CT

2.4.4.2 Performance of a CAD Scheme with MTANN Lesion Enhancer

The MTANN lesion enhancement filter followed by thresholding identified 97 % (67/69) of cancers with 6.7 FPs per section. The six classification-MTANNs were applied to the nodule candidates (true positives and FPs) for the classification of the candidates into nodules or non-nodules. The mixture of expert MTANNs was able to remove 60 % (8172/13,688) or 93 % (12,667/13,688) of non-nodules (FPs) with a

Table 2.1 Comparison of the performance of the previously reported CAD scheme with that of our MTANN-based CAD scheme at different stages

Previously reported CAD scheme		MTANN-based CAD scheme	
Nodule candidate detection by multiple thresholding	96 % sensitivity with 19.3 FPs/section	Nodule candidate detection by MTANN	97 % sensitivity with 6.7 FPs/section
Future analysis and rule-based scheme	96 % sensitivity with 9.3 FPs/section	Classification by MTANN	96 % sensitivity with 2.7 FPs/section
Classification by LDA	84 % sensitivity with 1.4 FPs/section		84 % sensitivity with 0.5 FPs/section

loss of 1 true positive or 10 true positives, respectively. Thus, our MTANN-based CAD scheme achieved a 96 % (66/69) or 84 % (57/69) sensitivity with 2.7 (5516/2052) or 0.5 (1021/2052) FPs per section, respectively, as shown in Table 2.1. The remaining true-positive nodules included a ground-glass opacity, cancer overlapping vessels, and a cancer touching the pleura. In contrast, the difference image technique followed by multiple thresholding in the previously reported CAD scheme detected 96 % (66/69) of cancers with 19.3 FPs per section. Thus, the MTANN lesion enhancement filter was effective for improving the sensitivity and specificity of a CAD scheme. The feature analysis and the rule-based scheme removed FPs further and achieved 9.3 FPs per section. Finally, with LDA, the previously reported CAD scheme yielded a sensitivity of 84 % (57/69) with 1.4 (2873/2052) FPs per section (the difference between the specificity of the previously reported CAD scheme and that of our new MTANN-based CAD scheme at the 84 % sensitivity level was statistically significant ($P < 0.05$) (Edwards et al. 2002)). Table 2.1 summarizes the comparison of the performance of the previously reported CAD scheme with that of the MTANN-based CAD scheme at different stages. Therefore, MTANNs were effective for improving the sensitivity and specificity of a CAD scheme.

2.4.5 Results for CAD for Thin-Slice CT

Recent technology of multidetector-row CT (MDCT) can provide thinner CT slices; and thus, quasi-isotropic or isotropic volume data are available. Consequently, nodules are more continuous in MDCT volumes. To process 3D MDCT volumes effectively, the development of a 3D technique for the reduction of FPs is necessary. Therefore, we developed a CAD scheme for nodule detection for thin-slice CT, which consisted of the detection of initial nodule candidates based on a selective enhancement filter (Li et al. 2003) and classification of the nodule candidates into nodules and non-nodules based on a rule-based scheme with image features. For handling MDCT slices with different slice thickness, we converted original CT data to isotropic volumes. We applied the selective enhancement filter to the isotropic volumes for enhancing nodules and suppressing vessels. Thresholding followed by the rule-based scheme was applied to the filtered volumes to classify candidates into nodules and non-nodules.

Our database contained 62 nodules in 32 scans acquired from 32 patients with an MDCT system with a four-detector scanner. The MDCT scan consisted of an average of 186 thin-slice CT images (slice thickness ranged from 1.0 to 2.5 mm). Each CT slice had an image matrix size of 512 × 512 pixels. Nodule sizes ranged from 5 to 30 mm. All nodules were confirmed by consensus between two chest radiologists.

With our initial CAD scheme, a sensitivity of 97 % (60/62 nodules) together with an average of 15 (476/32) false positives per patient was achieved. The trained multi-3D MTANN was applied for reduction of the FPs. Each 3D MTANN in the multi-3D MTANN was able to enhance nodules and suppress non-nodules representing the particular non-nodule type with which the 3D MTANN was trained, namely, various nodules in the output volumes of the 3D MTANN were represented by light distributions, whereas the eight different types of non-nodules were almost dark. Although the distribution of scores for nodules and non-nodules obtained by use of the scoring method overlapped, each 3D MTANN was able to distinguish nodules from each type of non-nodule; therefore, the multi-3D MTANN was able to remove many non-nodules. The performance of the multi-3D MTANN was evaluated by FROC analysis. Results indicated that 66 % (315/476) of FPs were removed with a loss of only two true positives by the multi-3D MTANN, as shown in Fig. 2.12. Thus, the FP rate of our CAD scheme was improved to 5.0 (161/32) FPs per patient at an overall sensitivity of 94 % (58/62 nodules).

2.5 Conclusion

In this chapter, CADe of lung cancer in thoracic CT is overviewed. In CADe schemes, machine learning plays an essential role, because accurate detection of lung cancer thus classification between lung cancer and other normal structures requires learning from image data/examples. Among various machine learning techniques, image-based machine learning such as the MTANNs is one of the most promising techniques in CADe schemes. There are two types of MTANNs used in CADe schemes: a supervised lesion enhancer and an FP reducer. The MTANN lesion enhancer improves the sensitivity of a CADe scheme substantially, whereas the MTANN FP reducer improves the specificity substantially. With the MTANN technology, both sensitivity and specificity of a CADe scheme were improved substantially, and the MTANN CADe scheme for lung nodule detection in thin-slice CT achieved 94 % sensitivity with 5.0 FPs per patient.

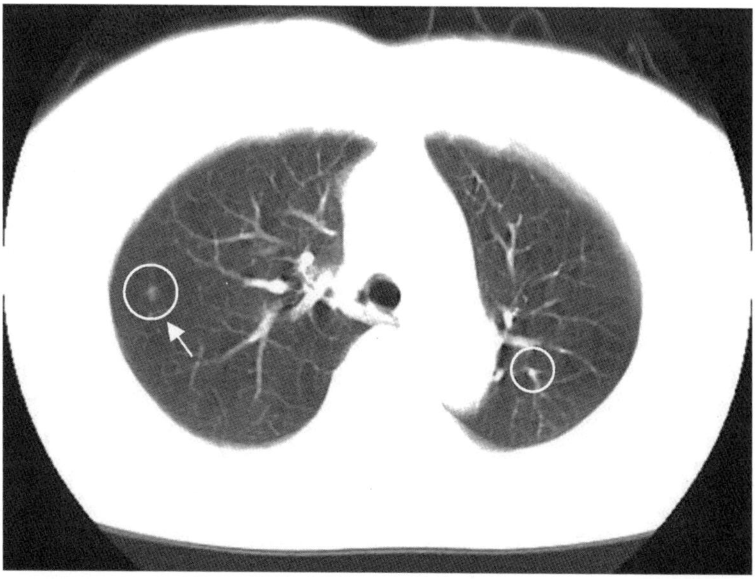

Fig. 2.12 CADe outputs (indicated by *circles*) on an axial CT slice of the lungs. A lung nodule (indicated by an *arrow*) was detected correctly by a CADe scheme with one FP detection (branch of lung vessels) on the *right*

Recently, convolutional neural networks and deep learning gained attentions from the computer vision community as well as medical image analysis community, because they outperformed feature-based machine learning (or simply classifiers) that had been dominant in the past three decades, in various computer vision competitions. The same observation was seen in the MTANN applications to CADe, namely, MTANNs were able to remove "difficult" FPs that had not been removed by feature-based machine learning, and the performance of CADe schemes was substantially improved by using the MTANNs. Thus, CADe schemes with the MTANN technology offer high performance in the detection and diagnosis of lesions in medical images, such as lung nodules in CT. I expect MTANN CAD schemes will be useful for improving the diagnostic performance of radiologists/physicians in early detection of lung cancer and, thus, potentially reducing the mortality of lung cancer.

Acknowledgments The author is grateful to all members of the Suzuki laboratory, i.e., postdoctoral scholars, computer scientists, visiting scholars/professors, medical students, graduate/undergraduate students, research technicians, research volunteers, and support staff, in the Department of Radiology at the University of Chicago and in the Medical Imaging Research Center at the Illinois Institute of Technology, for their valuable suggestions and support. Computer-aided diagnosis and machine learning technologies developed at the University of Chicago have been licensed to companies including R2 Technology (Hologic), Riverain Medical (Riverain Technologies), AlgoMedica, Deus Technology, Median Technologies, Mitsubishi Space Software, General Electric, and Toshiba.

References

Aoyama M, Li Q, Katsuragawa S, MacMahon H, Doi K (2002) Automated computerized scheme for distinction between benign and malignant solitary pulmonary nodules on chest images. Med Phys 29:701–708

Arimura H, Katsuragawa S, Suzuki K, Li F, Shiraishi J, Sone S, Doi K (2004) Computerized scheme for automated detection of lung nodules in low-dose computed tomography images for lung cancer screening. Acad Radiol 11:617–629

Armato SG 3rd, Giger ML, Moran CJ, Blackburn JT, Doi K, MacMahon H (1999) Computerized detection of pulmonary nodules on CT scans. Radiographics 19:1303–1311

Armato SG 3rd, Giger ML, MacMahon H (2001) Automated detection of lung nodules in CT scans: preliminary results. Med Phys, 28:1552–1561

Armato SG 3rd, Mclennan G, Mcnitt-Gray MF, Meyer CR, Yankelevitz D, Aberle DR, Henschke CI, Hoffman EA, Kazerooni EA, MacMahon H, Reeves AP, Croft BY, Clarke LP (2004) Lung image database consortium: developing a resource for the medical imaging research community. Radiology 232:739–748

Bae KT, Kim JS, Kim JH, Na Y (2002) Automatic detection of pulmonary nodules in multi-slice CT: performance of 3D morphologic matching algorithm. Radiology 225(P):476

Becker HC, Nettleton WJ Jr, Meyers PH, Sweeney JW, Nice Jr CM (1964) Digital computer determination of a medical diagnostic index directly from chest X-Ray images. IEEE Trans Biomed Eng 11:67–72

Chan HP, Doi K, Galhotra S, Vyborny CJ, MacMahon H, Jokich PM (1987) Image feature analysis and computer-aided diagnosis in digital radiography. I. Automated detection of microcalcifications in mammography. Med Phys 14:538–548

Chan HP, Sahiner B, Wagner RF, Petrick N (1999) Classifier design for computer-aided diagnosis: effects of finite sample size on the mean performance of classical and neural network classifiers. Med Phys 26:2654–2668

Chen H, Xu Y, Ma Y, Ma B (2010) Neural network ensemble-based computer-aided diagnosis for differentiation of lung nodules on CT images: clinical evaluation. Acad Radiol 17:595–602

Chen S, Suzuki K (2013) Computerized detection of lung nodules by means of “virtual dual-energy” radiography. IEEE Trans Biomed Eng 60:369–378

Chen S, Suzuki K (2014) Separation of bones from chest radiographs by means of anatomically specific multiple massive-training ANNs combined with total variation minimization smoothing. IEEE Trans Med Imaging 33:246–257

Chen S, Zhong S, Yao L, Shang Y, Suzuki K (2016) Enhancement of chest radiographs obtained in the intensive care unit through bone suppression and consistent processing. Phys Med Biol 61:2283–2301

Doi K (2005) Current status and future potential of computer-aided diagnosis in medical imaging. Br J Radiol 78(Spec No 1):S3–S19

Doi K (2007) Computer-aided diagnosis in medical imaging: Historical review, current status and future potential. Comput Med Imaging Graph 31:198–211

Duda RO, Hart PE, Stork DG (2001) Pattern recognition, 2nd edn. Wiley Interscience, Hoboken

Edwards DC, Kupinski MA, Metz CE, Nishikawa RM (2002) Maximum likelihood fitting of FROC curves under an initial-detection-and-candidate-analysis model. Med Phys 29:2861–2870

Farag AA, EL-Baz A, Gimelfarb G, EL-Ghar MA, Eldiasty T (2005) Quantitative nodule detection in low dose chest CT scans: new template modeling and evaluation for CAD system design. Med Image Comput Comput Assist Interv 8:720–728

Frangi AF, Niessen WJ, Hoogeveen RM, Van Walsum T, Viergever MA (1999) Model-based quantitation of 3-D magnetic resonance angiographic images. IEEE Trans Med Imaging 18:946–956

Fujita H, Doi K, Fencil LE, Chua KG (1987) Image feature analysis and computer-aided diagnosis in digital radiography. 2. Computerized determination of vessel sizes in digital subtraction angiography. Med Phys 14:549–556

Fukunaga K (1990) Introduction to statistical pattern recognition. Academic, San Diego

Ge Z, Sahiner B, Chan HP, Hadjiiski LM, Cascade PN, Bogot N, Kazerooni EA, Wei J, Zhou C (2005) Computer-aided detection of lung nodules: false positive reduction using a 3D gradient field method and 3D ellipsoid fitting. Med Phys 32:2443–2454

Giger ML, Suzuki K (2007) Computer-Aided Diagnosis (CAD). In: Feng DD (ed) biomedical information technology. Academic

Giger ML, Doi K, MacMahon H (1988) Image feature analysis and computer-aided diagnosis in digital radiography. 3. Automated detection of nodules in peripheral lung fields. Med Phys 15:158–166

Giger ML, Bae KT, MacMahon H (1994) Computerized detection of pulmonary nodules in computed tomography images. Investig Radiol 29:459–465

Giger ML, Chan HP, Boone J (2008) Anniversary paper: history and status of CAD and quantitative image analysis: the role of Medical Physics and AAPM. Med Phys 35:5799–5820

Golosio B, Masala GL, Piccioli A, Oliva P, Carpinelli M, Cataldo R, Cerello P, De Carlo F, Falaschi F, Fantacci ME, Gargano G, Kasae P, Torsello M (2009) A novel multithreshold method for nodule detection in lung CT. Med Phys 36:3607–3618

Gurcan MN, Sahiner B, Petrick N, Chan HP, Kazerooni EA, Cascade PN, Hadjiiski L (2002) Lung nodule detection on thoracic computed tomography images: preliminary evaluation of a computer-aided diagnosis system. Med Phys 29:2552–2558

Hanley JA, Mcneil BJ (1983) A method of comparing the areas under receiver operating characteristic curves derived from the same cases. Radiology 148:839–843

Hanson AJ (1992) The rolling ball. Graphics Gems III. Academic, Cambridge, MA

He L, Chao Y, Suzuki K, Wu K (2009) Fast connected-component labeling. Pattern Recogn 42:1977–1987

Henschke CI, Mccauley DI, Yankelevitz DF, Naidich DP, Mcguinness G, Miettinen OS, Libby DM, Pasmantier MW, Koizumi J, Altorki NK, Smith JP (1999) Early Lung Cancer Action Project: overall design and findings from baseline screening. Lancet 354:99–105

Henschke CI, Yankelevitz DF, Naidich DP, Mccauley DI, Mcguinness G, Libby DM, Smith JP, Pasmantier MW, Miettinen OS (2004) CT screening for lung cancer: suspiciousness of nodules according to size on baseline scans. Radiology 231:164–168

Iwano S, Nakamura T, Kamioka Y, Ikeda M, Ishigaki T (2008) Computer-aided differentiation of malignant from benign solitary pulmonary nodules imaged by high-resolution CT. Comput Med Imaging Graph 32:416–422

Kaneko M, Eguchi K, Ohmatsu H, Kakinuma R, Naruke T, Suemasu K, Moriyama N (1996) Peripheral lung cancer: screening and detection with low-dose spiral CT versus radiography. Radiology 201:798–802

Katsuragawa S, Doi K, MacMahon H (1988) Image feature analysis and computer-aided diagnosis in digital radiography: detection and characterization of interstitial lung disease in digital chest radiographs. Med Phys 15:311–319

Krizhevsky A, Sutskever I, Hinton GE (2012) Imagenet classification with deep convolutional neural networks. Adv Neural Inf Proces Syst 1097-1105

Lecun Y, Bengio Y, Hinton G (2015) Deep learning. Nature 521:436–444

Lee Y, Hara T, Fujita H, Itoh S, Ishigaki T (2001) Automated detection of pulmonary nodules in helical CT images based on an improved template-matching technique. IEEE Trans Med Imaging 20:595–604

Lee MC, Boroczky L, Sungur-Stasik K, Cann AD, Borczuk AC, Kawut SM, Powell CA (2010) Computer-aided diagnosis of pulmonary nodules using a two-step approach for feature selection and classifier ensemble construction. Artif Intell Med 50:43–53

Li F, Sone S, Abe H, MacMahon H, Armato SG 3rd, Doi K (2002) Lung cancers missed at low-dose helical CT screening in a general population: comparison of clinical, histopathologic, and imaging findings. Radiology 225(3):673–683

Li Q, Sone S, Doi K (2003) Selective enhancement filters for nodules, vessels, and airway walls in two- and three-dimensional CT scans. Med Phys 30:2040–2051
Lusted LB (1955) Medical electronics. N Engl J Med 252:580–585
Matsuki Y, Nakamura K, Watanabe H, Aoki T, Nakata H, Katsuragawa S, Doi K (2002) Usefulness of an artificial neural network for differentiating benign from malignant pulmonary nodules on high-resolution CT: evaluation with receiver operating characteristic analysis. AJR Am J Roentgenol 178:657–663
Matsumoto S, Kundel HL, Gee JC, Gefter WB, Hatabu H (2006) Pulmonary nodule detection in CT images with quantized convergence index filter. Med Image Anal 10:343–352
Mcnitt-Gray MF, Hart EM, Wyckoff N, Sayre JW, Goldin JG, Aberle DR (1999) A pattern classification approach to characterizing solitary pulmonary nodules imaged on high resolution CT: preliminary results. Med Phys 26:880–888
Messay T, Hardie RC, Rogers SK (2010) A new computationally efficient CAD system for pulmonary nodule detection in CT imagery. Med Image Anal 14:390–406
Metz CE (1986) ROC methodology in radiologic imaging. Investig Radiol 21:720–733
Meyers PH, Nice CM Jr., Becker H. C, Nettleton WJ, Jr., Sweeney JW, Meckstroth GR (1964) Automated computer analysis of radiographic images. Radiology 831029–1034.
Miettinen OS, Henschke CI (2001) CT screening for lung cancer: coping with nihilistic recommendations. Radiology 221:592–596
Mnih V, Kavukcuoglu K, Silver D, Rusu AA, Veness J, Bellemare MG, Graves A, Riedmiller M, Fidjeland AK, Ostrovski G, Petersen S, Beattie C, Sadik A, Antonoglou I, King H, Kumaran D, Wierstra D, Legg S, Hassabis D (2015) Human-level control through deep reinforcement learning. Nature 518:529–533
Mori K, Niki N, Kondo T, Kamiyama Y, Kodama T, Kawada Y, Moriyama N (2005) Development of a novel computer-aided diagnosis system for automatic discrimination of malignant from benign solitary pulmonary nodules on thin-section dynamic computed tomography. J Comput Assist Tomogr 29:215–222
Murphy K, Van Ginneken B, Schilham AM, De Hoop BJ, Gietema HA, Prokop M (2009) A large-scale evaluation of automatic pulmonary nodule detection in chest CT using local image features and k-nearest-neighbour classification. Med Image Anal 13:757–770
Otsu N (1979) A threshold selection method from gray level histograms. IEEE Trans Syst Man Cyber 9:62–66
Pu J, Zheng B, Leader JK, Wang XH, Gur D (2008) An automated CT based lung nodule detection scheme using geometric analysis of signed distance field. Med Phys 35:3453–3461
Retico A, Delogu P, Fantacci ME, Gori I, Preite Martinez A (2008) Lung nodule detection in low-dose and thin-slice computed tomography. Comput Biol Med 38:525–534
Riccardi A, Petkov TS, Ferri G, Masotti M, Campanini R (2011) Computer-aided detection of lung nodules via 3D fast radial transform, scale space representation, and Zernike MIP classification. Med Phys 38:1962–1971
Roellinger FX Jr, Kahveci AE, Chang JK, Harlow CA, Dwyer SJ III, Lodwick GS (1973) Computer analysis of chest radiographs. Comp Graph Image Process 2:232–251
Rumelhart DE, Hinton GE, Williams RJ (1986) Learning representations by back-propagating errors. Nature 323:533–536
Sahiner B, Chan HP, Hadjiiski L (2008) Classifier performance prediction for computer-aided diagnosis using a limited dataset. Med Phys 35:1559–1570
Shah SK, Mcnitt-Gray MF, Rogers SR, Goldin JG, Suh RD, Sayre JW, Petkovska I, Kim HJ, Aberle DR (2005) Computer aided characterization of the solitary pulmonary nodule using volumetric and contrast enhancement features. Acad Radiol 12:1310–1319
Sone S, Takashima S, Li F, Yang Z, Honda T, Maruyama Y, Hasegawa M, Yamanda T, Kubo K, Hanamura K, Asakura K (1998) Mass screening for lung cancer with mobile spiral computed tomography scanner. Lancet 351(9111):1242–1245
Sone S, Li F, Yang ZG, Honda T, Maruyama Y, Takashima S, Hasegawa M, Kawakami S, Kubo K, Haniuda M, Yamanda T (2001) Results of three-year mass screening programme for lung cancer using mobile low-dose spiral computed tomography scanner. Br J Cancer 84(1):25–32

Suzuki K (2004) Determining the receptive field of a neural filter. J Neural Eng 1:228–237

Suzuki K (2009) A supervised 'lesion-enhancement' filter by use of a massive-training artificial neural network (MTANN) in computer-aided diagnosis (CAD). Phys Med Biol 54:S31–S45

Suzuki K (2012a) Pixel-based Machine Learning (PML) in medical imaging. Int J Biomed Imag 2012 Article ID 792079, 18 pages

Suzuki K (2012b) A review of computer-aided diagnosis in thoracic and colonic imaging. Quant Imaging Med Surg 2:163–176

Suzuki K (2013) Machine learning in computer-aided diagnosis of the thorax and colon in CT: a survey. IEICE Trans Inf Syst E96-D:772–783

Suzuki K, Doi K (2005) How can a massive training artificial neural network (MTANN) be trained with a small number of cases in the distinction between nodules and vessels in thoracic CT? Acad Radiol 12:1333–1341

Suzuki K, Horiba I, Ikegaya K, Nanki M (1995) Recognition of coronary arterial stenosis using neural network on DSA system. Syst Comput Japan 26:66–74

Suzuki K, Horiba I, Sugie N (2001) A simple neural network pruning algorithm with application to filter synthesis. Neural Process Lett 13:43–53

Suzuki K, Horiba I, Sugie N (2002a) Efficient approximation of neural filters for removing quantum noise from images. IEEE Trans Signal Process 50:1787–1799

Suzuki K, Horiba I, Sugie N, Nanki M (2002b) Neural filter with selection of input features and its application to image quality improvement of medical image sequences. IEICE Trans Inf Syst E85-D:1710–1718

Suzuki K, Armato SG 3rd, Li F, Sone S, Doi K (2003a) Massive training artificial neural network (MTANN) for reduction of false positives in computerized detection of lung nodules in low-dose computed tomography. Med Phys 30:1602–1617

Suzuki K, Horiba I, Sugie N (2003b) Linear-time connected-component labeling based on sequential local operations. Comput Vis Image Underst 89:1–23

Suzuki K, Horiba I, Sugie N (2003c) Neural edge enhancer for supervised edge enhancement from noisy images. IEEE Trans Pattern Anal Mach Intell 25:1582–1596

Suzuki, K., Abe, H., Li, F. & Doi, K. (2004a) Suppression of the contrast of ribs in chest radiographs by means of massive training artificial neural network. In: Proceedings of the SPIE Medical Imaging (SPIE MI), May San Diego, CA, pp 1109–1119

Suzuki K, Horiba I, Sugie N, Nanki M (2004b) Extraction of left ventricular contours from left ventriculograms by means of a neural edge detector. IEEE Trans Med Imaging 23:330–339

Suzuki K, Li F, Sone S, Doi K (2005a) Computer-aided diagnostic scheme for distinction between benign and malignant nodules in thoracic low-dose CT by use of massive training artificial neural network. IEEE Trans Med Imaging 24:1138–1150

Suzuki K, Shiraishi J, Abe H, MacMahon H, Doi K (2005b) False-positive reduction in computer-aided diagnostic scheme for detecting nodules in chest radiographs by means of massive training artificial neural network. Acad Radiol 12:191–201

Suzuki K, Abe H, MacMahon H, Doi K (2006a) Image-processing technique for suppressing ribs in chest radiographs by means of massive training artificial neural network (MTANN). IEEE Trans Med Imaging 25:406–416

Suzuki K, Yoshida H, Nappi J, Dachman AH (2006b) Massive-training artificial neural network (MTANN) for reduction of false positives in computer-aided detection of polyps: Suppression of rectal tubes. Med Phys 33:3814–3824

Suzuki K, Shi Z, Zhang J (2008a) Supervised enhancement of lesions by use of a massive-training artificial neural network (MTANN) in computer-aided diagnosis (CAD). Proc. Int. Conf. Pattern Recognition (ICPR), December 2008, Tampa, FL. MoCT6.3

Suzuki K, Yoshida H, Nappi J, Armato SG 3rd, Dachman AH (2008b) Mixture of expert 3D massive-training ANNs for reduction of multiple types of false positives in CAD for detection of polyps in CT colonography. Med Phys 35:694–703

Suzuki K, Rockey DC, Dachman AH (2010a) CT colonography: advanced computer-aided detection scheme utilizing MTANNs for detection of "missed" polyps in a multicenter clinical trial. Med Phys 37:12–21

Suzuki K, Zhang J, Xu J (2010b) Massive-training artificial neural network coupled with Laplacian-eigenfunction-based dimensionality reduction for computer-aided detection of polyps in CT colonography. IEEE Trans Med Imaging 29:1907–1917

Swensen SJ, Jett JR, Hartman TE, Midthun DE, Sloan JA, Sykes AM, Aughenbaugh GL, Clemens MA (2003) Lung cancer screening with CT: Mayo Clinic experience. Radiology 226:756–761

Tan M, Deklerck R, Jansen B, Bister M, Cornelis J (2011) A novel computer-aided lung nodule detection system for CT images. Med Phys 38:5630–5645

Toriwaki J, Suenaga Y, Negoro T, Fukumura T (1973) Pattern recognition of chest x-ray images. Computer Graphics and Image Processing 2:252–271

Vapnik VN (1995) The Nature of Statistical Learning Theory. Springer, Berlin

Way TW, Sahiner B, Chan HP, Hadjiiski L, Cascade PN, Chughtai A, Bogot N, Kazerooni E (2009) Computer-aided diagnosis of pulmonary nodules on CT scans: improvement of classification performance with nodule surface features. Med Phys 36:3086–3098

Winsberg F, Elkin M, Macy J, Bordaz V, Weymouth W (1967) Detection of radiographic abnormalities in mammograms by means of optical scanning and computer analysis. Radiology 89:211–&

Xu JW, Suzuki K (2014) Max-AUC feature selection in computer-aided detection of polyps in CT colonography. IEEE J Biomed Health Inform 18:585–593

Xu XW, Doi K, Kobayashi T, MacMahon H, Giger ML (1997) Development of an improved CAD scheme for automated detection of lung nodules in digital chest images. Med Phys 24:1395–1403

Ye X, Lin X, Dehmeshki J, Slabaugh G, Beddoe G (2009) Shape-based computer-aided detection of lung nodules in thoracic CT images. IEEE Trans Biomed Eng 56:1810–1820

Yuan R, Vos PM, Cooperberg PL (2006) Computer-aided detection in screening CT for pulmonary nodules. AJR Am J Roentgenol 186:1280–1287

Chapter 3
Computer-Aided Detection and Differentiation of Breast Cancer on Mammograms

Ryohei Nakayama

Abstract Mammography is the most sensitive method available for early detection of breast cancer. However, approximately 10–30 % of breast cancer incidents are not detected using mammograms because of the size and location of a lesion, density of the breast tissue, and interpretation ability of radiologists. It is also difficult for radiologists to determine whether a detected lesion is malignant or benign. The positive predictive value of mammography is typically between 15 and 30 %, which is rather low. To overcome these problems, many investigators have developed computer-aided diagnosis (CAD) schemes for identifying regions of potential lesions in mammograms and for evaluating the malignancy of a detected lesion. CAD is defined as a diagnosis performed by a radiologist who considers the computer output as a second opinion. The purpose of CAD is to improve the diagnostic accuracy and consistency of image interpretation by radiologists. In this chapter, we provide a brief summary of some works, development examples, and potential usefulness of CAD in clinical practice.

Keywords Computer-aided diagnosis • Mammogram • Breast cancer • Detection aid • Differentiation aid

3.1 Introduction

Breast cancer has the highest incidence rate in females (World Health Organization 2006). As with cancer of other organs, early detection and early treatment can help to reduce the rates of breast cancer mortality. Mammography is the most sensitive method available for early detection of breast cancer. Therefore, it is widely used for breast cancer screening in many developed countries (Dowling et al. 2010; Smith et al. 2014). When interpreting mammograms, it is important to detect

R. Nakayama, Ph.D. (✉)
Department of Electronic and Computer Engineering, Ritsumeikan University,
1-1-1 Noji-higashi, Kusatsu, Shiga 525-8577, Japan
e-mail: ryohei@fc.ritsumei.ac.jp

H. Arimura (ed.), *Image-Based Computer-Assisted Radiation Therapy*,
DOI 10.1007/978-981-10-2945-5_3

radiographic indications of breast cancer such as clustered microcalcifications, masses, architectural distortions, and bilateral asymmetries (Kopans 2006). However, approximately 10–30 % of breast cancer incidents are not detected using mammograms because of the size and location of a lesion, density of the breast tissue, and interpretation ability of radiologists (Bird et al. 1992; Burhenne et al. 1994; Kolb et al. 2002). It is also difficult for radiologists to determine whether a detected lesion is malignant or benign. The positive predictive value of mammography, i.e., the ratio of the number of found breast cancers to the number of biopsies, is typically between 15 and 30 % (Adler and Helvie 1992; Kopans 1992), which is rather low. Unnecessary biopsies are physical and psychological burden for patients.

To overcome these problems, many investigators have developed computer-aided diagnosis (CAD) schemes for identifying regions of potential lesions in mammograms and for evaluating the malignancy of a detected lesion over the past two decades. The former is frequently called the computer-aided detection (CADe) scheme as a detection aid, whereas the latter is called the computer-aided differentiation (CADx) scheme as a differentiation aid. CAD is defined as a diagnosis performed by a radiologist who considers the computer output as a second opinion (Doi 2005, 2007). The purpose of CAD is to improve the diagnostic accuracy and consistency of image interpretation by radiologists. In this chapter, we provide a brief summary of some works, development examples, and potential usefulness of CADe and CADx in clinical practice.

3.2 CADe Schemes

Many investigators studied CADe schemes for clustered microcalcifications, masses, architectural distortions, and bilateral asymmetries. Most of them have been focused on clustered microcalcifications and masses, which are more common radiographic indications. These CADe schemes consist of two main steps: lesion image enhancement and false-positive (FP) reduction.

3.2.1 CADe Schemes for Clustered Microcalcifications

Conventional methods used in CADe schemes for clustered microcalcifications are based on image enhancement and the segmentation of regions of interest (ROIs). Chan et al. (1988) developed a difference-image approach using a combination of a matched filter and a box-rim filter. They removed the structured background of a mammogram by subtracting a signal-suppressed image from a signal-enhanced image. Romualdo et al. (2013) proposed restoration methodology to enhance mammographic images by improving contrast features and suppressing noise simultaneously. Using the Anscombe transformation, a signal-dependent quantum noise was converted into an approximately signal-independent Gaussian additive noise. In the Anscombe domain, noise was filtered using an adaptive Wiener filter. A filter based on the modulation transfer function of the imaging system was employed for image enhancement. Gulsrud and Husøy (2001) proposed a texture feature extraction method based on a single filter optimized with respect to the Fisher criterion. The texture features were employed to differentiate an ROI with clustered microcalcifications from that with normal tissue. Bocchi et al. (2004) used a fractal model to describe the background of a mammogram. They showed that the fractal model coupled with matched filtering could enhance microcalcification images with respect to the background. Yoshida et al. (1996) multiplied every scale by a weight factor and then reconstructed the enhanced images of microcalcifications by applying the inverse transform for a discrete wavelet transform. The weights were determined through supervised learning, using a set of training cases.

As other approaches, many CADe schemes based on machine learning for detecting and classifying microcalcifications were reported by investigators. Cheng et al. (2004) proposed an approach based on fuzzy logic and scale-space techniques. A mammogram was fuzzified using fuzzy entropy principle and the fuzzy set theory, and then scale-space and Laplacian-of-Gaussian filter techniques were applied to detect the locations of microcalcifications. They showed that fuzzy logic systems can detect microcalcifications accurately even in mammograms of very dense breasts. Lee and Chen (1996) showed that in the wavelet analysis, the multiresolution information related to the contextual information, which was extracted from the Gaussian Markov random field, provided a useful technique for detecting microcalcifications. Zhang and Gao (2012) proposed a novel framework using twin support vector machine (SVM). Microcalcification images were enhanced using an artifact removal filter and a high-pass filter. Subspace learning algorithms were embedded into this framework for subspace selection of each image block to be handled. A twin SVM classifier was employed to distinguish the blocks with microcalcifications from other blocks. Hernandez-Cisneros and Terashima-Marin (2006) proposed a procedure for classifying clustered microcalcifications in mammograms using the sequential difference of Gaussian filters and three evolutionary artificial neural networks (ANNs).

Some studies reported that CADe-assisted reading in screening mammography increases sensitivity, but decreases specificity. A decrease in specificity causes an increase of the recall rate. Therefore, CADe schemes which detect only clustered microcalcifications with high likelihood of malignancy have been developed in recent years.

3.2.2 *CADe Schemes for Masses*

The mass detection and the identification of the margin of mass using mammograms are difficult processes for radiologists. Two types of CADe schemes for masses have been proposed: schemes for detecting masses and schemes for detecting and segmenting them.

As one of the studies aimed at only detection, Herredsvela et al. (2005) proposed the detection process using morphological hierarchical watersheds. A mammogram image was simplified using a reconstructive open/close alternating sequential filter while the object shapes and edges were maintained. Then the regional maxima of the simplified image were extracted as internal markers for the hierarchical watershed transform. Rojas-Domínguez and Nandi (2008) developed an enhancement algorithm that improved the image contrast based on local statistical measures of mammograms. Mass candidate regions were segmented through thresholding at multiple levels, and objective features were determined. A region-ranking system identified the candidate with the highest likelihood of abnormality based on the objective features. Sakellaropoulos et al. (2006) showed the usefulness of the wavelet-based feature analysis for identifying spiculated and circumscribed masses in dense breast regions. Dense parenchyma was first labeled using Gaussian mixture modeling. Orientation features were extracted from large-scale and small-scale subimages obtained using the wavelet decomposition. The logistic regression analysis was employed to differentiate spiculated and circumscribed masses from normal dense parenchyma. Oliver et al. (2006) reported that mass candidate regions were detected using a deformable template matching approach, in which a template was constructed using the eigenimages of masses. An algorithm adapted from the eigenface approach was then used to reduce detected FP regions. Li et al. (2015) developed a bilateral image analysis scheme for reducing FP regions during the detection of masses in dense mammograms. A matching cost was defined to quantify the credibility of the corresponding region in a pair of bilateral mammograms. The similarity measurement was employed to distinguish masses from normal tissues in a pair of bilateral regions based on global and local image appearances.

As one of the studies aimed at both detection and segmentation, Wei et al. (2005) combined the gradient field analysis with the gray-level information to identify mass candidates. The morphological and spatial gray-level-dependent texture features were extracted for each candidate. Linear discriminant analysis classifiers were employed to differentiate masses from normal tissues. Eltonsy et al. (2007) proposed a technique based on the concentric layers surrounding a focal area with suspicious morphological characteristics and low relative incidence in the breast region. The mammographic regions with a high concentration of the concentric layers with a progressively lower average intensity were assumed mass candidates. Petrick et al. (1996) detected masses automatically by applying a Gaussian–Laplacian edge detector to an image, whose regions of potential masses were enhanced using an adoptive density-weighted contrast enhancement filter. Fauci et al. (2004) proposed a detection method of ROIs with masses using a supervised neural network. Some objective features related to the geometrical information and the shape parameters were determined in each ROI. A supervised neural network using objective features differentiated ROIs with masses from those with normal tissue. Yin et al. (2003) presented a method for robustly located mass areas even in noisy mammograms using the so-called intelligent mesh. Varela et al. (2007) applied an iris filter at different scales to enhance mass regions. Mass candidate regions were segmented using an adaptive threshold. Mass regions were characterized using a neural network classifier based on the iris filter output, gray level, texture, and contour-related and morphological features. Abdel-Dayem and El-Sakka (2005) proposed a detection/segmentation method based on the optimal threshold determined by minimizing the fuzzy entropy. Moreover, they employed a block-based performance criterion; thus, radiologists could compare segmented mass regions using a computer.

As with clustered microcalcifications, CADe schemes focused on masses with high likelihood of malignancy only have been developed in recent years.

3.2.3 CADe Schemes for Architectural Distortions

Most CADe schemes are focused on clustered microcalcifications and masses, which are detected easily than architectural distortions (Burrell et al. 2001; Bird et al. 1992). Using even commercial CADe systems, the sensitivities of architectural distortions were from 21 to 38 % (Baker et al. 2003). Therefore, a high-performance CADe scheme for architectural distortions has been desired.

Matsubara et al. (2015) developed an automated method for the direction analysis of linear structures. The direction of the linear structures in each ROI was defined by a direction filter and a background filter, which determined one of eight directions. The concentration and the isotropic indexes were evaluated using the determined direction of the linear structures to detect architectural distortion candidates. Karssemeijer and Te-Brake (1996) proposed a method based on the statistical analysis of the map of pixel orientations using a multiscale approach. Line-based orientations were evaluated from the output values of three-directional, second-order, and Gaussian derivative operators at each scale. A classifier with the output of these operators was employed to detect stellate patterns such as architectural distortions. Guo et al. (2005) investigated a detection method based on SVM with the Hausdorff dimension, which characterized the texture feature. When compared to radial basis function neural networks, they showed more accurate classification results produced using the SVM in distinguishing architectural distortion abnormality from normal breast parenchyma. Rangayyan et al. (2010) presented a detection method using Gabor filters, phase portrait analysis, fractal analysis, and texture analysis. Using this method, initial architectural distortion candidates were detected in prior mammograms of interval cancer and in normal control cases. Tourassi et al. (2006) investigated the application of the fractal analysis to detection of architectural distortions. The fractal dimension of mammographic ROIs was calculated using the circular average power spectrum technique. They showed that the average fractal dimension of normal ROIs was statistically significantly higher than that of ROIs with architectural distortions. Yoshikawa et al. (2014) detected the mammary gland structures using an adaptive Gabor filter.

The adaptive Gabor filter consisted of three Gabor filters, which were manufactured by changing the combination of parameters. A concentrated region, such as an architectural distortion, was enhanced based on the detected mammary gland.

In the described studies, the sensitivities of architectural distortions were approximately 70–90 %, which were lower than those of clustered microcalcifications and masses. The improvement of the detection accuracy has been desired to apply a CADe scheme for architectural distortions to clinical practice.

3.2.4 CADe Schemes for Bilateral Asymmetries

Although bilateral asymmetry is not a common radiographic indication like clustered microcalcifications and masses, its detection is important in mammography. This is because bilateral asymmetry may be the only clue to breast cancer when clustered microcalcifications, masses, and architectural distortions are not visible (Sickles 2011). Bilateral asymmetry can be caused by physiological processes or projection artifacts. Therefore, radiologists have to diagnose the cause of bilateral asymmetry. However, it can be overlooked or misinterpreted even by experienced radiologists (Majid et al. 2003; Burrell et al. 2001; Venkatesan et al. 2009).

Although a CADe scheme for bilateral asymmetry is desired, a limited number of studies were conducted. Ferrari et al. (2001) proposed a procedure based on the detection of linear directional components using a multiresolution representation through Gabor wavelets. The filter responses for different scales and orientations were analyzed using the Karhunen–Loeve transform to select the principal components. Rose diagrams computed from the phase images and statistical measures computed thereof were used for quantitative and qualitative analyses of the oriented patterns. Rangayyan et al. (2007) analyzed bilateral asymmetry in mammograms by combining the directional information, morphological measures, and geometric moments related to the density distributions. The difference of the rose diagrams was obtained using the directional data of the aligned left and right breasts. The directional features in the difference of the rose diagrams were employed to identify the changes caused by breast cancer. Tzikopoulos et al. (2011) presented a fully automated segmentation scheme based on breast density estimation. SVMs with some features, such as a fractal dimension-related feature for breast density categorization, classified bilateral asymmetry areas. Wang et al. (2010, 2011) developed a method for detecting asymmetry of the mammographic tissue density represented by the related feature differences from bilateral images. A genetic algorithm was applied to select a set of optimal features from 20 features and build an ANN for distinguishing between the positive and negative cases.

In described studies, sensitivity and specificity of bilateral asymmetry are insufficient. We hope that the detection accuracy will be improved in further studies.

3.3 Example of CADe Scheme

3.3.1 Summary

The detection performances of clustered microcalcifications in the CADe schemes based on the wavelet transform are relatively higher than those in other methods without implementing the wavelet transform (Yoshida et al. 1994, 1996; Clarke et al. 1994; Qian et al. 1994, 1995; Laine et al. 1994, 1995). The results indicate that the multiresolution analysis on the wavelet transform is useful for detecting microcalcifications with various sizes. However, using most of the CADe schemes based on the wavelet transform, the shape of microcalcifications is not analyzed in detail. In this section, we provide a novel filter bank based on the concept of the Hessian matrix for classifying nodular and linear structures. Then we attempt to detect ROIs with clustered microcalcifications using the nodular features (N features) and the nodular and linear features (NL features) obtained through this filter bank.

3.3.2 Materials

Our database consists of 1200 standard-view mammograms obtained from 300 patients in the DDSM (Digital Database for Screening Mammography, University of South Florida) (Heath et al. 1998). In these mammograms, the total number of clustered microcalcifications is 610 (239 malignant lesions and 371 benign lesions). All mammograms were digitized to a pixel size of 0.0435 mm $\times$ 0.0435 mm in a 12-bit gray scale.

3.3.3 Methods

3.3.3.1 Overall Scheme for Detecting Clustered Microcalcifications

Figure 3.1 shows the schematics of the method for detecting ROIs with clustered microcalcifications in mammograms. First, the mammogram images were decomposed into several subimages at different scales from 1 to 4 using a novel filter bank. These subimages were horizontal, vertical, and diagonal subimages for the second difference. The subimages for nodular component (NC) and the subimages for nodular and linear component (NLC) were obtained using the analysis of the Hessian matrix consisted of the subimages for the second difference. ROIs with a size of 5 mm $\times$ 5 mm were then selected automatically from the mammogram images in increments of 1 mm, so that one ROI would overlap with the adjacent ROIs. In each ROI, eight features were determined from the subimages

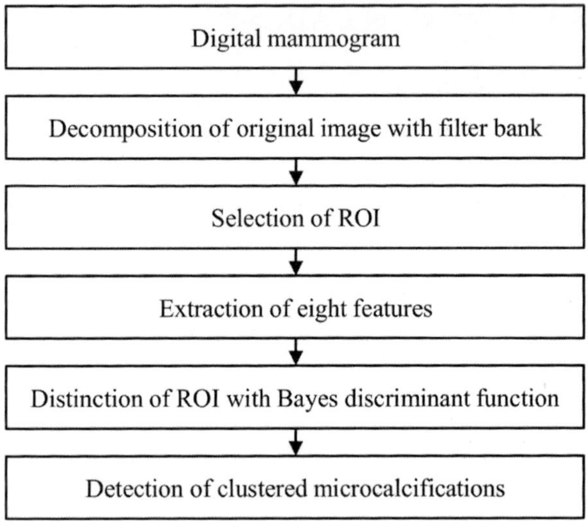

Fig. 3.1 Schematics of the method for detecting ROIs with clustered microcalcifications in mammograms

for NC at scales from 1 to 4 and the subimages for NLC at scales from 1 to 4. The Bayes discriminant function with these eight features was employed for distinguishing abnormal ROIs with clustered microcalcifications from two different types of normal ROIs without clustered microcalcifications. The region connecting the ROIs classified as abnormal was considered to be the region with potential clustered microcalcifications.

3.3.3.2 Filter Bank for Detecting NC and NLC

1. Hessian matrix classifying nodular and linear structures

For the distinction of clustered microcalcifications from normal tissues in mammograms, both NCs, such as microcalcifications, and LCs, such as blood vessels and mammary ducts, are important to be detected. To detect these components, we can employ the second derivative (Shimizu et al. 1994, 1995). The values of the second derivatives for nodular structure in all directions are negative. However, the value of the second derivative for the linear structure is zero along the direction of the axis of the linear structure, whereas it is negative along the direction perpendicular to the axis of the linear structure. Therefore, filters based on the second derivatives can be used for the detection or enhancement of nodular and linear structures. On the other hand, the minimal and maximal values of the second derivatives in all directions can be calculated using small eigenvalue λ_1 and large eigenvalue λ_2 of the Hessian matrix, because the second derivative of function $f(x, y)$ in arbitrary direction θ is given by

$$\frac{\partial^2 f}{\partial x^2}\cos^2\theta + 2\frac{\partial^2 f}{\partial x \partial y}\cos\theta\sin\theta + \frac{\partial^2 f}{\partial y^2}\sin^2\theta$$
$$= (\cos\theta \quad \sin\theta)\begin{pmatrix} \frac{\partial^2 f}{\partial x^2} & \frac{\partial^2 f}{\partial x \partial y} \\ \frac{\partial^2 f}{\partial x \partial y} & \frac{\partial^2 f}{\partial y^2} \end{pmatrix}\begin{pmatrix} \cos\theta \\ \sin\theta \end{pmatrix}.$$

Therefore, the following formulas indicate the conditions that must be satisfied by two eigenvalues λ_1 and λ_2 for nodular and linear structures, respectively:

For a nodular structure: $\lambda_1 \cong \lambda_2 < 0$.
For a linear structure: $\lambda_1 < 0,\ \lambda_2 \cong 0$.

2. Filter bank for detecting NC and NLC

Figure 3.2 shows the filter bank based on the concept of the Hessian matrix for classifying nodular and linear structures. To obtain each element of the Hessian matrix using this filter bank, high-pass filter $H_H(z)$, high-pass filter $F_H(z)$, high-pass filter $H_H(z)F_H(z)$, and smoothing filter $H_L(z)F_L(z)$ at scale j are given by

$$\begin{aligned} H_H(z) &= 1/2\left(-z^j + z^{-j}\right), \\ F_H(z) &= 1/2\left(z^j - z^{-j}\right), \\ H_H(z)F_H(z) &= 1/4\left(-z^{2j} + 2 - z^{-2j}\right), \\ H_L(z)F_L(z) &= 1/4\left(z^{2j} + 2 + z^{-2j}\right). \end{aligned}$$

By applying the smoothing filter $H_L(z)F_L(z)$ to original image S_0f, smoothed subimage S_1f at the next scale, i.e., a scale of 1, is obtained. Horizontal subimage W_f^H is obtained by applying high-pass filter $H_H(z)F_H(z)$ at vertical direction, whereas vertical subimage W_f^V is obtained by applying high-pass filter $H_H(z)$ $F_H(z)$ at horizontal direction. Diagonal subimage W_f^D is obtained by applying high-pass filter $H_H(z)$ at vertical direction followed by high-pass filter $H_H(z)$ at horizontal direction.

In the filter bank shown in Fig. 3.2, $NC_j(x, y)$ (the subimage for NC at scale j) was defined by the absolute value of large eigenvalue λ_2 of the Hessian matrix at scale j. Here, if $\lambda_2 > 0$, the pixels were zero because the eigenvalues for the nodular structure tend to become negative. $NLC_j(x, y)$ (the subimage for NLC at the scale j) was defined by the absolute value of small eigenvalue λ_1 of the Hessian matrix at the scale j. Here, if $\lambda_1 > 0$, the pixels were zero.

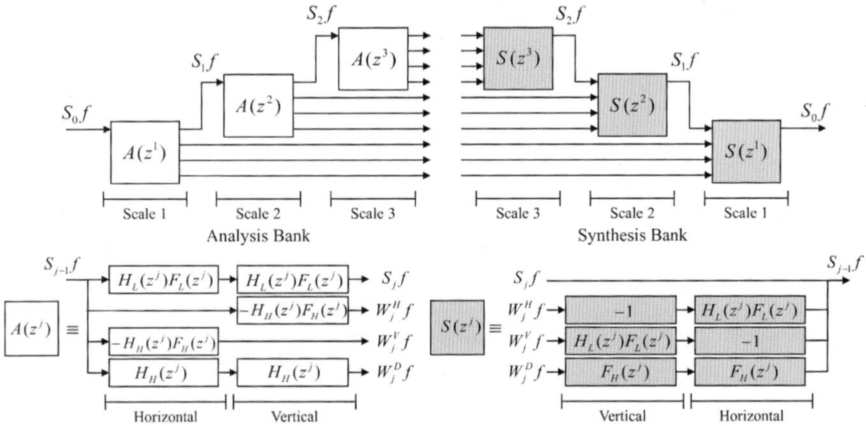

Fig. 3.2 Filter bank based on the concept of the Hessian matrix for classifying nodular and linear structures

3.3.3.3 Extraction of the Features for Detecting Clustered Microcalcifications

We determined the eight features for distinguishing abnormal ROIs with clustered microcalcifications from two different types of normal ROIs without clustered microcalcifications (normal ROIs with blood vessels and normal ROIs without blood vessels). These eight features were extracted from the subimages for NC at scales from 1 to 4 and the subimages for NLC at scales from 1 to 4. Figure 3.3 shows the subimages for NC and for NLC, which were obtained from an abnormal ROI with clustered microcalcifications, normal ROI with blood vessels, and normal ROI without blood vessels. As shown in the subimages for NC, some pixel values for abnormal ROI were higher than those for two normal ROIs. As shown in the subimages for NLC, some pixel values for normal ROI without blood vessels were lower than those for abnormal ROI and normal ROI with blood vessels. The N features at each scale from 1 to 4 were determined using the average value of the pixel values higher than 97 % of the cumulative histograms of the subimage for NC at each scale from 1 to 4. The NL features at each scale from 1 to 4 were also determined using the average value of the pixel values higher than 97 % of the cumulative histograms of the subimage for NLC at each scale from 1 to 4.

3.3.3.4 Detection of ROIs with Clustered Microcalcifications

To detect clustered microcalcifications, we employed the Bayes discriminant function (Duda et al. 2000) for distinguishing three classes ω_i $(i = 1, 2, 3)$. Classes ω_1, ω_2, and ω_3 corresponded to abnormal ROI with clustered microcalcifications, normal ROI with blood vessels, and normal ROI without blood vessels, respectively. We divided our database into a training set and a test set. Each set included

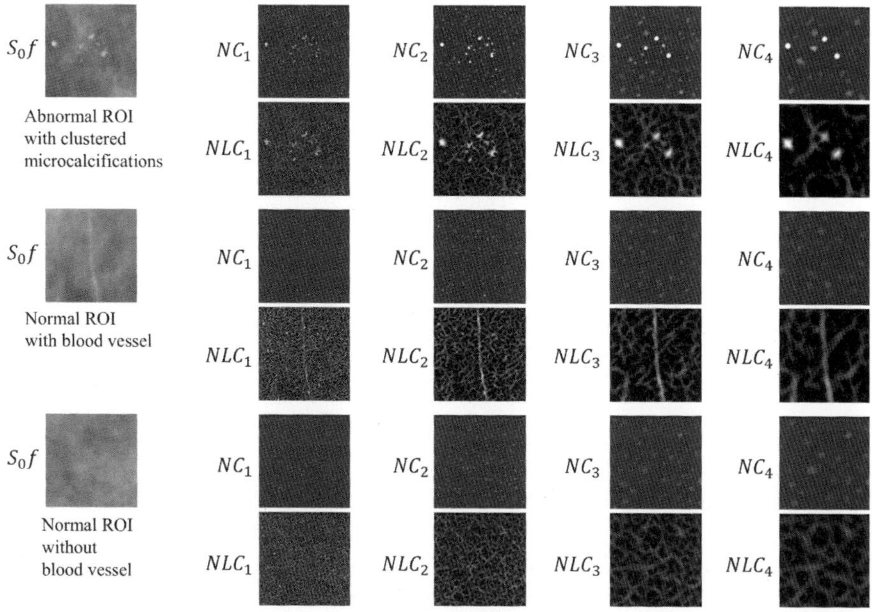

Fig. 3.3 Subimages for NC and for NLC, which were obtained from an abnormal ROI with clustered microcalcifications, normal ROI with blood vessel, and normal ROI without blood vessel

600 mammograms obtained from 150 patients. We then trained the Bayes discriminant function using three different types of ROIs selected from the training set. The studied ROIs were 300 abnormal ROIs with clustered microcalcifications, 300 normal ROIs with blood vessels, and 300 normal ROIs without blood vessels. The normal ROIs were randomly selected from normal mammograms without clustered microcalcifications. In each of these three classes, the N and NL feature vector $\boldsymbol{x}$ at scales from 1 to 4 which were determined from each ROI were used for calculating mean vector $\boldsymbol{m}_i$ and covariance matrix $\boldsymbol{V}_i$. Mean vector $\boldsymbol{m}_i$ and covariance matrix $\boldsymbol{V}_i$ are defined as

$$\boldsymbol{m}_i = \frac{1}{n_i} \sum_{x \in X_i} \boldsymbol{x},$$

$$\boldsymbol{V}_i = \frac{1}{n_i} \sum_{x \in X_i} (\boldsymbol{x} - \boldsymbol{m}_i)(\boldsymbol{x} - \boldsymbol{m}_i)^t.$$

Here, n_i and X_i are the number of patterns and the pattern set in class ω_i, respectively. The Bayes discriminant function for distinguishing three classes ω_i $(i = 1, 2, 3)$ is given by

$$g_i(\boldsymbol{x}) = -\frac{1}{2}(\boldsymbol{x} - \boldsymbol{m}_i)^t \boldsymbol{V}_i^{-1}(\boldsymbol{x} - \boldsymbol{m}_i) - \frac{1}{2}\log|\boldsymbol{V}_i|,$$

where $|\cdot|$ is the determinant. Then we then selected the ROIs at intervals of approximately 1 mm in the test set. To distinguish the three types of ROIs, the eight features determined from the selected ROIs were inputted to the Bayes discriminant function as feature vector $\boldsymbol{x}$. Bayes discriminant function $g_i(\boldsymbol{x})$ outputted three values indicating the likelihood of each class. The class yielding the largest output value was considered as the result of the distinction of the three types of ROIs. Regions connecting the ROIs, which were classified as abnormal, were considered as regions with potential clustered microcalcifications.

3.3.3.5 Evaluation of the Detection Performance

A free-response receiver operating characteristic (FROC) curve (Metz 1989) is usually used to summarize the detection performance of a CADe scheme quantitatively. An FROC curve is a plot of the true-positive (TP) fraction achieved by a computerized scheme with respect to the average number of FPs per image varied over the continuum of a given threshold. In our case, the FROC curve is not easy to be calculated because the Bayes discriminant function output three values indicating the likelihood of each class. Therefore, first, we multiplied output value $g_1(x)$, indicating the likelihood of an ROI with clustered microcalcifications, by a coefficient before comparing $g_1(x)$, $g_2(x)$, and $g_3(x)$. Next, the ROI was considered abnormal when $g_1(x)$ was the highest value among the three output values. When the center of the region connecting the ROIs, which were classified as abnormal, was within a true cluster identified by an experienced radiologist, this region was considered "truly" detected. In this study, the coefficient was varied from 0.5 to 1.5.

3.3.4 Detection Performance

Figure 3.4 shows the relationship between the TP and the FPs obtained by applying the Bayes discriminant function with the eight features. For detecting clustered microcalcifications, many investigators have developed CADe schemes using the features related to the nodular structure only. Therefore, to investigate the usefulness of the NL features, the relationship between the TP and the FPs for the Bayes discriminant function with the four features, i.e., all features except for the NL feature, is also shown in Fig. 3.4. The detection performance of the Bayes discriminant function with the eight features is much higher than that of the Bayes discriminant function with the four features. The points, at which the blood vessels intersect, tended to become nodular in structure. Therefore, they were detected as FP candidates in many other algorithms for the detection of clustered

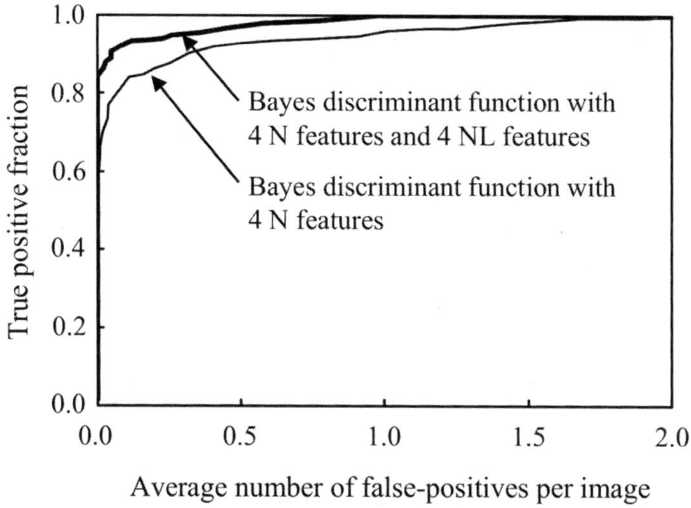

Fig. 3.4 Comparison of relationships between the TP and the FPs obtained by applying the Bayes discriminant functions with the eight features and with the four features

microcalcifications. This result indicates that the number of these FP candidates is reduced by identifying the ROIs with blood vessels.

A CADe scheme based on the Bayes discriminant function with the eight features for distinguishing the three types of ROIs identifies 310 of the 310 clustered microcalcifications in the test set, yielding a sensitivity of 100.0 % and a false-positive rate of 0.98 per mammogram. Please refer to the paper (Nakayama et al. 2006a) for the details.

3.4 Usefulness of CADe

Freer and Ulissey (2001) prospectively assessed the effect of CADe on the interpretation of screening mammograms. In this study, 12,860 screening mammograms over a 12-month period were interpreted using a CADe system. The use of the CADe system resulted in the following: an increase in the recall rate from 6.5 to 7.7 %, no change in the positive predictive value for biopsy (38 %), an increase in the number of detected cancer incidents of 19.5 %, and an increase in the rate of detected early-stage cancer incidents from 73 to 78 %. Birdwell et al. (2005) studied prospectively 8682 women during a 19-month period. Approximately 10 % of 8682 patients were recalled using a CADe scheme. CAD-prompted recalls contributed to 8 % of total recalled findings and 7 % of detected cancer incidents. Ko et al. (2006) prospectively interpreted 5016 screening mammograms over a 26-month period without and with the use of a CADe system. With the CADe system, the recall rate increased from 12 to 14 %. The use of the CADe system had no significant effect on the positive predictive value for biopsy and could increase the cancer detection rate by at least 4.7 % and the sensitivity by at least 4 %. Gur et al. (2004) interpreted 115,571 screening mammograms with ($n = 59{,}139$) or without ($n = 56{,}432$) the use of a CADe system in an academic setting. They presented that the recall and breast cancer detection rates did not change significantly if the CADe system was used. Fenton et al. (2007) analyzed 429,345 mammograms for 222,135 women without and with the use of a CADe system. The use of the CADe system decreased the specificity from 90.2 to 87.2 %, increased the rate of biopsies by 19.7 %, and decreased the rate of the detection of invasive cancer by 12 %. They concluded that the CADe system reduces the accuracy of interpretation of screening mammograms. However, in this study, the use of the CADe system increased the sensitivity from 80.4 to 84 % ($P = 0.32$) and increased the rate of the detection of ductal carcinomas in situ by 34 %.

Even the same CADe schemes will demonstrate different sensitivities and specificities depending on the practice setting, number of the interpreted cases, experience of radiologists in mammogram interpretation, and experience of radiologists in the usage of the CADe scheme. These results are associated with an increase in sensitivity and with a decrease in specificity in screening mammography if a CADe scheme is used.

3.5 CADx Schemes

Most of the studies of CADx schemes focus on clustered microcalcifications and masses. There are few studies of CADx schemes for architectural distortions or bilateral asymmetries. Therefore, we only provide the information on CADx schemes for clustered microcalcifications and masses in this section. A CADx scheme consists of four main steps: image segmentation, feature extraction, feature selection, and classification.

Jiang et al. (1996) developed a method for differentiating malignant clustered microcalcifications from those benign. An ANN with eight computer-extracted features of clustered microcalcifications was employed to identify breast cancer. Computer analysis allowed to identify malignant clustered microcalcifications in 100 % cases and those benign in 82 % cases. The accuracy of computer analysis was statistically significantly better than that of five radiologists. Jiang et al. (1999) also extended this method of the classification of lesions as malignant or benign to multiple-view mammograms. Markopoulos et al. (2001) analyzed the malignancy of clustered microcalcifications using an ANN with eight features of the calcifications (density, number, area, brightness, diameter average, distance average, proximity average, and perimeter compacity average). They showed a statistically significant difference in the area under the ROC curve (AUC) values between the ANN (0.937) and the performance of physicians (0.810). Kallergi (2004) selected 13 classification features from descriptors of the morphology of the individual calcifications and the cluster distribution. The 13 features were combined with the age of patients and were given as inputs to an ANN. The classification performance reached a sensitivity of 100 % for a specificity of 85 %. Chan et al. (1998) developed computerized feature extraction of morphological features (size, contrast, and shape) and the texture features derived from the spatial gray-level dependence matrices. Linear discriminant classifiers with the features selected from the morphological features and the texture features were employed to evaluate the malignancy of clustered microcalcifications. They reported that the classifier could identify 50 % of the benign clusters at a sensitivity of 100 % for malignancy.

Huo et al. (1998, 2000) developed a computerized method for the classification of benign and malignant masses. The inputs to an ANN included four characteristics of masses (margin, sharpness, density, and texture) that were automatically extracted using an image-processing algorithm. The categorization of lesions as malignant or benign using the ANN achieved an AUC value of 0.90. Bilska-Wolak et al. (2003) compared the performance of a likelihood ratio-based algorithm (LRb) with respect to a case-based reasoning (CBR) classifier, which provided a solution to a new problem using past similar cases. The difference in the estimation of the probability density functions results in a very small difference in the performance. They reported that using both classifiers in approximately half of cases of benign mammographic masses, biopsy could be avoided at a sensitivity of 98 %. Brake et al. (2000) defined a number of features related to the image characteristics that radiologists use to distinguish real lesions from normal tissue. An ANN was used to map the computed features to a measure of suspiciousness of each region that was found suspicious using a mass detection method. Approximately 75 % of all cancer incidents were detected at a specificity level of 0.1 false positive per image. Floyd et al. (2000) proposed a case-based reasoning approach for the classification based on the ratio of the number of matched malignant cases to the number of total matches in the database. When 98 % of the malignancies would be biopsied, the number of benign biopsies would be decreased by 41 %.

3.6 Examples of CADx Schemes

3.6.1 Summary

Many investigators reported that the performance of radiologists was improved significantly when they used the computer output indicating the likelihood of malignancy for clustered microcalcifications, as shown in Sect. 3.7. However, the performance level of the computerized schemes was considerably greater than that of radiologists using the computer output. This result implies that radiologists cannot rely on the computer output completely even if the computerized scheme has a high-performance level.

To make clinical decisions to perform biopsy or follow-up on clustered microcalcifications by considering possible histological classifications of magnification mammograms may reduce the number of unnecessary biopsies. Invasive carcinoma and noninvasive carcinoma of the comedo type usually grow rapidly (Kopans 2006; Morimoto and Sasa 1996; Sakamoto and Haga 2001). Noninvasive carcinoma of the noncomedo type, which presents a lower risk than noninvasive carcinoma of the comedo type, grows relatively slowly (Kopans 2006; Morimoto and Sasa 1996; Sakamoto and Haga 2001). Mastopathy and fibroadenoma expand very slowly (Kopans 2006; Morimoto and Sasa 1996; Sakamoto and Haga 2001). Therefore, the computerized analysis of microcalcifications on determining the likelihood of histological classifications and the likelihood of malignancy may help radiologists to make a decision on patient treatment. In this section, we provide a CADx scheme for identifying histological classifications of clustered microcalcifications on magnification mammograms.

3.6.2 Materials

Our database consists of 58 magnification mammograms that were obtained from 35 patients. It includes 35 malignant clustered microcalcifications (9 invasive carcinomas, 12 noninvasive carcinomas of the comedo type, and 14 noninvasive carcinomas of the noncomedo type) and 23 benign clustered microcalcifications (17 mastopathies and 6 fibroadenomas). The histological classifications of all clustered microcalcifications were proved using stereotaxic core needle biopsy.

These magnification mammograms were obtained using Kodak MinR-2000/MinR-2000 screen/film system. The magnification factor of the magnification mammograms was 1.8. The mammographic X-ray system included an X-ray tube with a focal spot of 0.1 mm and a molybdenum anode, 0.03-mm-thick molybdenum filter, and 5:1 reciprocating grid. These mammograms were digitized to a matrix size of 512×512 with a pixel size of 0.0275 mm in a 12-bit gray scale using EPSON ES-8000 digitizer (the optical resolution is 800×1600 dpi; the optical density range is 0.0–3.3D).

3.6.3 Methods

3.6.3.1 Segmentation of Microcalcifications and the Determination of the Cluster Margin

Figure 3.5 shows an example of the segmentation of microcalcifications and the determination of the cluster margin. For the segmentation of individual microcalcifications within a cluster on mammograms, first, we enhanced the microcalcifications using the filter bank described in Sect. 3.3.3. Then a gray-level thresholding technique (Gonzales and Woods 2007) was applied to the enhanced

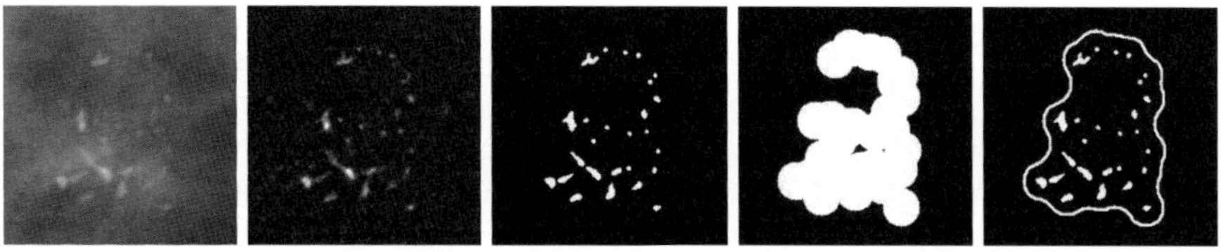

(a) (b) (c) (d) (e)

Fig. 3.5 Example of the segmentation of microcalcifications and the definition of cluster margin. (**a**) The original ROI containing clustered microcalcifications; (**b**) the microcalcifications enhanced by a novel filter bank; (**c**) the microcalcifications segmented by a *gray-level* thresholding technique; (**d**) the candidate for the cluster margin yielded by drawing the circles at the center of gravity of each microcalcifications; (**e**) the cluster margin determined by smoothing the shape of the candidate for the cluster margin

image. To segment all microcalcifications in our database, we empirically used a 600-pixel value as a threshold value.

For obtaining information about the distribution of microcalcifications within a cluster, the cluster margin was determined automatically. First, we drew circles at the center of gravity of each microcalcification. The diameters of these circles were increased from 20 to 60 pixels until all circles within a cluster were connected. Then the region of the connected circles was considered as a candidate for the cluster margin. The shape of the cluster margin could not be estimated accurately when the candidate for the cluster margin had a large indentation, as shown in Fig. 3.5d. Therefore, we employed a binary morphologic closing operator (Sera 1988) to smooth the shape of the candidate for the cluster margin. The structure element for this binary morphologic closing operator was given by the circle with half the diameter of the circle, which was used for determining the candidate for the cluster margin. Finally, the edge of the smoothed candidate was determined as the cluster margin.

3.6.3.2 Extraction of Five Objective Features

We selected five objective features to identify histological classification by considering the differences in image features among five histological classifications. These objective features were (i) variation in the size of microcalcifications within a cluster, (ii) variation in the pixel values of microcalcifications within a cluster, (iii) shape irregularity of microcalcifications within a cluster, (iv) extent of the linear and branching distributions of microcalcifications, and (v) distribution of microcalcifications toward the nipple.

(i) The variation in the size: The variation in the size of microcalcifications was determined using the relative standard deviation in the areas of microcalcifications within a cluster. The area of each microcalcification was defined as the number of pixels within the segmented microcalcification.

(ii) The variation in the pixel values: The variation in the pixel values of the microcalcifications was determined using the standard deviation in the pixel values of microcalcifications within a cluster. The pixel value of each microcalcification was defined as the mean value of the five largest pixel values in the segmented microcalcification of the original image.
(iii) Shape irregularity: To determine the shape irregularity of microcalcifications, first, we defined the irregularity index for each microcalcification as the standard deviation of 16 shape factors. The 16 shape factors consisted of eight minimal distances and eight maximal distances between the center of a microcalcification and its edges. The minimal and maximal distances were obtained in the eight regions located at intervals of 45°. Then the shape irregularity of microcalcifications was determined using the mean value of the five largest irregularity indices of individual microcalcifications within a cluster.
(iv) The extent of the linear and branching distributions: The extent of the linear and branching distributions was determined using the standard deviation of the 16 shape factors. These 16 shape factors were not applied to individual microcalcifications but to the cluster margins defined in the previous section.
(v) The distribution toward the nipple: To determine the distribution of microcalcifications toward the nipple, first, we drew a straight line from the center of the nipple to the center of a cluster. Then we drew a straight line perpendicular to this line through the cluster center. The first line is called the main straight line, and the second line is called the substraight line. Next, the distances of all microcalcifications from these two lines were determined, and the two mean values were calculated. The distribution of microcalcifications toward the nipple was determined using the ratio of the mean distance of the substraight line to the mean distance of the main straight line.

3.6.3.3 Identification of the Histological Classifications

A classifier based on the Bayes decision function (Duda et al. 2000) was employed for distinguishing between the five different types of histological classifications. The probability density function for each histological classification was assumed to be approximated using the normal distribution. The mean vector and the covariance matrix of the normal distributions were obtained from all data in our database. The prior probabilities were assumed equal. A leave-one-out testing method was used for training and testing the Bayes decision function. In this method, training was carried out for all cases except for one case in the database. The case not used for training was used for testing through the trained Bayes decision function. This procedure was repeated until every case in our database was used once. The five output values obtained using the trained Bayes decision function indicated the likelihood of each histological classification. The output value yielding the largest value was considered as the result of the classification.

3.6.4 Classification Performance

Figure 3.6 shows the mean values and the standard deviations of each objective feature of the five different types of histological classifications. These objective features were normalized using all cases in the database. The values on the vertical axis may correspond to the likelihood of malignancy because the five objective features have large values in case of malignant microcalcifications. The five objective features of invasive carcinoma and noninvasive carcinoma of the comedo type have large values. However, invasive carcinoma can be distinguished from noninvasive carcinoma of the comedo type using the two features related to the extent of the linear and branching distributions and the distribution toward the nipple. The five objective features of mastopathy and fibroadenoma have low values. Fibroadenoma can be distinguished from mastopathy because the five objective features of fibroadenoma have lower values than those of mastopathy.

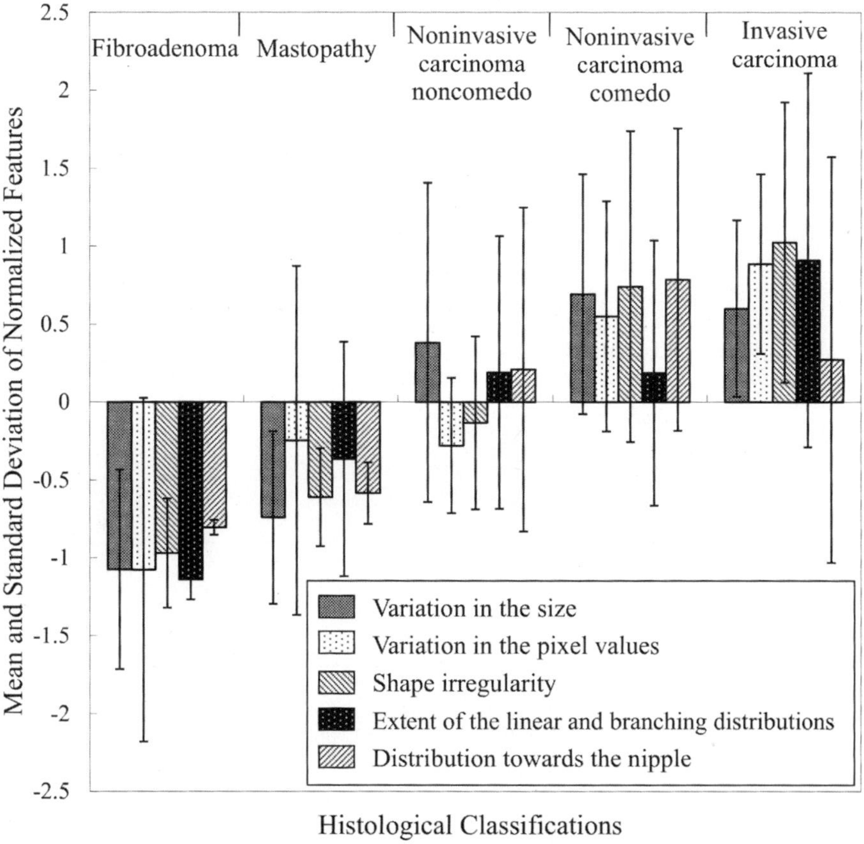

Fig. 3.6 Mean values and the standard deviations of each objective feature of the five different types of histological classifications

The five objective features of noninvasive carcinoma of the noncomedo type are nearly zero. It is difficult to distinguish noninvasive carcinoma of the noncomedo type from mastopathy. Therefore, these cases should undergo follow-up at a short interval in clinical practice. Table 3.1 shows the results of tests for univariate equality of group means. The Wilk's lambda (Johnson and Wichern 2007) for the shape irregularity was smaller than any other features, and the F value (Johnson and Wichern 2007) for the shape irregularity was larger than any other features. Therefore, the shape irregularity made a larger contribution to identifying five histological classifications of clustered microcalcifications. The distribution toward the nipple made some contributions to the classification. However, the p value for the distribution toward the nipple satisfied the significance level ($p < 0.001$). Therefore, the five objective features were statistically significant for identifying histological classifications of clustered microcalcifications.

Table 3.2 shows the results of the distinction of the five histological classifications by use of the classifier based on a Bayes decision function. The classification accuracies of this CADx scheme for distinguishing between the three malignant

Table 3.1 Results of tests for univariate equality of group means

	Wilk's lambda	*F* value	*p* value
Variation in the size	0.52	12.19	< 0.001
Variation in the pixel values	0.65	07.04	< 0.001
Shape irregularity	0.50	13.00	< 0.001
Extent of linear and branching distributions	0.68	06.32	< 0.001
Distribution toward the nipple	0.69	06.05	< 0.001

Table 3.2 Results of the distinction of the five histological classifications by use of the classifier based on a Bayes decision function

	Computer output				
Pathological diagnosis	Invasive carcinoma	Noninvasive carcinoma of comedo type	Noninvasive carcinoma of noncomedo type	Mastopathy	Fibroadenoma
Invasive carcinoma (9)	7(77.8 %)	1(11.1 %)	0(0.0 %)	1(11.1 %)	0(0.0 %)
Noninvasive carcinoma of comedo type (12)	2(16.7 %)	9(75.0 %)	1(8.3 %)	0(0.0 %)	0(0.0 %)
Noninvasive carcinoma of noncomedo type (14)	0(0.0 %)	2(14.2 %)	12(85.8 %)	0(0.0 %)	0(0.0 %)
Mastopathy (17)	0(0.0 %)	1(5.9 %)	1(5.9 %)	14(82.3 %)	1(5.9 %)
Fibroadenoma (6)	0(0.0 %)	0(0.0 %)	0(0.0 %)	1(16.7 %)	5(83.3 %)

histological classifications were 77.8 % (7/9) for invasive carcinoma, 75.0 % (9/12) for noninvasive carcinoma of the comedo type, and 85.8 % (12/14) for noninvasive carcinoma of the noncomedo type. The classification accuracies for distinguishing between the two benign histological classifications were 82.3 % (14/17) for mastopathy and 83.3 % (5/6) for fibroadenoma. The sensitivity and the specificity were 97.1 % (34/35) and 91.3 % (21/23), respectively. The positive predictive value was 94.4 % (34/36), whereas the negative predictive value was 95.4 % (21/22). Please refer to papers (Nakayama et al. 2004, 2006a, b, 2007) for the details.

3.7 Usefulness of CADx

An observer study of most of the studies for evaluating the usefulness of CADx was carried out retrospectively. Jiang et al. (1999) tested whether CADx can improve the performance of radiologists in the diagnosis of clustered microcalcifications in mammograms. The average AUC increased from 0.61 without the use of CADx to 0.75 with the use of CADx ($P < .0001$). On average, using the computer aid, each observer recommended 6.4 additional biopsies for malignant lesions and 6.0 fewer biopsies for benign lesions. Jiang et al. (2001) also evaluated whether CADx can reduce the interobserver variation in the accuracy of radiologists. As measured using the SD of the AUC, it was reduced by 46 % if the computer aid was used.

Huo et al. (2002) evaluated the effectiveness of CADx as an aid to radiologists reviewing clinical mammograms. When CADx was used, the average performance of radiologists improved, as indicated by an increase in the AUC from 0.93 to 0.96 and by an increase in the sensitivity from 94 to 98 %. Chan et al. (1999) evaluated the effects of using CADx on the classification of malignant and benign masses seen on mammograms by radiologists. The AUC values of radiologists varied from 0.79 to 0.92 without implementing CADx and improved to 0.87–0.96 if CADx was used. An improved positive predictive value as a function of the false-negative fraction was predicted using the improved ROC curves.

These results are associated with an increase in both sensitivity and specificity in retrospective observer studies using the CADx schemes for clustered microcalcifications and masses. We look forward to the introduction of an integrated CAD scheme with the combination of a CADe scheme and a CADx scheme to clinical practice with no further delay.

References

Abdel-Dayem AR, El-Sakka MR (2005) Fuzzy entropy based detection of suspicious masses in digital mammogram images. In: Proceedings of 27th Annual International Conference of the Engineering in Medicine and Biology Society, vol 4. IEEE, Shanghai, pp 4017–4022

Adler DD, Helvie MA (1992) Mammographic biopsy recommendations. Curr Opin Radiol 4 (5):123–129

Baker JA, Rosen EL, Lo JY, Gimenez EI, Walsh R, Soo MS (2003) Computer-aided detection (CAD) in screening mammography: sensitivity of commercial CAD systems for detecting architectural distortion. AJR Am J Roentgenol 181(4):1083–1088

Bilska-Wolak AO, Floyd CE Jr, Nolte LW, Lo JY (2003) Application of likelihood ratio to classification of mammographic masses; performance comparison to case-based reasoning. Med Phys 30(5):949–958

Bird RE, Wallace TW, Yankaskas BC (1992) Analysis of cancers missed at screening mammography. Radiology 184(3):613–617

Birdwell RL, Bandodkar P, Ikeda DM (2005) Computer-aided detection with screening mammography in a university hospital setting. Radiology 236(2):451–457

Bocchi L, Coppini G, Nori J, Valli G (2004) Detection of single and clustered microcalcifications in mammograms using fractals models and neural networks. Med Eng Phys 26(4):303–312

Brake GM, Karssemeijer N, Hendriks JH (2000) An automatic method to discriminate malignant masses from normal tissue in digital mammograms. Phys Med Biol 45(10):2843–2857

Burhenne HJ, Burhenne LW, Goldberg F, Hislop TG, Worth AJ, Rebbeck PM, Kan L (1994) Interval breast cancers in the Screening Mammography Program of British Columbia: analysis and classification. AJR Am J Roentgenol 162(5):1067–1071

Burrell HC, Evans AJ, Wilson AR, Pinder SE (2001) False-negative breast screening assessment: what lessons can we learn? Clin Radiol 56(5):385–388

Chan HP, Doi K, Vyborny CJ, Lam KL, Schmidt RA (1988) Computer-aided detection of microcalcifications in mammograms. Methodology and preliminary clinical study. Investig Radiol 23(9):664–671

Chan HP, Sahiner B, Lam KL, Petrick N, Helvie MA, Goodsitt MM, Adler DD (1998) Computerized analysis of mammographic microcalcifications in morphological and texture feature spaces. Med Phys 25(10):2007–2019

Chan HP, Sahiner B, Helvie MA, Petrick N, Roubidoux MA, Wilson TE, Adler DD, Paramagul C, Newman JS, Sanjay-Gopal S (1999) Improvement of radiologists' characterization of mammographic masses by using computer-aided diagnosis: an ROC study. Radiology 212 (3):817–827

Cheng HD, Wang J, Shi X (2004) Microcalcification detection using fuzzy logic and scale space approaches. Pattern Recogn 37(2):363–375

Clarke LP, Kallergi M, Qian W, Li HD, Clark RA, Silbiger ML (1994) Tree-structured non-linear filter and wavelet transform for microcalcification segmentation in digital mammography. Cancer Lett 77(2–3):173–181

Doi K (2005) Current status and future potential of computer-aided diagnosis in medical imaging. Br J Radiol 78(1):S3–S19

Doi K (2007) Computer-aided diagnosis in medical imaging: historical review, current status and future potential. Comput Med Imaging Graph 31(4–5):198–211

Dowling EC, Klabunde C, Patnick J, Ballard-Barbash R (2010) Breast and cervical cancer screening programme implementation in 16 countries. J Med Screen 17(3):139–146

Duda RO, Hart PE, Stork DG (2000) Pattern classification. Wiley-Interscience, New York

Eltonsy NH, Tourassi GD, Elmaghraby AS (2007) A concentric morphology model for the detection of masses in mammography. IEEE Trans Med Imaging 26(6):880–889

Fauci F, Bagnasco S, Bellotti R, Cascio D, Cheran SC, De Carlo F, De Nunzio G, Fantacci ME, Forni G, Lauria A, Lopez-Torrez E, Magro R, Masala GL, Oliva P, Quarta M, Raso G, Retico A, Tangaro S (2004) Mammogram segmentation by contour searching and massive lesion classification with neural network. In: Proceedings of the 2004 I.E. Nuclear Science Symposium. IEEE, Rome, pp 2695–2699

Fenton JJ, Taplin SH, Carney PA, Abraham L, Sickles EA, D'Orsi C, Berns EA, Cutter G, Hendrick RE, Barlow WE, Elmore JG (2007) Influence of computer-aided detection on performance of screening mammography. N Engl J Med 356(14):1399–1409

Ferrari RJ, Rangayyan RM, Desautels JE, Frère AF (2001) Analysis of asymmetry in mammograms via directional filtering with Gabor wavelets. IEEE Trans Med Imaging 20(9):953–964
Floyd CE Jr, Lo JY, Tourassi GD (2000) Case-based reasoning computer algorithm that uses mammographic findings for breast biopsy decisions. AJR Am J Roentgenol 175(5):1347–1352
Freer TW, Ulissey MJ (2001) Screening mammography with computer-aided detection: prospective study of 12,860 patients in a community breast center. Radiology 220(3):781–786
Gonzales RC, Woods RE (2007) Digital image processing. Prentice Hall, New Jersey
Gulsrud TO, Husøy JH (2001) Optimal filter-based detection of microcalcifications. IEEE Trans Biomed Eng 48(11):1272–1281
Guo Q, Shao J, Ruiz V (2005) Investigation of support vector machine for the detection of architectural distortion in mammographic images. J Phys Conf Ser 15:88–94
Gur D, Sumkin JH, Rockette HE, Ganott M, Hakim C, Hardesty L, Poller WR, Shah R, Wallace L (2004) Changes in breast cancer detection and mammography recall rates after the introduction of a computer-aided detection system. J Natl Cancer Inst 96(3):185–190
Heath M, Bowyer K, Kopans D, Kegelmeyer P Jr, Moore R, Chang K, Munishkumaran S (1998) Current status of the digital database for screening mammography. Digit Mammography Comput Imaging Vis 13:457–460
Hernandez-Cisneros RR, Terashima-Marin H (2006) Evolutionary neural networks applied to the classification of microcalcification clusters in digital mammograms. In: Proceedings of the 2006 I.E. Congress on Evolutionary Computation. IEEE, Vancouver, pp 2459–2466
Herredsvela J, Gulsrud TO, Engan K (2005) Detection of circumscribed masses in mammograms using morphological segmentation. In: Fitzpatrick JM, Reinhardt JM (eds) Medical imaging 2005: image processing: proceedings of SPIE 5747. SPIE, San Diego, pp 902–913
Huo Z, Giger ML, Vyborny CJ, Wolverton DE, Schmidt RA, Doi K (1998) Automated computerized classification of malignant and benign masses on digitized mammograms. Acad Radiol 5(3):155–168
Huo Z, Giger ML, Vyborny CJ, Wolverton DE, Metz CE (2000) Computerized classification of benign and malignant masses on digitized mammograms: a study of robustness. Acad Radiol 7 (12):1077–1084
Huo Z, Giger ML, Vyborny CJ, Metz CE (2002) Breast cancer: effectiveness of computer-aided diagnosis observer study with independent database of mammograms. Radiology 224 (2):560–568
Jiang Y, Nishikawa RM, Wolverton DE, Metz CE, Giger ML, Schmidt RA, Vyborny CJ, Doi K (1996) Malignant and benign clustered microcalcifications: automated feature analysis and classification. Radiology 198(3):671–678
Jiang Y, Nishikawa RM, Schmidt RA, Metz CE, Giger ML, Doi K (1999) Improving breast cancer diagnosis with computer-aided diagnosis. Acad Radiol 6(1):22–33
Jiang Y, Nishikawa RM, Schmidt RA, Toledano AY, Doi K (2001) Potential of computer-aided diagnosis to reduce variability in radiologists interpretations of mammograms depicting microcalcifications. Radiology 220(3):787–794
Johnson RA, Wichern DW (2007) Applied multivariate statistical analysis. Prentice Hall, London
Kallergi M (2004) Computer-aided diagnosis of mammographic microcalcification clusters. Med Phys 31(2):314–326
Karssemeijer N, Te-Brake GM (1996) Detection of stellate distortions in mammograms. IEEE Trans Med Imaging 15(5):611–619
Ko JM, Nicholas MJ, Mendel JB, Slanetz PJ (2006) Prospective assessment of computer-aided detection in interpretation of screening mammography. AJR Am J Roentgenol 187 (6):1483–1491
Kolb TM, Lichy J, Newhouse JH (2002) Comparison of the performance of screening mammography, physical examination, and breast US and evaluation of factors that influence them: an analysis of 27,825 patient evaluations. Radiology 225(1):165–175
Kopans DB (1992) The positive predictive value of mammography. AJR Am J Roentgenol 158 (3):521–526

Kopans DB (2006) Breast imaging. Lippincott Williams & Wilkins, Philadelphia
Laine AF, Schuler S, Fan J, Huda W (1994) Mammographic feature enhancement by multiscale analysis. IEEE Trans Med Imaging 13(4):725–740
Laine AF, Fan J, Yang W (1995) Wavelets for contrast enhancement of digital mammography. IEEE Eng Med Biol Mag 14(5):536–550
Lee GG, Chen CH (1996) A multiresolution wavelet analysis and Gaussian Markov random field algorithm for breast cancer screening of digital mammography. In: Del Guerra A (ed) Proceedings of the 1996 I.E. Nuclear Science Symposium. IEEE, Anaheim, pp 1737–1741
Li Y, Chen H, Yang Y, Cheng L, Cao L (2015) A bilateral analysis scheme for false positive reduction in mammogram mass detection. Comput Biol Med 57:84–95
Majid AS, de Paredes ES, Doherty RD, Sharma NR, Salvador X (2003) Missed breast carcinoma: pitfalls and pearls. Radiographics 23(4):881–895
Markopoulos C, Kouskos E, Koufopoulos K, Kyriakou V, Gogas J (2001) Use of artificial neural networks (computer analysis) in the diagnosis of microcalcifications on mammography. Eur J Radiol 39(1):60–65
Matsubara T, Ito A, Tsunomori A, Hara T, Muramatsu C, Endo T, Fujita H (2015) An automated method for detecting architectural distortions on mammograms using direction analysis of linear structures. In: Proceedings of 37th Annual International Conference of Engineering in Medicine and Biology Society. IEEE, Milan, pp 2661–2664
Metz CE (1989) Some practical issues of experimental design and data analysis in radiological ROC studies. Investig Radiol 24(3):234–245
Morimoto T, Sasa M (1996) Atlas of screening mammography. Digital-Press, Tokyo
Nakayama R, Uchiyama Y, Watanabe R, Katsuragawa S, Namba K, Doi K (2004) Computer-aided diagnosis scheme for histological classification of clustered microcalcifications on magnification mammograms. Med Phys 31(4):789–799
Nakayama R, Uchiyama Y, Yamamoto K, Watanabe R, Namba K (2006a) Computer-aided diagnosis scheme using a filter bank for detection of microcalcification clusters in mammograms. IEEE Trans Biomed Eng 53(2):273–283
Nakayama R, Watanabe R, Namba K, Takeda K, Yamamoto K, Katsuragawa S, Doi K (2006b) Computer-aided diagnosis scheme for identifying histological classification of clustered microcalcifications by use of follow-up magnification mammograms. Acad Radiol 13 (10):1219–1228
Nakayama R, Watanabe R, Namba K, Takeda K, Yamamoto K, Katsuragawa S, Doi K (2007) An improved computer-aided diagnosis scheme using the nearest neighbour criterion for determining histological classification of clustered microcalcifications. Methods Inf Med 46 (6):716–722
Oliver A, Freixenet J, Marti R, Denton ERE, Zwiggelaar R (2006) Mammographic mass eigendetection. In: Proceedings of Medical Image Understanding and Analysis Conference 2006. MIUA, Manchester, pp 71–75
Petrick N, Chan HP, Sahiner B, Wei D (1996) An adaptive density-weighted contrast enhancement filter for mammographic breast mass detection. IEEE Trans Med Imaging 15(1):59–67
Qian W, Clarke LP, Kallergi M, Clark RA (1994) Tree-structured nonlinear filters in digital mammography. IEEE Trans Med Imaging 13(1):25–36
Qian W, Clarke LP, Zheng B, Kallergi M, Clark RA (1995) Computer assisted diagnosis for digital mammography. IEEE Eng Med Biol Mag 14(5):561–569
Rangayyan RM, Ferrari RJ, Frère AF (2007) Analysis of bilateral asymmetry in mammograms using directional, morphological, and density features. J Electron Imaging 16(1):12
Rangayyan RM, Banik S, Desautels JE (2010) Computer-aided detection of architectural distortion in prior mammograms of interval cancer. J Digit Imaging 23(5):611–631
Rojas-Domínguez A, Nandi AK (2008) Detection of masses in mammograms via statistically based enhancement, multilevel-thresholding segmentation, and region selection. Comput Med Imaging Graph 32(4):304–315

Romualdo LC, Vieira MA, Schiabel H, Mascarenhas ND, Borges LR (2013) Mammographic image denoising and enhancement using the Anscombe transformation, adaptive wiener filtering, and the modulation transfer function. J Digit Imaging 26(2):183–197
Sakamoto G, Haga S (2001) Fundamental and clinic of ductal carcinoma in situ. Shinoharashinsha, Tokyo
Sakellaropoulos F, Skiadopoulos S, Karahaliou A, Costaridou L, Panayiotakis G (2006) Using wavelet-based features to identify masses in dense breast parenchyma. Digital Mammography in Lect Notes Comput Sci 4046:557–564
Sera J (1988) Image analysis and mathematical morphology. Academic Press, London
Shimizu A, Toriwaki J, Hasegawa J (1994) Characteristics of minimum directional difference filter which extracts circumscribed shadows in chest x-ray images. Syst Comput Jpn 25 (2):56–66
Shimizu A, Toriwaki J, Hasegawa J (1995) Characteristics of rotatory second order difference filter for computer aided diagnosis of medical images. Systems and Computers in Japan 26 (11):38–51
Sickles EA (2011) Mammography: asymmetries, masses, and architectural distortion. In: Diseases of the heart and chest, including breast 2011–2014, pp 255–258
Smith RA, Manassaram-Baptiste D, Brooks D, Cokkinides V, Doroshenk M, Saslow D, Wender RC, Brawley OW (2014) Cancer screening in the United States, 2014: a review of current American Cancer Society guidelines and current issues in cancer screening. CA Cancer J Clin 64(1):30–51
Tourassi GD, Delong DM, Floyd CE Jr (2006) A study on the computerized fractal analysis of architectural distortion in screening mammograms. Phys Med Biol 51(5):1299–1312
Tzikopoulos SD, Mavroforakis ME, Georgiou HV, Dimitropoulos N, Theodoridis S (2011) A fully automated scheme for mammographic segmentation and classification based on breast density and asymmetry. Comput Methods Prog Biomed 102(1):47–63
Varela C, Tahoces PG, Méndez AJ, Souto M, Vidal JJ (2007) Computerized detection of breast masses in digitized mammograms. Comput Biol Med 37(2):214–226
Venkatesan A, Chu P, Kerlikowske K, Sickles EA, Smith-Bindman R (2009) Positive predictive value of specific mammographic findings according to reader and patient variables. Radiology 250(3):648–657
Wang X, Lederman D, Tan J, Wang XH, Zheng B (2010) Computerized detection of breast tissue asymmetry depicted on bilateral mammograms: a preliminary study of breast risk stratification. Acad Radiol 17(10):1234–1241
Wang X, Lederman D, Tan J, Wang XH, Zheng B (2011) Computerized prediction of risk for developing breast cancer based on bilateral mammographic breast tissue asymmetry. Med Eng Phys 33(8):934–942
Wei J, Sahiner B, Hadjiiski LM, Chan HP, Petrick N, Helvie MA, Roubidoux MA, Ge J, Zhou C (2005) Computer-aided detection of breast masses on full field digital mammograms. Med Phys 32(9):2827–2838
World Health Organization, World Health Organization Statistical Information System (2006) Available from: http://www.who.int/whosis/mort/en/index.html
Yin L, Deshpande S, Chang JK (2003) Automatic lesion/tumor detection using intelligent mesh-based active contour. In: Proceedings of 15th IEEE International Conference on Tools with Artificial Intelligence. IEEE, Sacramento, pp 390–397
Yoshida H, Doi K, Nishikawa RM (1994) Automated detection of clustered microcalcifications in digital mammograms using wavelet processing techniques. In: Loew MH (ed) Medical Imaging 1994: image processing: proceedings of SPIE 2167. SPIE, Newport Beach, pp 868–886
Yoshida H, Doi K, Nishikawa RM, Giger ML, Schmidt RA (1996) An improved computer-assisted diagnostic scheme using wavelet transform for detecting clustered microcalcifications in digital mammograms. Acad Radiol 3(8):621–627

Yoshikawa R, Teramoto A, Matsubara T, Fujita H (2014) Automated detection of architectural distortion using improved adaptive Gabor filter. Breast Imaging in Lect Notes Comput Sci 8539:606–611

Zhang X, Gao X (2012) Twin support vector machines and subspace learning methods for microcalcification clusters detection. Eng Appl Artif Intell 25(5):215–221

Chapter 4
Computer-Aided Differentiation for Pathology Images

Masahiro Yamaguchi

Abstract The evolution of whole slide imaging (WSI) technology promotes the pathology environment based on digital imaging, called "digital pathology," and enables monitor-based diagnosis instead of conventional diagnosis based on microscopic observation, as well as the application of computer image analysis to pathology practice. This chapter introduces the background, basic techniques, and examples of image analysis technology for digital pathology. Computer-aided diagnosis with quantifying morphological and molecular features will be a significant tool for diagnostic pathology such as cancer detection, grade differentiation, and the decision of therapeutic plan. Some systems for automated processing of WSI data are also presented including the systems that have been employed in practice. The color correction, which is one of the most important issues in the pathological image analysis, is also addressed.

Keywords Digital pathology • Whole slide imaging • Quantitative pathology • Nuclear atypia • Structural atypia • Morphological feature • Color correction • Spectral imaging

4.1 Introduction

In diagnostic pathology, pathologists examine the tissue taken from the lesion through macroscopic and microscopic observations, to determine the type of disease or to make a decision if the tumor is malignant or benign. The result directly contributes to the decision of therapeutic plan. Thus pathology plays an essential role in cancer diagnosis and treatment, and it is often called "definitive diagnosis" or "final diagnosis." Molecular and genetic analyses are extensively used presently, such as for subtype classification. Even so, the observation of tissue and cell morphology is still a fundamental and important part in diagnostic pathology. Since diagnosis is done by direct observation under a microscope, digital imaging

M. Yamaguchi (✉)
School of Engineering, Tokyo Institute of Technology, 4259-G2-28, Nagatsuta, Midori-ku, Yokohama 226-8503, Japan
e-mail: yamaguchi.m.aa@m.titech.ac.jp

H. Arimura (ed.), *Image-Based Computer-Assisted Radiation Therapy*,
DOI 10.1007/978-981-10-2945-5_4

technology has not been introduced in routine practice, in contrast to radiology field. However, recently emerging technology called "digital slide" or whole slide imaging (WSI) (Pantanowitz et al. 2011; Gilbertson et al. 2006) allows the full introduction of digital imaging in diagnostic pathology. In WSI, the specimen on a glass slide is scanned in very high resolution, and huge-size image data thus obtained can be observed on a monitor with changing the field and magnification interactively.

Once the tissue specimens are digitized, they can be exploited not only for making a diagnosis by observing images on a monitor but also for diagnostic support system based on image analysis technology (Meijer et al. 1997; Gurcan et al. 2009; Saito et al. 2013; Kothari et al. 2013; Kayser et al. 2009; He et al. 2012). In this chapter, the application of digital image analysis and pattern recognition technology to the advancement of diagnostic pathology is described, along with some challenges in this field.

When applying the digital imaging technology to pathology domain, the practice in the radiology imaging is useful; computer-aided diagnosis (CAD) is one of them. Although the methodology in radiology CAD can be applied, some differences should be noted. In radiology CAD, screening or the detection of tumor was one of the main targets, while differential or qualitative diagnosis is a major part in pathology since the tissue under examination is acquired from a lesion. Not only the detection of abnormality but the decision of malignancy or the classification of grades or subtype is needed as well in pathology CAD. Moreover, the performance of pathology CAD should be evaluated based on the therapeutic effectiveness, which is an actual outcome of diagnostic pathology.

In the microscopic observation in histopathology and cytology, the color of tissue plays significant role. In histopathology, the tissue acquired from the human body is fixed with formalin, embedded in paraffin block, cut to thin sections, and then colorized with staining for visualizing the tissue structure. There are roughly three types of staining techniques: hematoxylin and eosin (HE) stain that is often called general stain, special stains that visualize specific tissue element depending on the purpose of observation, and immunohistochemistry (IHC) stain useful for visualizing the protein expressions. Figure 4.1 shows the example of images of HE-stained, special-stained, and IHC-stained tissues. Accordingly, the color information is very important in the pathology image analysis (Yagi and Gilbertson 2005; Rabinovich et al. 2004; Abe et al. 2005; Murakami et al. 2012). In Sect. 4.4, some issues related to color in pathology imaging are also discussed.

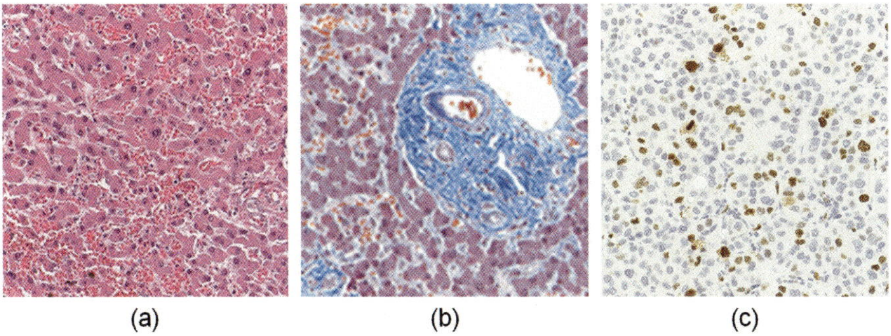

Fig. 4.1 Examples of images of histological stained tissues. (**a**) HE, (**b**) Masson's trichrome (special stain), and (**c**) IHC

4.2 Digital Imaging Technology in Diagnostic Pathology

4.2.1 Evolution of WSI Technology

The introduction of digital imaging technology started with telepathology (Weinstein et al. 2009). A remote pathologists support clinicians through network by observing the digital image in telepathology. A pathologist can also be supported by another pathologist at remote site with different specialty, and double-check can be performed in efficient manner by employing telepathology system. There have been different types of telepathology systems used—store-forward, video, robotic, and WSI. The development of telepathology system has greatly contributed to the advancement of pathology imaging technology.

The research and development of WSI have been made since late 1990s, but practical deployment was difficult because it needs to deal with huge amount of data. The pixel pitch should be smaller than 1 μm or even 0.3 μm, and the size of a specimen is typically 20~30 mm, that is, the image size becomes 20,000×20,000 ~ 100,000×100,000 pixels. Then the corresponding data amount is 1.2 GB~30 GB per image in uncompressed case. The scanning time, data transfer, and interactive display as well as image quality were difficult problems for practical use. Nevertheless, now the technologies for WSI scanner and viewer have been greatly evolved, such as the systems of optics, mechanical controlling, digital image interface, and fast computing. Advanced scanner system now enables the scan of a single slide in 1 minute and comfortable interactive display. Figure 4.2 shows the schematic drawing of WSI technology. In this example shown in Fig. 4.2b, the area in 25.2 mm × 22.7 mm was scanned with 0.23 μm pixel pitch, and an image in 110,592×99,840 pixels was obtained.

Still it is expected to address some issues related to image quality and focusing. Since a tissue sample on a glass slide is not completely flat, it is necessary to adjust the focus of the objective lens depending on the location on the specimen, but the autofocusing occasionally fails. In addition, when the tissue section is relatively

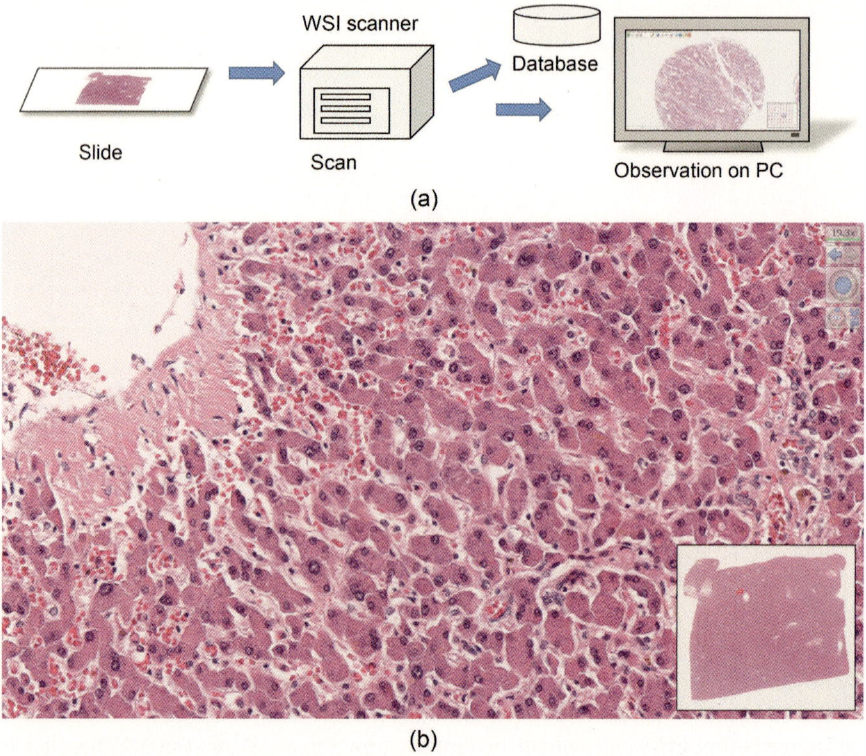

Fig. 4.2 (**a**) The concept of WSI system. Tissue specimen on a glass slide is digitized by a WSI scanner, and the image is reproduced on a monitor. (**b**) An example of observation. The whole specimen is shown in the window at bottom right, and the image scanned with using a 40x objective lens is displayed on the entire screen

thick, or in the case of cytology samples, the focus position needs to be changed during observation. The images of different focus positions can be acquired by state-of-the-art scanners, called "z-stack." However, much larger amount of data and longer acquisition time are required, and z-stack is currently used in limited cases. As an effort related to the image quality control, some techniques (Hashimoto et al. 2012) are developed for automatic detection of the area suffered by image blur due to focusing error as well as strong noise generated during the scanning process. The detected areas are re-scanned so that good quality WSI can be obtained.

So far, WSI has been used in practice mainly in telepathology, education, conference, and research applications. Moreover, it is being also adopted to primary diagnosis and clinical use (Pantanowitz et al. 2011; Gilbertson et al. 2006). WSI technology will significantly contribute to the introduction of information technology in pathology division, the connection and integration with PACS or EMR, and the deployment of pathology CAD based on digital image analysis.

The lineup of WSI apparatus includes a small-scale research-purpose device and a large-scale system suitable for hospital clinical use that automatically process a large number of slides. This practical WSI technology promotes the revolution of pathology field, referred to as "digital pathology." The Food and Drug Administration (FDA) of the USA established a WSI working group, and the issues toward clinical use are discussed in the working group (Center for Devices and Radiological Health 2016).

In pathology department, traditionally the diagnostic workflow is based on the exchange of tissue block or biopsy samples taken from lesion, or specimens on glass slides. If all pathological specimens are digitized and managed as digital data, the need of handling "things" like tissue samples is minimum, and overall workflow of pathology department can be integrated into a computerized management system. It will promote more efficient diagnosis process; thereby the diagnosis results will be informed sooner to the patient, and the patient treatment will start earlier. Besides, the management of "things" will also be improved, e.g., reducing the risk of mixing-up samples and shortening turnaround time. The discipline on this subject is recognized as pathology informatics, and digital pathology is a key technology in this field.

4.2.2 Application of Image Analysis Technology

Since the diagnosis in pathology is carried out by visual observation of the tissue morphology, cell arrangement, and color, it is sometimes pointed out that there is a problem in the observer variability and reproducibility. In some cases, the morphological feature is represented by several levels of numbers, but it is based on visual determination and said to be qualitative or semiquantitative diagnosis rather than quantitative. Although counting the number of IHC stained cells is done as well, the manual counting is inaccurate and troublesome.

The progress of digital image analysis, pattern recognition, and machine learning is remarkable, such as face recognition. By measuring the image features by applying such a digital image analysis technology, it becomes possible to quantify the morphological features of tissue specimen. Then it will enable more detailed lesion classification, accuracy improvement in the determination of the degree of malignancy, and better diagnostic report which is more useful for clinicians. Under this background, active research is being carried out on the application of image analysis technology to the pathology diagnosis.

Tissue architecture and cell morphology have been studied long regarding the relation between the morphological features and the type of disease or the degree of malignancy. It is known as pathological morphology or morphometry, and computerized analysis has been also applied (Meijer et al. 1997). For example, the shape features of cell nuclei are measured, such as the diameter, area, and circularity, or the nuclear-cytoplasmic ratio (N/C ratio). Those morphological features are compared with other pathological indices, clinical course, or prognostic indications.

However, even though using a computer, the measurement is based on manual process using general-purpose image processing software, and the results are rather affected by the operator judgment. Then it is still considered as "semiquantitative." Moreover, as it requires labor and time, full application to routine practice is difficult, and the use has been limited mainly for research purpose.

Recently, the development of molecular-targeted therapy is remarkable in cancer treatment. The effectiveness of such therapy is completely different depending on the target molecule expression, and the determination of applicability is extremely important. The image analysis technology of IHC-stained tissue is getting attention as a tool for the objective assessment of applicability and the improved accuracy and efficiency (Gurcan et al. 2009; Irshad et al. 2014). The molecular expression is also important in subtype classification and evaluation of tumor grade. It is evaluated by IHC-stained samples and more recently fluorescent staining. Some examples of image analysis for molecular expression are introduced in the Sect. 4.3.2.

On the other hand, HE staining which is a routine staining technique has long history, and pathologists acquire considerable information from the observation of HE-stained samples. Thus it is promising to apply computerized image analysis to HE-stained samples. Although there have been many reports on the image analysis of HE-stained tissue specimen, most of them need manual process as mentioned above (Meijer et al. 1997). The region of interest is determined manually; the tissue elements such as nuclei are extracted with adjusting threshold, or the contour is traced by hand; then morphological features are measured; and statistical analysis is applied. As it needs laborious process, it is difficult to be employed in routine diagnosis. But the emergence of WSI is changing the situation. A completely automated system is developed for the analysis of HE-stained specimens, in which the WSI data is processed without human interaction, and the malignant regions are automatically detected (Gurcan et al. 2009; Wienert et al. 2012; Kiyuna et al. 2008). The system has been put into practice in laboratory test company for quality control and quality assurance by double-check. It is a CAD in pathology field and is expected to be applied to the system that will provide more useful information for pathologists and clinical practice.

4.3 Examples of Computer-Aided Analysis

4.3.1 Analysis of HE-Stained Image

Cancer cells have features such as nuclear enlargement, chromatin increase, cell atypia, and cell disarrangement. Since cell nuclei are stained with hematoxylin and observed clearly in HE-stained tissue, most of the techniques first extract cell nuclei, and the morphological features are calculated using extracted nuclei (Gurcan et al. 2009; Atupelage et al. 2014; Cataldo et al. 2012). Figure 4.3a

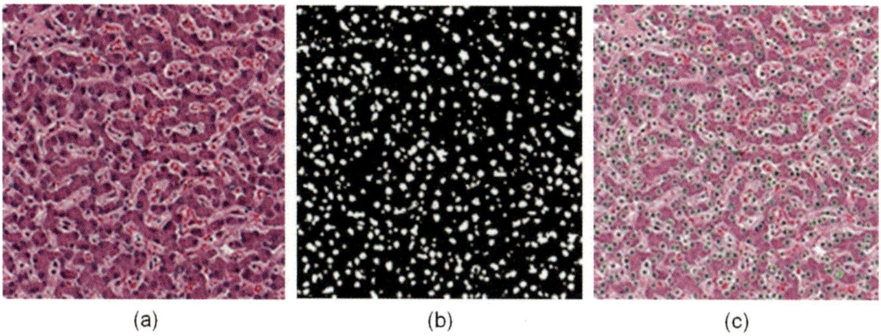

Fig. 4.3 Nuclei detection from a color image of HE-stained liver tissue. (**a**) Original color image; (**b**) after thresholding R channel component; (**c**) detected nuclei are marked with *circles*

Fig. 4.4 Spectral absorbance of hematoxylin and eosin

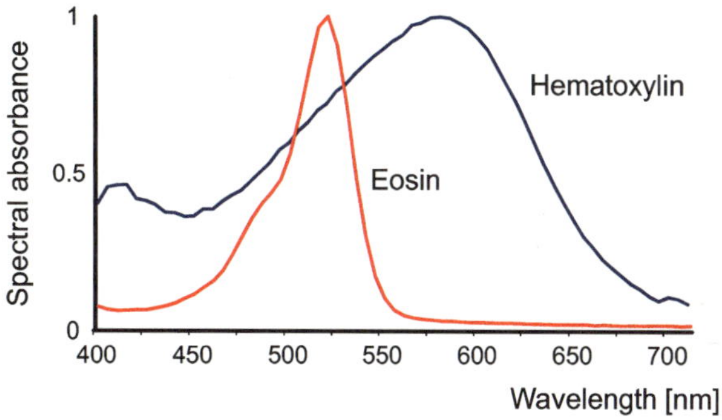

shows an example color image of HE-stained tissue of the liver, where the nuclei and cytoplasm are stained in blue and pink, respectively. The spectral absorption coefficients of hematoxylin and eosin are shown in Fig. 4.4. The hematoxylin absorbs light in 550~650 nm wavelength range, and the eosin has strong absorption peak around 530 nm. Therefore, in a color image consisting of red, green, and blue (R, G, and B) components, the R channel image holds the information of hematoxylin absorption, and the contrast of nuclei is high. Thus an approach to extract nuclei is thresholding R channel image as shown in Fig. 4.3b, but binarization is not enough for nucleus identification, since there is density variation inside a nucleus because of the chromatin distribution and nucleolus. For identifying each nucleus, image processing technique based on mathematical morphology is often applied, such as opening and closing, or distance transformation, and local maximum can be considered as the candidate of the nucleus location. When the nuclear density is high and adjacent cells are attached, they are separated by some image processing technique such as mathematical morphology. Besides, since the nuclei are often circular, it is advantageous to combine pattern matching technique such as normalized cross correlation using disk-shaped template.

In HE staining, lymphocytes are also stained in blue in addition to the nuclei of parenchymal and stromal cells and need to be removed from the extracted nuclei. Using the features of lymphocytes, e.g., darker than other nuclei, smaller, and circular, lymphocytes are identified and removed from the nucleus list detected in the previous step. Figure 4.3c is an example of nuclear detection. After the extraction of nuclei, the contour of nucleus is derived, and morphological features of cell nuclei are calculated using the contour shape and other parameters of the nucleus.

As the feature that represents nuclear shape, following indices are often used: area, perimeter, circularity, and long/short axis (after ellipse fitting). The N/C ratio mentioned before is also used commonly in morphometry. Moreover, as the chromatin texture is related to cell proliferation, the texture features inside a nucleus are often evaluated, e.g., mean and standard deviation of pixel values inside nucleus region, textural features derived from gray-level co-occurrence function, Gabor features, wavelet, and fractal/multifractal and contour complexity (Atupelage et al. 2014; Doyle et al. 2012; Yamashita et al. 2014). These indices are calculated for each nucleus, and the feature index for each tissue is obtained as statistics such as mean, standard deviation, median, or percentiles. Then various studies using those morphological indices have been reported. For example, the discriminability of benign and malignant tissue from a certain set of features is evaluated, or the feature set that has correlation with prognostic outcome indicators is investigated.

Using the locations of extracted nuclei and connecting neighboring nuclei, graph-based analysis is also applied (Sharma et al. 2015). Region partitioning is also utilized, and the tissue structure is characterized using the areas or perimeters of the partitioned regions. In intestinal organs, breast, or prostate, the gland structure is important, and nuclear arrangement is also useful to analyze the gland structure.

For the automatic detection or grading of cancer, multivariate analysis or machine learning techniques are employed. Discriminant analysis, neural network, support vector machine (SVM), random forest, and deep learning techniques are common examples that can be exploited to detection or classification (Gurcan et al. 2009; Saito et al. 2013; Kothari et al. 2013; Kayser et al. 2009).

In histopathology diagnosis of breast cancer, nuclear grade is usually used for characterizing the tumor. The nuclear grade is determined based on nuclear atypia and mitotic activity. For the assessment of nuclear atypia, nuclei are firstly detected, and the features related to the size and shape of each nucleus are measured (Petushi et al. 2006; Veta et al. 2014; Dong et al. 2014). Then mean or median of those features represents the regularity of nuclei in the tissue, and their standard deviation shows the uniformity of the same features. In addition, the detection of mitotic nuclei is important. From the texture inside the nuclei, the mitotic cells are discriminated. The count of mitosis cells in a certain view field is an important index that signifies the aggressiveness of the cancer. It is also reported that the computer image analysis enables the differentiation of malignant tumor such as noninvasive ductal carcinoma in situ (DCIS) from a benign, low-risk lesion, such as usual ductal hyperplasia. DCIS is considered to be preinvasive malignant type and should be treated rapidly. The differentiation is difficult even in visual observation, and computer analysis can provide valuable information for differentiation.

Researches are also conducted for prostate cancer application (Wienert et al. 2012; Wetzel et al. 1999; Tabesh et al. 2007; Mosquera-Lopez et al. 2015). In prostate biopsy examination, firstly cancer regions that have characteristic gland formation must be detected from the tissue, and Gleason score, which is widely used to assess the aggressiveness of the cancer, is determined. The score strongly connected to the selection of treatment. The treatment options include surgery, external or internal radiation, hormone therapy, and follow-up. Accurate classification allows patients better treatment selection for superior quality of life. In conventional visual diagnosis, two most predominant cancer regions are selected, and the gland pattern is classified into five-level grades. The classification is performed with structure or texture analysis. The Gleason score is the sum of the grades for two regions. Automated grading techniques for prostate cancer have been studied long, but most of them were using single microscopic field and determined the grade for the given image. Most recently, using WSI data, full automation is being explored by implementing two steps, cancer detection and grading (Wienert et al. 2012). The computer analysis will facilitate more accurate and quantitative grading system rather than old scoring system which is limited by visual observation.

CAD tool for lymphoma has been also developed (Sertel et al. 2010; Belkacem-Boussaid et al. 2011; Kornaropoulos et al. 2014). Follicular lymphoma is one type of slowly glowing non-Hodgkin lymphoma, and its treatment is selected from some options, i.e., radiation therapy, chemotherapy or immunotherapy that includes molecular-targeted medicine, and follow-up. It is important to distinguish indolent case, and histopathological observation plays a crucial part of the differentiation. In the diagnosis, the number of centroblast cells must be counted in high-magnification image. It is pointed out that the number obtained through visual observation is affected by some factors related to human operation, such as the limited selection of test fields, fatigue, and observer variation. The CAD system first identifies the follicles from the tissue in WSI. To count centroblasts, the technique similar to nuclear detection is used, and the discrimination of centroblast and non-centroblast follows.

4.3.2 Image Analysis of IHC-Stained Tissue

IHC staining technique visualizes the expression of specific antigen in the tissue. In breast cancer, the subtype classification is done based on the presence of estrogen receptor ER), progesterone receptor (PR), human epidermal growth factor 2 (HER2), and Ki-67 protein, and they are assessed by IHC-stained specimen. Most of IHC test is done by using 3,3′-diaminobenzodine (DAB) staining, in which positively stained region appeared in brown, and hematoxylin is used as counter-stain, and the negative nuclei becomes blue.

In conventional pathological examination, the expression of protein is evaluated visually by microscopic observation. In the case of quantifying a receptor present in nuclei, such as ER, PR, and Ki-67, the numbers of positive and negative nuclei are counted in the cancer tissue, and the percentage of positive nuclei is used as the index. HER2 is localized in the membrane, and the staining strength in cell membrane is classified into 0, 1+, 2+, and 3+. The issue of observer variability is pointed out, namely, the score is sometimes affected by inter- and intra-observer variation.

The development of molecular-targeted therapy is actively studied, and promising developments have been done. One of the significant examples is Trastuzumab (known as its brand name Herceptin). It is proved to be effective for breast and gastric cancers in which HER2 receptor is overexpressed. Such type of cancer is poor prognosis, but the targeted medicine is applicable. When determining the applicability of HER2, firstly IHC staining of HER2 is used in histopathological examination. If the result of IHC test is equivocal, additional fluorescent in situ hybridization (FISH) test is performed for final decision. Computerized image analysis (Gurcan et al. 2009; Irshad et al. 2014) is applied to the first-step IHC test, for the purpose of automated, reproducible, and quantitative examination. Detection of positive region is not difficult by automated image analysis, though the determination of threshold is necessary, but in contrast, the selection of region for examination is difficult to be automated. The region of interest (ROI) must be cancer tissue, while stromal region should be excluded, which is difficult to be automated. Therefore in the current systems, the ROI is manually specified, and the system automatically extract cell membrane, and the staining strength is quantified by an image analysis software.

Ki-67 protein, which represents the proliferation characteristics of cells, is evaluated by the ratio of positive nuclei against all nuclei. The ratio is called "labeling index." Thus the image analysis is basically the detection of nuclei and the classification of positive/negative nuclei. Again the ROI selection is a difficult issue, and mostly the automatic counting system is semiautomatic. Ki-67 is used in cancer diagnosis of many different types, because it is considerably related to the malignancy of the cancer.

For the selection of ROI, the cancer detection technique is needed. Sometimes the selection is not easy from IHC DAB-stained image, and HE-stained tissue of serial section is used. The removal of non-tissue regions is also needed for the IHC quantification.

4.3.3 Automated WSI Analysis System for Quantitative Pathology

It is necessary to automatically process whole slide image data for deployment of image analysis technology in routine diagnosis. Most of the technologies described

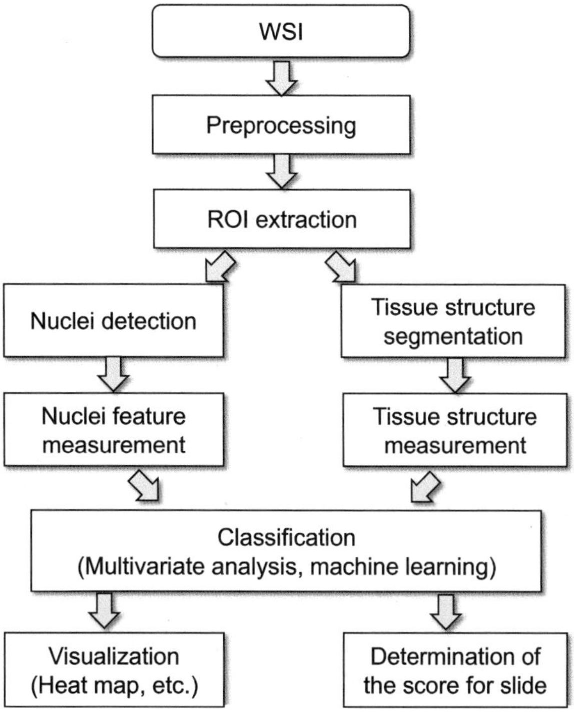

Fig. 4.5 The flowchart of typical automated system of WSI analysis

above are applied after some manual adjustment or ROI selection. Additional procedures are required for automation.

Figure 4.5 shows an example of the system overview of automatic WSI analysis system (Saito et al. 2013; Kothari et al. 2013; Kayser et al. 2009; Doyle et al. 2012; Yamashita et al. 2014; Samsi et al. 2012; Yeh et al. 2014). Initially, tissue is detected from the whole slide image, because the tissue occupies limited area on a glass slide. After tissue area is determined, many ROIs are extracted from the tissue area in the very large-size WSI. The ROI size is fixed and the following processing is applied to the extracted ROIs. The color correction is applied to the ROI data, since the image is affected by color variability as explained in the Sect. 4.4. Sometimes it is needed to detect the area of tissue fold, bubbles, or artifact where tissue is partly crushed and to exclude those regions from the analysis (Bautista and Yagi 2010).

The analysis of each ROI is done in the same way as the approach explained in Sect. 4.3.1. Nuclei and other tissue elements are identified and segmented, and the shape and texture features are measured in each segmented tissue elements. The statistics in each ROI is calculated if needed, and a feature vector which encompasses those statistics and other morphological indices is used in multivariate analysis or machine learning technique.

To use the image analysis results in diagnosis, the results for all ROIs should be summarized. For example, in the quantification of IHC-stained slide, the score is calculated for a slide. The score that represents a slide is obtained as mean, median, or maximum depending on clinical requirements.

As an example, an automated image analysis system has been developed recently for quantifying fibrosis from WSI of Elastica van Gieson (EVG) stained biopsy tissue (Abe et al. 2013). The quantification of liver fibrosis is important in the diagnosis of chronic liver disease. In EVG staining, the collagen and elastic fibers are stained in red and black, respectively. Then the area ratios of collagen and elastic fiber against whole tissue are used as the scores. In this system, ROIs are extracted from tissue region, the collagen and elastin scores are calculated in each ROI, and the total score for the slide is determined as the representative values of the scores in all ROIs. Quantification of fiber is valuable in the assessment of hepatitis and other disorders in various organs, the prediction of cancer risk, and the evaluation of new treatment methodologies.

Another example of fully automated system is WSI-CAD system, which has been applied to gastric, colorectal, and breast cancers (Saito et al. 2013). In the system, after the preprocessing including artifact removal and color balancing, the tissue structure is analyzed using low-magnification image so as to detect abnormal gland formation and other structural abnormality. The detected regions are ROIs for further analysis, in which the nuclear features are analyzed using high-magnification images. Then benign and malignant lesions are automatically discriminated. The system is used in practice at clinical test laboratory for the purpose of QC/QA. The automatic cancer detection is also worthy for quantification of IHC-stained tissue, since the score must be calculated in the cancer tissue.

The automated WSI analysis system is applied to hepatocellular carcinoma as well (Yamashita et al. 2014; Ishikawa et al. 2016; Aziz et al. 2015). After preprocessing such as color correction, the nuclear detection and nuclear feature measurement are employed. Also, stromal areas, sinusoids, and fat droplets are segmented for the structural feature measurements. The system shows the quantification results as a heat map. Moreover, the cancer discrimination is performed by SVM using the feature vector composed of nuclear and structural features. The result of feature measurement and SVM classification are also visualized as a heat map as shown in Fig. 4.6. The accuracy of classification was tested by fivefold cross validation using about 1000 ROIs. As a result, both the sensitivity and specificity were almost 90 % (Aziz et al. 2015). The heat map of the possibility of malignancy will support pathologists to pick up the regions that should be observed carefully, and the heat map of each feature provides pathologists supportive information for subtype classification, grading, treatment selection, and reasoning of the diagnosis.

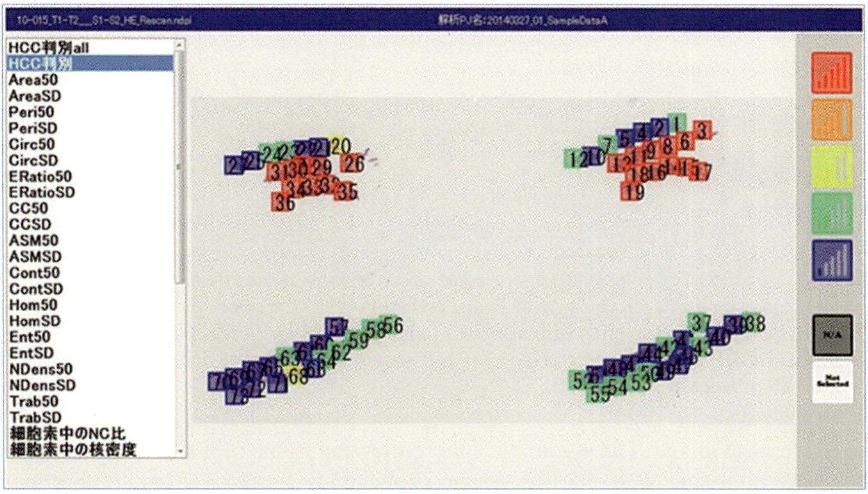

Fig. 4.6 Heat map visualization of the probability of cancer. Four biopsy samples are shown, and red regions show high possibility of cancer. Other features automatically calculated by the system can be selected to be visualized as a similar heat map

4.4 Color and Spectral Information Processing

4.4.1 Color Correction

The color of histological tissue specimen is determined by the staining and sometimes affected by the staining process, such as the selection of recipe, reagent condition, temperature, PH, and staining time. In addition, the color sometimes faded after some time passed. Additionally, the color of WSI is affected by the characteristics of imaging device, such as illuminant spectrum; spectral sensitivities of R, G, B components; and tone reproduction curve (gamma characteristics). Plus, image handling software and display monitor influence the color visualized on a monitor screen (Yagi and Gilbertson 2005). Such color variation affects the diagnosis using a color display and, moreover, causes a serious issue in image analysis.

In HE-stained specimen, the color is mostly determined by H and E dyes, and approximately the absorbance can be modeled by Beer-Lambert law based on a simple model as shown in Fig. 4.7. Although it is not exactly linear in the case of RGB color image, a linear model is often applied after tone reproduction curve correction (Rabinovich et al. 2004; Abe et al. 2005; Murakami et al. 2012).

An advantage of the model based on Beer-Lambert law is to enable color unmixing for separating H and E components from an RGB color image. Then the segmentation of nuclei and other tissue elements can be implemented using the dye component images. This model can also be applied to the color correction. In the color correction technique in the liver biopsy image analysis system (Yamashita et al. 2014), RGB values are log-transformed, and the color distribution is adjusted

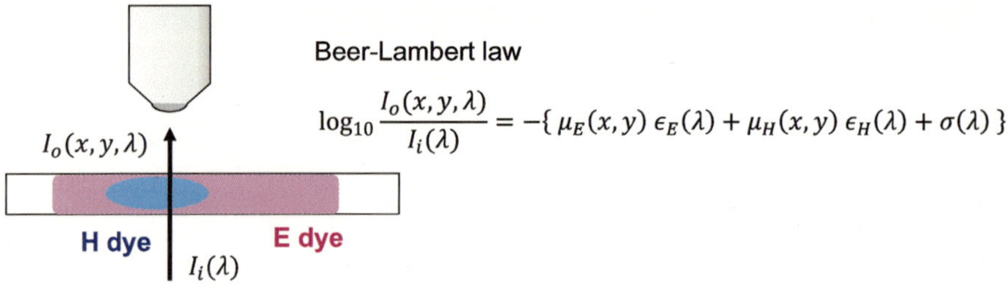

Fig. 4.7 The model of color in the microscopic observation of stained tissue specimen (example of HE-stained case). In the equation of Beer-Lambert law, $I_i(\lambda)$, spectral distribution of incident light; $I_o(\lambda)$, spectral distribution of transmitted light; $\epsilon_E(\lambda)$ and $\epsilon_H(\lambda)$, spectral absorption coefficients of E and H dyes; $\mu_E(x, y)$ and $\mu_H(x, y)$, dye amount distribution of E and H dyes; and $\sigma(\lambda)$, spectral absorbance of tissue

to a reference image. The automatic color correction is one of the key technologies for fully automatic WSI analysis system explained in Sect. 4.3. Similar algorithm was developed for other staining techniques, such as DAB and EVG as well.

The technology for the correction of the difference in color reproduction characteristics depending on devices is called color management. The RGB values captured by an imaging device usually depend on the device characteristics, and color management technology enables the exchange of color information between different devices consistently. One method for color management is to use a standard color space, such as sRGB, where it is easy to be implemented, but the color gamut and the quantization levels are limited, resulting in the loss of color information during data exchange. Another method is a color management using ICC (International Color Consortium) profile. ICC profile describes the characteristics of a device and enables the exchange of color without loss of color information. ICC recently started a working group for the discussion on the application of color management technology in medical imaging including digital pathology (ICC 2016). The method for color quality evaluation is under discussion, and a color chart for the evaluation of WSI scanner is proposed. The standardized way for color management in digital pathology will be established in the near future, and it will be beneficial not only for the diagnosis using display monitor but also the application of digital image analysis.

4.4.2 Spectral Imaging Application

Pathology image obtained by color camera or WSI scanner is normally constituted of RGB three-primary color channels, but the application of spectral imaging technology is also investigated. If the spectrum of light is divided into multiple components (usually more than three), it is called multispectral imaging (Levenson et al. 2004; Fuji et al. 2002). It allows the visualization of the information that is invisible by direct observation, using higher wavelength resolution or invisible wavelength range. Multispectral imaging was shown to be effective in the classification of melanoma or eosinophilic cells.

"Digital staining" using multispectral image is the technology that imitates physical staining process by digital image processing (Bautista et al. 2005; Bautista and Yagi 2012). For example, it is applied to digital Masson's trichrome (MT) staining from multispectral image of HE-stained tissue. MT staining is usually used to visualize fiber region, in which the color is similar to cytoplasm region in HE-stained case. Using the spectral characteristics of fiber tissue, it is possible to visualize fiber area from the multispectral image of HE-stained tissue. Similarly using digital staining technique, eosin component can be digitally added to the image of DAB with hematoxylin counterstain. It helps the quantification of IHC-stained tissue, because eosin visualizes cytoplasm, and the tissue structure becomes clearer so that the observer can easily understand the cell is included in the target cancer tissue or not. Physical stain requires lengthy time, and digital staining technique will facilitate rapid and efficient examination.

Multispectral imaging is also effective for accurate color unmixing, or called spectral unmixing (Levenson et al. 2004; Fuji et al. 2002). In addition to the fact that the accuracy of unmixing of HE staining is improved, multiple chromogen can be used in the imaging. In visualization step, spectral unmixing and synthesis will provide richer information from a single tissue specimen.

Unmixing technique is advantageous in fluorescence imaging as well (Kraus et al. 2007). Fluorescence observation is done more frequently in recent times, for examining protein expressions in high accuracy. However, autofluorescence and cross talk are sometimes mingled, and they are troublesome in quantification. The unmixing technique is promising for removing such autofluorescence and cross talk.

4.5 Summary

The status of introduction of digital technology and the possibility of computer-aided differentiation in diagnostic pathology are presented. The pattern recognition technology is ultimately advancing recently, such as big data analysis or deep learning. Once it becomes possible to provide quantitative feature of tissues and cells by computer-based analysis, such feature can be exploited as a new biomarker, which is considered to be morphological marker, or phenotype marker. Such biomarker will be employed along with gene or protein markers for determining the treatment method that is most suitable for the specific patient. For this purpose, it is necessary to realize the image analysis technology that provides reliable and versatile morphological features even from the capture by different scanners and the analysis of the relationship between those morphological markers and prognosis or effectiveness of therapy selection.

Acknowledgments The author sincerely expresses his acknowledgment to the collaborators of the work introduced in this chapter: Prof. Michiie Sakamoto, Dr. Akinori Hashiguchi, and Dr. Tokiya Abe in Keio University, Dr. Akira Saito in Tokyo Medical University; Dr. Ken-ichi Kamijo, Dr. Tomoharu Kiyuna, and Ms. Yoshiko Yamashita in NEC Corporation; Prof. Naoki Kobayashi and Dr. Masahiro Ishikawa in Saitama Medical University; Prof. Hiroshi Nagahashi, Dr. Fumikazu Kimura, and Dr. Yuri Murakami in Tokyo Institute of Technology; and Dr. Yukako Yagi in Massachusetts General Hospital. Some of the works introduced in this chapter is supported by New Energy and Industrial Technology Development Organization (NEDO), Japan.

References

Abe T, Hashiguchi A, Yamazaki K, Ebinuma H, Saito H, Kumada H, Izumi N, Masaki N, Sakamoto M (2013) Quantification of collagen and elastic fibers using whole-slide images of liver biopsy specimens. Pathol Int 63(6):305–310

Abe T, Murakami Y, Yamaguchi M, Ohyama N, Yagi Y (2005) Color correction of pathological images based on dye amount quantification. Opt Rev 12(4):293–300

Atupelage C, Nagahashi H, Kimura F, Yamaguchi M, Abe T, Hashiguchi A, Sakamoto M (2014) Computational hepatocellular carcinoma tumor grading based on cell nuclei classification. J Med Imag 1(3):034501

Aziz MA, Kanazawa H, Murakami Y, Kimura F, Yamaguchi M, Kiyuna T, Yamashita Y, Saito A, Ishikawa M, Kobayashi N, Abe T, Hashiguchi A, Sakamoto M (2015) Enhancing automatic classification of hepatocellular carcinoma images through image masking, tissue changes and trabecular features. J Pathol Inform 6:26

Bautista PA, Yagi Y (2010) Improving the visualization and detection of tissue folds in whole slide images through color enhancement. J Pathol Inform 1:25

Bautista PA, Yagi Y (2012) Digital simulation of staining in histopathology multispectral images: enhancement and linear transformation of spectral transmittance. J Biomed Opt 17(5):056013

Bautista PA, Abe T, Yamaguchi M, Yagi Y, Ohyama N (2005) Digital staining for multispectral images of pathological tissue specimens based on combined classification of spectral transmittance. Comput Med Imaging Graph 29(8):649–657

Belkacem-Boussaid K, Samsi S, Lozanski G, Gurcan MN (2011) Automatic detection of follicular regions in H&E images using iterative shape index. Comput Med Imaging Graph 35 (7–8):592–602

Cataldo SD, Ficarra E, Macii E (2012) Computer-aided techniques for chromogenic immunohistochemistry: status and directions. Comput Biol Med 42(10):1012–1025

Center for Devices and Radiological Health, U.S. Food and Drug Administration (2016) Technical performance assessment of digital pathology whole slide imaging devices, guidance for Industry and Food and Drug Administration Staff, the activity of WSI working group is available at https://nciphub.org/groups/wsi_working_group. 30 August 2016

Dong F, Irshad H, Oh E-Y, Lerwill MF, Brachtel EF, Jones NC, Knoblauch NW, Montaser-Kouhsari L, Johnson NB, Rao LKF, Faulkner-Jones B, Wilbur DC, Schnitt SJ, Beck AH (2014) Computational Pathology to Discriminate Benign from Malignant Intraductal Proliferations of the Breast. PLoS One 9(12):e114885

Doyle S, Feldman MD, Shih N, Tomaszewski J, Madabhushi A (2012) Cascaded discrimination of normal, abnormal, and confounder classes in histopathology: Gleason grading of prostate cancer. BMC Bioinform 13:282

Fuji K, Yamaguchi M, Ohyama N, Mukai K (2002) Development of support system for pathology using spectral transmittance—the quantification method of stain conditions. SPIE Med Imag Proc SPIE 4684:1516–1523

Gilbertson JR, Ho J Anthony L, Jukic DM, Yagi Y, Parwani AV (2006) Primary histologic diagnosis using automated whole slide imaging: a validation study. BMC Clin Pathol 6:4

Gurcan MN, Laura EB, Madabhushi A, Can A, Rajpoot NM, Yener B (2009) Histopathological image analysis: a review. IEEE Rev Biomed Eng 2:147–171

Hashimoto N, Bautista PA, Yamaguchi M, Ohyama N, Yagi Y (2012) Referenceless image quality evaluation for whole slide imaging. J Pathol Inform 3:9

He L, Long LR, Antani S, Thoma GR (2012) Histology image analysis for carcinoma detection and grading. Comput Methods Prog Biomed 107(3):538–556

ICC: International Color Consortium (2016) Medical imaging working group. Available from: http://www.color.org/groups/medical/medical_imaging_wg.xalter. 30 August 2016

Irshad H, Veillard A, Roux L, Racoceanu D (2014) Methods for nuclei detection, segmentation, and classification in digital histopathology: a review—current status and future potential. IEEE Rev Biomed Eng 7:97–114

Ishikawa M, Murakami Y, Ahi ST, Yamaguchi M, Kobayashi N, Kiyuna T, Yamashita Y, Saito A, Abe T, Hashiguchi A, Sakamoto M (2016) Automatic quantification of morphological features for hepatic trabeculae analysis in stained liver specimens. J Med Imag (to appear)

Kayser K, Görtler J, Bogovac M, Bogovac A, Goldmann T, Vollmer E, Kayser G (2009) AI (artificial intelligence) in histopathology--from image analysis to automated diagnosis. Folia Histochem Cytobiol 47(3):355–361

Kiyuna T, Saito A, Kerr E, Bickmore W (2008) Characterization of chromatin texture by contour complexity for cancer cell classification. 8th IEEE international conference on BioInformatics and BioEngineering, 2008. (BIBE 2008), pp 1–6

Kornaropoulos EN, Niazi MKK, Lozanski G, Gurcan MN (2014) Histopathological image analysis for centroblasts classification through dimensionality reduction approaches. Cytometry A 85(3):242–255

Kothari S, Phan JH, Stokes TH, Wang MD (2013) Pathology imaging informatics for quantitative analysis of whole-slide images. J Am Med Inform Assoc 20(6):1099–1108

Kraus B, Ziegler M, Wolff H (2007) Linear fluorescence unmixing in cell biological research. Mod Res Educ Top Microsc 863–872

Levenson R, Cronin PJ, Pankratov KK (2004) Spectral imaging for brightfield microscopy. Proc SPIE 4959:27–33

Meijer GA, Beliën JA, van Diest PJ, Baak JP (1997) Origins of ... image analysis in clinical pathology. J Clin Pathol 50(5):365–370

Mosquera-Lopez C, Agaian S, Velez-Hoyos A, Thompson I (2015) Computer-aided prostate cancer diagnosis from digitized histopathology: a review on texture-based systems. IEEE Rev Biomed Eng 8:98–113

Murakami Y, Gunji H, Kimura F, Yamaguchi M, Yamashita S, Saito A, Abe T, Sakamoto M, Bautista PA, Yagi Y (2012) Color correction in whole slide digital pathology. In: Proceedings of the 20th color imaging conference, pp 253–258

Pantanowitz L, Valenstein PN, Evans AJ, Kaplan KJ, Pfeifer JD, Wilbur DC, Collins LC, Colgan TJ (2011) Review of the current state of whole slide imaging in pathology. J Pathol Inform 2:36

Petushi S, Garcia FU, Haber MM, Katsinis C, Tozeren A (2006) Large-scale computations on histology images reveal grade-differentiating parameters for breast cancer. BMC Med Imaging 6:14

Rabinovich A, Laris CA, Agarwal S, Price JH, Belongie S (2004) Unsupervised color decomposition of histologically stained tissue samples. In: Thrun S, Saul LK, Schölkopf B (eds) Advances in neural information processing systems, vol 16. MIT Press, Cambridge, pp 667–674

Saito A, Cosatto E, Kiyuna T, Sakamoto M (2013) Dawn of the digital diagnosis assisting system, can it open a new age for pathology? In: Proceedings of the SPIE: medical imaging 2013, digital pathology, vol 8676 867602-1-16

Samsi S, Krishnamurthy AK, Gurcan MN (2012) An efficient computational framework for the analysis of whole slide images: application to follicular lymphoma immunohistochemistry. J Comput Sci 3(5):269–279

Sertel O, Lozanski G, Shana'ah A, Gurcan MN (2010) Computer-aided detection of centroblasts for follicular lymphoma grading using adaptive likelihood based cell segmentation. IEEE Trans Biomed Eng 57(10):2613–2616

Sharma H, Zerbe N, Lohmann S, Kayser K, Hellwich O, Hufnagl P (2015) A review of graph-based methods for image analysis in digital histopathology. Diagn Pathol 1:61

Tabesh A, Teverovskiy M, Pang H, Kumar VP, Verbel D, Kotsianti A, Saidi O (2007) Multifeature prostate cancer diagnosis and Gleason grading of histological images. IEEE Trans Med Imag 26(10):1366–1378

Veta M, Pluim JP, Diest PJ, Viergever MA (2014) Breast cancer histopathology image analysis: a review. IEEE Trans Biomed Eng 61(5):1400–1411

Weinstein RS, Graham AR, Richter LC, Barker GP, Krupinski EA, Lopez AM, Erps KA, Bhattacharyya AK, Yagi Y, Gilbertson JR (2009) Overview of telepathology, virtual microscopy, and whole slide imaging: prospects for the future. Hum Pathol 40:1057–1069

Wetzel AW, Crowley R, Kim S, Dawson R, Zheng L, Joo YM, Yagi Y, Gilbertson J, Gadd C, Deerfield DW, Becich MJ (1999), Evaluation of prostate tumor grades by content-based image retrieval. 27th AIPR workshop: advances in computer-assisted recognition. Proceedings of the SPIE, vol 3584, pp 244–252

Wienert S, Heim D, Saeger K, Stenzinger A, Beil M, Hufnagl P, Dietel M, Denkert C, Klauschen F (2012) Detection and segmentation of cell nuclei in virtual microscopy images: a minimum-model approach. Scientific Rep 2:503

Yagi Y, Gilbertson JR (2005) Digital imaging in pathology: the case for standardization. J Telemed Telecare 11(3):109–116

Yamashita Y, Kiyuna T, Sakamoto M, Hashiguchi A, Ishikawa M, Murakami Y, Yamaguchi M (2014) Development of a prototype for hepatocellular carcinoma classification based on morphological features automatically measured in whole slide images. Analyt Cell Pathol 2014:817192

Yeh F-C, Parwani AV, Pantanowitz L, Ho C (2014) Automated grading of renal cell carcinoma using whole slide imaging. J Pathol Inform 5:23

Part II
Computer-Assisted Radiation Treatment Planning

Chapter 5
Computer-Assisted Target Volume Determination

Hidetaka Arimura, Yusuke Shibayama, Mohammad Haekal, Ze Jin, and Koujiro Ikushima

Abstract The gross tumor volume (GTV) regions are the fundamental regions used to determine the clinical target volumes (CTVs) and planning target volume (PTV). The accuracy of the GTVs may affect tumor control and adverse events related to organs at risk or normal tissue. The PTV is the volume that includes the CTV plus CTV-to-PTV margin including the internal margin (IM) and the setup margin (SM). This chapter introduces the computational segmentation approaches for GTV and computational determination of the CTV-to-PTV margin.

Keywords Gross tumor volume (GTV) • Clinical target volume (CTV) • Segmentation • Planning target volume (PTV) • CTV-to-PTV margin

5.1 Introduction

In general, radiation treatment planning (RTP) starts from the delineation of gross tumor volumes (GTVs), which are the fundamental regions used for determination of the clinical target volumes (CTVs) and planning target volumes (PTVs). The accuracy of GTVs may affect the tumor control and adverse events related to organs at risk or normal tissue. The GTV is the gross palpable or visible/demonstrable extent and location of malignant growth based on the multifaceted information obtained from a combination of imaging modalities (computed tomography (CT), magnetic resonance imaging (MRI), positron emission tomography (PET), ultrasound, etc.), diagnostic modalities (pathology and histological reports, etc.), and clinical examination (ICRU 1993). Figure 5.1 illustrates the definitions of the target volumes including the GTV, CTV, and PTV (ICRU 1999). The CTV is the tissue

H. Arimura (✉)
Division of Medical Quantum Science, Department of Health Sciences, Faculty of Medical Sciences, Kyushu University, 3-1-1 Maidashi, Higashi-ku, Fukuoka 812-8582, Japan
e-mail: arimurah@med.kyushu-u.ac.jp

Y. Shibayama • M. Haekal • Z. Jin • K. Ikushima
Division of Medical Quantum Science, Department of Health Sciences, Graduate School of Medical Sciences, Kyushu University, 3-1-1 Maidashi, Higashi-ku, Fukuoka 812-8582, Japan

H. Arimura (ed.), *Image-Based Computer-Assisted Radiation Therapy*,
DOI 10.1007/978-981-10-2945-5_5

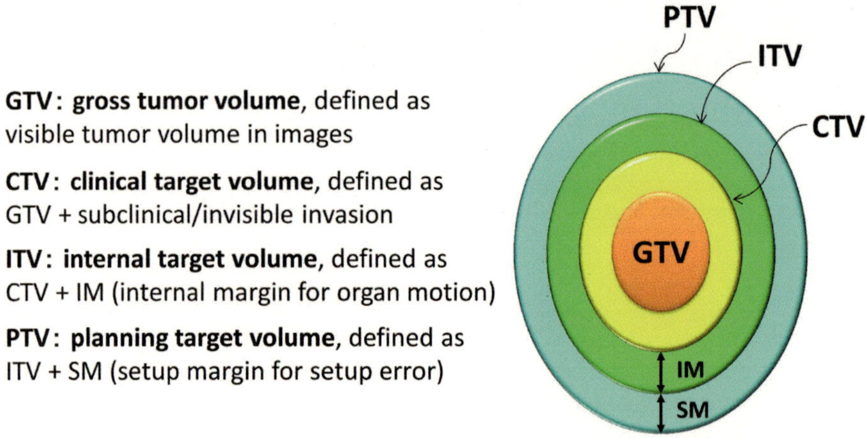

Fig. 5.1 Definitions of target volumes

volume that contains a demonstrable GTV and/or subclinical microscopic involvement. This volume has to therefore be treated adequately in order to achieve the aim of therapy: cure or palliation. The PTV is originally a geometrical concept taking into consideration the net effect of all possible geometrical variations, in order to ensure that the prescribed dose is actually absorbed in the CTV. The PTV is the practical volume that includes the CTV plus the CTV-to-PTV margin including the internal margin (IM) and setup margin (SM). The IM is designed to take into account variations in the size and position of the CTVs relative to the patient's reference frames (usually defined by the bone anatomy), i.e., variations due to organ motions such as breathing, bladder or rectal contents, etc. The SM allows for setup uncertainties such as machine tolerances and intra-treatment variations. The margin must be added to account specifically for uncertainties (inaccuracies and lack of reproducibility) in patient positioning and alignment of the therapeutic beams during treatment planning and through all treatment sessions. The CTV-to-PTV margins are calculated using the van Herk's margin model (van Herk et al. 2000; van Herk 2004), which has been widely used in clinical practice.

This chapter introduces the automated segmentation approaches for the GTV, the basics of CTV-to-PTV margins, and computational determination of the CTV-to-PTV margin based on statistical shape models.

5.2 Automated Segmentation of GTV

The uncertainties of GTV regions have a high impact on the precision of the entire radiation treatment course including treatment planning and patient positioning (Weiss and Hess 2003). The CTV and PTV in the RTP are determined based on the GTV regions. In particular, the GTV is critical in stereotactic body radiation therapy (SBRT), as highly precise positioning is required to deliver a higher dose per fraction to tumors. Once the GTV regions have been estimated, the CTVs are automatically determined based on the GTV itself or extending the GTV with microscopic invasion. The major reasons for the necessity of computer-assisted delineation of the GTV and CTV are given below:

1. Low reproducibility: There are large intra- and interobserver variabilities of GTV contours determined by radiation oncologists (Leunens et al. 1993; van de Steene et al. 2002; Bradley et al. 2004; Chao et al. 2007). Leunens et al. (1993) reported that the results of their study on brain tumors demonstrated that subjective interpretation (manual delineation) of the tumor extent might be one of the largest factors contributing to the overall uncertainty in radiation treatment planning.
2. Tedious and time-consuming manual contouring: According to Chao's study (Chao et al. 2007), the average percentage of time saved by contouring using a computer-assisted method is 26–29 % for experienced physicians and 38–47 % for less experienced physicians.

The GTVs are the fundamental regions used to determine the PTV regions, which are the actual target regions in radiation treatment planning and patient setup. Therefore, a number of automated segmentation approaches of the GTVs have been studied to mitigate the intra- and inter-planner variability, to reduce planning time, and to increase the segmentation accuracy of the GTV (Rousson et al. 2005; Biehl et al. 2006; Aristophanous et al. 2007; El Naqa et al. 2007; Geets et al. 2007; Day et al. 2009; Belhassen and Zaidi 2010; Kerhet et al. 2010; Zhang et al. 2010; Hatt et al. 2011; Niyazi et al. 2013; Jin et al. 2014).

The automated segmentation approaches can be categorized into two major types: positron emission tomography (PET)-based and PET/CT-based. PET-based approaches are based on model-based methods (Rousson et al. 2005), thresholding of the standardized uptake value (SUV) (Biehl et al. 2006; Zhang et al. 2010), region-growing methods using the SUV (Day et al. 2009), pixel-clustering-based segmentation (Aristophanous et al. 2007), gradient-based segmentation methods (Geets et al. 2007), the fuzzy locally adaptive Bayesian approach (Hatt et al. 2011), the fuzzy c-means algorithm (Belhassen and Zaidi 2010), the total lesion glycolysis (TLG) algorithm of PET Response Criteria in Solid Tumors (PERCIST) (Niyazi et al. 2013), and a machine-learning framework to assist in the threshold-based segmentation (Kerhet et al. 2010).

PET/CT-based approaches are based on a multivalued level set method that provides a feasible and accurate framework to combine imaging data obtained from different modalities (PET/CT) (El Naqa et al. 2007) and an optimum contour selection (OCS) method for segmentation of lung GTV regions using a level set method (Jin et al. 2014).

In this section, since the textbook focused on dealing with theoretically general approaches, the authors introduced pixel-clustering-based segmentation (Aristophanous et al. 2007), the OCS method (Jin et al. 2014), and the multivalued level set method (El Naqa et al. 2007).

5.2.1 Pixel-Clustering-Based Segmentation

Aristophanous et al. (2007) developed a pixel-clustering-based segmentation technique on selected PET tumor regions from non-small cell lung cancer patients. The general algorithm of the pixel-clustering-based segmentation approach with a Gaussian mixture model (GMM) to classify voxels into tumor and normal tissue voxels is described in this section. The clustering is referred to as "unsupervised learning" and does not require teacher signals (i.e., answers) as does "supervised learning" such as an artificial neural network. The basic idea of the pixel-clustering-based segmentation is to classify voxels into two classes, i.e., tumor and normal tissue voxels, by clustering the voxels according to the maximum a posteriori probability obtained by Bayes' theorem (Aristophanous et al. 2007).

Let a region of interest (ROI) in an objective image be a vector $\boldsymbol{x} = (x_1, x_2, \ldots, x_N)$, where x_i is the intensity at voxel i, and N is the number of voxels in the ROI. The voxel intensity is regarded as the random variable, which is assumed to be independent and identically distributed with a probability density function $f(x_i)$. Suppose that we have a set of K density functions, $f_k(x_i|\theta_k)$, parameterized by θ_k, where k is the class number ($k = 1, 2, \ldots, K$; K, the number of classes), called component densities (or classes). Let the probability density function of the voxel intensity x_i given by θ_k be a Gaussian function, which can be expressed by

$$f_k(x_i|\theta_k) = \frac{1}{\sqrt{2\pi\sigma_k^2}} \exp\left(-\frac{(x_i - \mu_k)^2}{2\sigma_k^2}\right), \quad \theta_k = (\mu_k, \sigma_k), \tag{5.1}$$

where μ_k and σ_k are the mean value and standard deviation in the kth class, respectively. Then, the probability density function of the voxel intensity x_i given by a parameter vector $\boldsymbol{\Psi} = (\pi_1, \pi_2, \ldots, \pi_K, \theta_1, \theta_2, \ldots, \theta_K)$($\pi_k$, mixing proportions) is defined by

$$f(x_i|\boldsymbol{\Psi}) = \sum_{k=1}^{K} \pi_k f_k(x_i|\theta_k). \tag{5.2}$$

The mixing proportion π_k, which is regarded as the probability of belonging to a class k, satisfies the following conditions:

$$0 \leq \pi_k \leq 1 \text{ and} \sum_{k=1}^{K} \pi_k = 1. \tag{5.3}$$

Let $\boldsymbol{Z}^{(i)} = \left(Z_1^{(i)}, Z_2^{(i)}, \ldots, Z_K^{(i)}\right)$ be a class random vector, where $Z_k^{(i)}$ is defined as

$$Z_k^{(i)} = \begin{cases} 1 & \text{if a voxel i belongs to a class } k \\ 0 & \text{otherwise.} \end{cases} \tag{5.4}$$

The class random vector $\mathbf{Z}^{(i)}$ follows a multinomial distribution. In accordance with Bayes' theorem, the posterior probability that $Z^{(i)} = k$ when a voxel intensity x_i and a parameter vector $\boldsymbol{\Psi}$ are given is calculated by

$$P\left(Z^{(i)} = k|x_i, \boldsymbol{\Psi}\right) = \frac{\pi_k f_k(x_i|\theta_k)}{\sum_{m=1}^{K} \pi_m f_m(x_i|\theta_m)} \tag{5.5}$$

This equation denotes the probability that the ith voxel belongs to the kth class. The final class of each voxel can be determined by the class, which has the maximum a posteriori probability among classes 1 to K. By using an expectation-maximization (EM) algorithm, from which the maximum likelihood parameters can be obtained, the parameter vector $\boldsymbol{\Psi}$ can be estimated by maximizing the following likelihood function:

$$L(\boldsymbol{\Psi}) = \prod_{i=1}^{N} f(x_i|\boldsymbol{\Psi}) = \prod_{i=1}^{N} \sum_{k=1}^{K} \frac{\pi_k}{\sqrt{2\pi\sigma_k^2}} \exp\left(-\frac{(x_i - \mu_k)^2}{2\sigma_k^2}\right). \tag{5.6}$$

At the Eth step, at first, the posterior probability $P(Z^{(i)} = k| x_i, \boldsymbol{\Psi})$ (Eq. 5.5) is calculated with the probability density function $f_k(x_i| \theta_k)$ based on the initially clustered regions. Second, the expectation of a natural logarithm of the likelihood is obtained by using Eq. (5.6). At the Mth step, the parameter vector $\boldsymbol{\Psi}$ is updated based on new clustered regions. This iteration of E- and M-steps is stopped when the change in the logarithm of the likelihood is smaller than a threshold value.

5.2.2 *Optimum Contour Selection Method*

The OCS method retrospectively determines a global optimum objective contour from multiple active delineations around a tumor. In addition, PET images are employed to determine the initial GTV regions to be used in the OCS method. First, the PET image is registered with the planning CT image through a diagnostic CT image of the PET/CT dataset by using an affine transformation (Jin et al. 2014). Initial GTV regions are obtained by thresholding the PET image at 80 % of the maximum standard uptake value (SUV_{max}) within a rectangular volume of interest (VOI), which has the same geometric position as the VOI in the planning CT image. Each initial GTV location is corrected in the VOI. Finally, the GTV region is segmented using the OCS method.

The SUV is employed for identification of the initial GTV regions, and is calculated as a ratio of the radioactivity concentration of tissue at a single time point to the injected dose of radioactivity concentration at that time point, divided by the body weight (Boellaard 2009):

$$SUV = \frac{C(\mathrm{kBq/ml})}{D(\mathrm{MBq})/W(\mathrm{kg})}, \tag{5.7}$$

where C represents the radioactivity concentration in kBq/ml obtained from the pixel value in the PET image multiplied by a cross calibration factor, D is the injected dose of 18-fluorodeoxyglucose (FDG) administered in MBq (decay corrected), and W is the body weight of the patient in kg.

The final GTVs are segmented by applying the OCS method to the initial regions, which are determined from the PET images. The basic concept of the OCS method is to retrospectively select a global optimum object contour from among multiple active delineations with a level set method around the tumors. In the OCS method, the level set method (LSM) (Sethian 1999) is employed for searching for the optimum object contour in the relationship between the average speed function value on an evolving curve and the evolution time.

An original level set equation of a partial differential equation (Sethian 1999) can be defined as

$$\frac{\partial \phi(\boldsymbol{r}(t), t)}{\partial t} + F \parallel \nabla \phi(\boldsymbol{r}(t), t) \parallel = 0, \tag{5.8}$$

where $\phi(\boldsymbol{r}(t), t)$ is the level set function, $\boldsymbol{r}(t)$ is the position vector at time t, and F is the speed function, which depends on circumstances on the evolution curve. The level set function is actually a distance image where the pixel values inside the initial curve are negative Euclidean distance values from each pixel to the closest pixel on the curve, but those outside the curve are positive distance values. The level set equation can be transformed into a Hamilton-Jacobi equation, which is equivalent to the Euler-Lagrange equation, as follows:

$$\frac{\partial \phi(\boldsymbol{r}(t), t)}{\partial t} + H(F, \phi(\boldsymbol{r}(t), t), t) = 0, \tag{5.9}$$

where $H(F, \phi(\boldsymbol{r}(t), t), t) = F\|\nabla \phi(\boldsymbol{r}(t), t)\|$, which is considered as a Hamiltonian. Solving (integration of a differential equation) a Hamilton-Jacobi equation of a contour involves the prediction of the contour with a minimum energy (possibly, a stable contour) from the analytical mechanics standpoint.

In the first step of the OCS method, the GTV contour and the speed function value obtained by the LSM are recorded at each evolution time from the initial GTV region until the evolution time reaches 10,000 or the evolving curve reaches the edge of the ROI in the planning CT image. The level set function $\varphi(x, y, t)$ is updated from the initial GTV contour by using the following discrete partial differential equation:

$$\phi^{n+1}(x,y,t) = \phi^{n}(x,y,t) - \Delta t F(x,y,t) \parallel \nabla \phi^{n}(x,y,t) \parallel, \qquad (5.10)$$

where n is the evolution number, t is the evolution time, Δt is the evolution time interval, and $F(x, y, t)$ is the speed function. The evolution time is the time of the contour deformation in updating the discrete partial differential equation. The zero level set of $\phi(x, y, t)$, which corresponds to the contour of the segmented region, moves according to the speed function $F(x, y, t)$ in the three-dimensional level set function. The zero level set function, i.e., the evolving curve, moves according to the following speed function $F(x, y, t)$:

$$F\ (x,y,t) = b(x,y)\{1 - \nu\kappa(x,y,t)\}, \qquad (5.11)$$

$$b(x,y) = \frac{1}{1+ \parallel \nabla\{G(x,y) * I(x,y)\} \parallel}, \qquad (5.12)$$

where $b(x, y)$ is the function of the edge indicator, $G(x, y)$ is the Gaussian function, $I(x, y)$ is the planning CT image to be processed, * denotes convolution, v is a constant, and $\kappa(x, y, t)$ is the curvature. The edge indicator function $b(x, y)$ and speed $F\ (x, y, t)$ would be small around the edge, whereas the functions $b(x, y)$ and $F\ (x, y, t)$ would be large in relatively homogeneous regions.

In the second step, the GTV contour is determined from the optimum contour derived using the LSM by searching for the minimum point in the relationship between the evolution time and the average speed function value on an evolving curve, based on the steepest descent method (SDM). To avoid local minimum traps, the average speed function is smoothed by a median filter, and the smoothed function is resampled by a larger interval than the original one, before applying the SDM.

Figure 5.2a shows the relationship in the LSM between the evolution time and the average speed function value on an evolving curve. Figure 5.2b illustrates GTV contours, which were multiply delineated by the proposed method on the planning CT image of a lung cancer case. The average speed function $\bar{F}(x, y, t)$ as a function of the evolution time t converges to a global minimum of 4803. Therefore, the optimum contour can be determined by detecting the minimum point in the relationship between the average speed function and the evolution time.

5.2.3 *Machine-Learning-Based Delineation*

The key idea of the machine-learning-based delineation (MLD) was to feed image features around GTV contours determined based on the knowledge or experiences of radiation oncologists into a machine learning classifier during the training step, after which the classifier produced the "degree of GTV" for each voxel in the testing step (Ikushima et al. 2016). The overall procedure of the MLD framework consists of the following four steps:

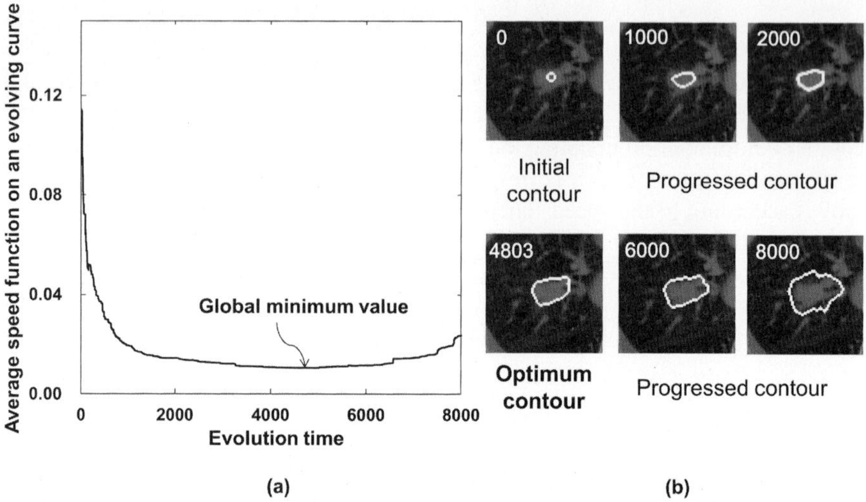

Fig. 5.2 Illustrations of (**a**) the relationship in the level set method between the evolution time and the average speed function on a moving front line and (**b**) contours on a planning CT image at evolution times

1. The PET and diagnostic CT images were aligned with planning CT images based on the centroid of lung regions in two CT images.
2. The morphological and biological image features were derived from planning CT, PET, and diagnostic CT images. The image features are pixels and gradient values of three types of images.
3. The initial GTV regions were obtained using one of machine learning techniques, i.e., a support vector machine (SVM), which learned the image features inside and outside each GTV region determined by radiation oncologists or radiologists.
4. Final GTV regions were determined by thresholding the SVM outputs and/or the OCS method.

The SVM (Vapnik 1999) is one of machine learning techniques that can classify data into several (generally two) categories based on the output of a discriminant function. The SVM constructs a discriminant function in a linearly separable space by applying a nonlinear kernel function to a given training dataset. We consider a training dataset of training data and teacher signals, $[\mathbf{x}_i, y_i]$ ($\mathbf{x}_i \in R^n$, i, data number; n, dimension; $i = 1, \ldots, l$, l, number of data, $y_i \in \{-1, 1\}$), which we would like to classify. The discriminant function $f(\mathbf{x})$ constructed by the SVM is expressed by (Vapnik 1999)

$$f(\boldsymbol{x}) = \sum_{i=1}^{N} y_i \alpha_i K(\boldsymbol{x}, \boldsymbol{x}_i) + b, \tag{5.13}$$

where $\boldsymbol{x}_i$ ($i = 1, \ldots, N, N$, number of support vectors) is the support vector, b and α_i are parameters that determine the discriminant function, and $K(\mathbf{x}, \boldsymbol{x}_i)$ is the nonlinear kernel function, which can map a linearly non-separable dataset to a linearly separable dataset. The output was referred to as "degree of GTV" in this study.

The training procedure of construction of the SVM is shown as follows:

Step 1: A training dataset of image features and teacher signals $[\mathbf{x}_i, y_i]$ is prepared, where $\mathbf{x}_i = (x_{1i}, x_{2i}, \ldots, x_{Fi})$ (F, number of image features). In this study, F is 6 or 4, which depends on lung tumor type.

Step 2: All parameters of the discriminant function are optimized by repeatedly calculating the parameters using image features of the training dataset based on a quadratic programming approach (Vapnik 1999).

The efficacy of the proposed framework was evaluated in 14 lung cancer cases (solid, 6; ground glass opacity (GGO), 4; mixed GGO, 4) using the three-dimensional Dice similarity coefficient (DSC), which denotes the degree of region similarity between the GTVs contoured by radiation oncologists and those determined using the proposed framework. Figure 5.3 shows the planning CT, PET, and SVM-output images for three types of lung tumors. A tumor of the solid type has a high intensity with SUV_{max} of 7.75, but the GGO and mixed GGO types of tumors show low intensities with SUV_{max} of 1.09 and 1.62, respectively. On the other hand, the SVM enhanced not only the solid type of tumor but also the GGO and mixed GGO types of tumors in spite of low SUV_{max}. The proposed framework including the SVM and OCS method achieved an average DSC of 0.777 for 14 cases, whereas the OCS-based framework produced 0.507. The average DSCs for GGO and mixed GGO were 0.763 and 0.701, respectively, obtained by the proposed framework.

5.2.4 Multivalued Level Set Method

El Naqa et al. (2007) demonstrated the multimodality segmentation approach for delineating target regions by combining complementary information from different imaging modalities such as PET, CT, and MR systems and thus identifying GTV regions by simultaneously using anatomical and functional information. Their method was based on an active contour model without edges for vector-valued images (such as RGB or multispectral images) (Chan et al. 2000). The advantage of this model is to segment objects with different missing parts in different channels in a mutually complementary manner. El Naqa et al. took advantage of mutually complementary functions of the active contour model for vector-valued images such as medical multimodality images in a same coordinate system.

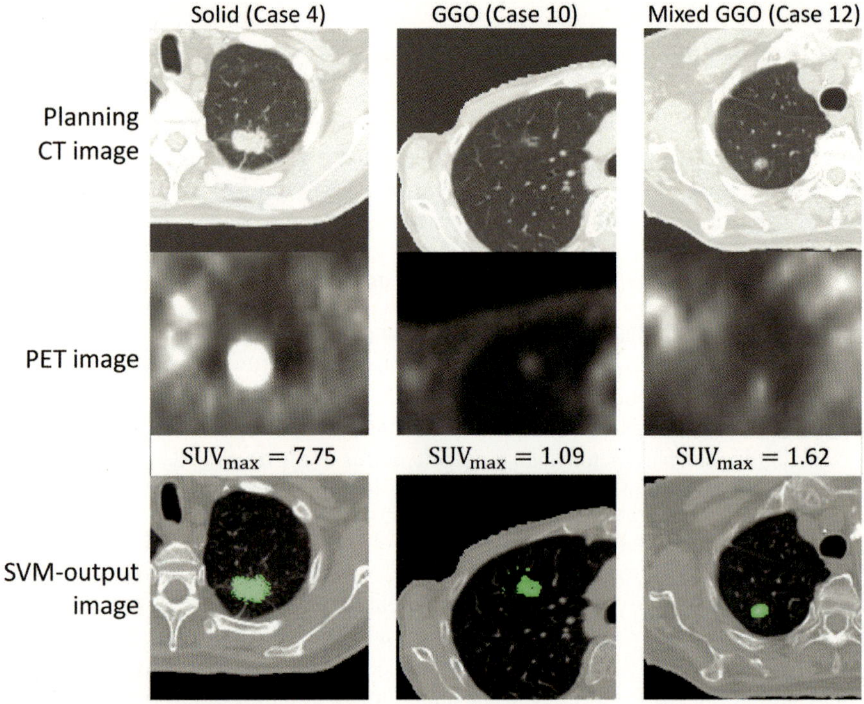

Fig. 5.3 shows the planning CT, PET, and SVM-output images for three types (solid, GGO, mixed GGO) of lung tumors

El Naqa et al. (2007) developed variational methods based on multivalued level set (MVLS) deformable models for simultaneous 2D or 3D segmentation of multimodality images consisting of combinations of coregistered PET, CT, or MR datasets. In their approach, a GTV region in an image $I_i(x, y)$ for the ith imaging modality is segmented by minimizing the following energy function E with information of N images $I_i(x, y)$ ($i = 1$ *to* N; N, number of imaging modalities):

$$E(C, c^+, c^-) = \mu \cdot \mathrm{length}(C) + \frac{1}{N}\sum_{i=1}^{N}\left\{\begin{array}{l}\lambda_i^+ \int_\Omega |I_i(x,y) - c_i^+|^2 H(\phi)dxdy + \\ \lambda_i^- \int_\Omega |I_i(x,y) - c_i^-|^2 (1 - H(\phi))dxdy + \gamma_i\left(\boldsymbol{c}_i^+ - \boldsymbol{c}_i^-\right)^2\end{array}\right\}, \tag{5.14}$$

where C is the parameterized evolving curve, c^+ and c^- are the average values of the image $I_i(x, y)$ inside and outside the curve C, respectively, and Ω is the bounded open subset of $\boldsymbol{R}^2$. $H(\phi)$ is the Heaviside function, which is defined as

$$H(x) = \begin{cases} 1 & x \geq 0 \\ 0 & \text{otherwise.} \end{cases} \tag{5.15}$$

The Heaviside function may be approximated by a smooth inverse tangent function in the implementation. $\mu, \lambda_i^+, \lambda_i^-, \gamma_i$ are parameters that should be determined by the users.

5.2.5 *Evaluation of Segmentation Accuracy of Developed Methods*

It is essential to evaluate the accuracy of the developed segmentation methods. The segmentation accuracy should be evaluated using indicators such as the Jaccard index (Crum et al. 2006), which denotes the degree of coincidence between the candidate region obtained by a developed method and the reference region obtained by a manual method, as follows:

$$\mathrm{JI} = \frac{n(T \cap C)}{n(T \cup C)}, \tag{5.16}$$

where T is the reference region manually determined by radiation oncologists, C is the region automatically determined by using a developed method, $n(T \cup C)$ is the number of logical OR pixels between T and C, and $n(T \cap C)$ is the number of logical AND pixels between T and C. The following Dice similarity coefficient (Crum et al. 2006) is also used for evaluation of segmentation accuracy:

$$\mathrm{DSC} = \frac{2 \cdot n(T \cap C)}{n(T) + n(C)}, \tag{5.17}$$

where $n(T)$ is the number of pixels in the reference region and $n(C)$ is the number of pixels in the automatically segmented region.

5.3 Basics of CTV-to-PTV Margin

In the clinical practice of radiation therapy, there are many uncertainties with respect to targeting tumors as follows:

- Intra- and interobserver variability of target delineations (observer errors or noise)
- Intra- and inter-fractional patient setup (positioning) errors (external errors)
- Intra- and inter-fractional variation of target position and shape (organ motion or internal errors)

- Additional undefined errors

A number of efforts to minimize these uncertainties have been performed to increase the accuracy of radiation therapy. Sophisticated immobilization devices, image-guided patient positioning systems, and real-time tumor tracking systems have been utilized in recent years. Nevertheless, safety margins, i.e., CTV-to-PTV margins, are required when delivering sufficient doses to target tumors. The margin is considered the *inevitable choice* for treating cancer even though the surrounding normal tissue is exposed to the *leaked dose*.

van Herk (2004) summarized a number of margin recipes published in past studies for target, respiration (target), and OAR. Gardner et al. (2015) evaluated the variability among human observers in delineating (delineation errors) the prostate, bladder, and rectum on planning CT and CBCT images. The contouring variation was evaluated using quantitative metrics, such as Dice coefficient, Hausdorff distance, contour distance, and center-of-mass deviation.

van Herk et al. (2000) proposed a CTV-to-PTV margin model, which has been widely used, as follows:

$$\boldsymbol{m}_{PTV} = \alpha\boldsymbol{\sigma}_s + \beta(\boldsymbol{\sigma} - \boldsymbol{\sigma}_p), \tag{5.18}$$

$$\boldsymbol{\sigma} = \sqrt{\boldsymbol{\sigma}_r^2 + \boldsymbol{\sigma}_p^2}, \tag{5.19}$$

where $\boldsymbol{\sigma}_s$ is the 3D vector with the square root of a quadratic sum of the SD vectors of all systematic errors, α is the coefficient of $\boldsymbol{\sigma}_s$ depending on confidence levels, β is the distance between the 95 and 50 % isodose surface of a blurred dose distribution, $\boldsymbol{\sigma}_r$ is the 3D vector with the square root of a quadratic sum of SD vectors of all random errors, and $\boldsymbol{\sigma}_p$ is the SD describing the width of the penumbra of a planned dose distribution, which may depend on the radiotherapy machines.

A one-dimensional CTV-to-PTV margin model in the x direction is given by

$$m(x)_{PTV} = \alpha\sigma_s(x) + \beta\{\sigma(x) - \sigma_p(x)\}. \tag{5.20}$$

The systematic errors are involved with the delineation errors, setup errors, organ motion errors (translation and rotation), and shape variations of the CTVs, whereas the random errors are involved with organ motion errors and shape variations of the CTVs. The systematic and random errors are described in the next section.

Figure 5.4 shows an illustration of the systematic and random errors of targets for a population of N patients. Let a target position vector of a patient i ($i = 1$ to N) at a kth fraction ($k = 1$ to M) be $\boldsymbol{p}_{i,k}$. The basic concept of this figure was extracted from a paper of Stroom and Heijmen (2002). The target mean position vector $\bar{\boldsymbol{p}}_i$ of a patient i for all fractions is calculated by

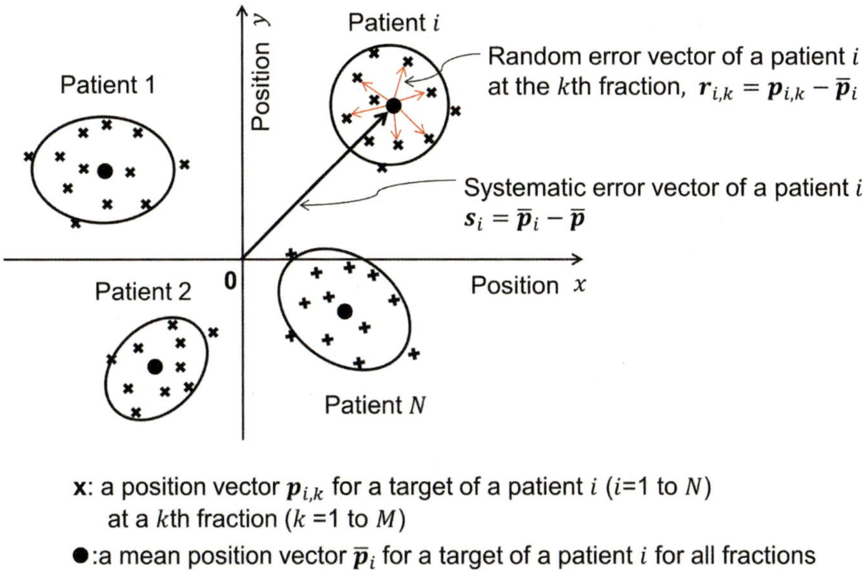

Fig. 5.4 An illustration of systematic and random errors of targets for a population for N patients

$$\bar{\boldsymbol{p}}_i = \frac{1}{M}\sum_{k=1}^{M}\boldsymbol{p}_{i,k}. \tag{5.21}$$

Furthermore, a mean vector $\bar{\boldsymbol{p}}$ of the target mean position vector $\bar{\boldsymbol{p}}_i$ for all patients is obtained by

$$\bar{\boldsymbol{p}} = \frac{1}{N}\sum_{i=1}^{N}\bar{\boldsymbol{p}}_i, \tag{5.22}$$

which could be close to a zero vector. Therefore, the systematic error vector $\boldsymbol{s}_i$ of a patient i is defined as

$$\boldsymbol{s}_i = \bar{\boldsymbol{p}}_i - \bar{\boldsymbol{p}}, \tag{5.23}$$

where the mean vector of the systematic error $\boldsymbol{s}_i$ for all patients is a zero vector. The systematic error $\sigma_s(x)$ in the x direction is calculated by

$$\sigma_s(x) = \sqrt{\frac{1}{N}\sum_{i=1}^{N}\{\bar{p}_i(x) - \bar{p}(x)\}^2}. \tag{5.24}$$

The random error vector $\boldsymbol{r}_{i,k}$ for the kth fraction of the ith patient is defined as

$$\boldsymbol{r}_{i,k} = \boldsymbol{p}_{i,k} - \bar{\boldsymbol{p}}_i, \tag{5.25}$$

and the random error $\sigma_{r,i}(x)$ of a patient i in the x direction is calculated by

$$\sigma_{r,i}(x) = \sqrt{\frac{1}{M}\sum_{k=1}^{M}\{p_{i,k}(x) - \bar{p}_i(x)\}^2}. \tag{5.26}$$

Therefore, the random error $\sigma_r(x)$ for all patients in the x direction is obtained by

$$\sigma_r(x) = \sqrt{\frac{1}{N}\sum_{i=1}^{N}\sigma^2{}_{r,i}(x)}. \tag{5.27}$$

The systematic and random errors in the y and z directions are calculated in the same way. If readers wish to consider several systematic errors $\sigma_{s,a}(x)$ ($a = 1$ to A; A, number of different systematic errors, e.g., delineation errors, setup errors, organ motion errors), which could be independent of each other, the total systematic error can be obtained by

$$\sigma_s(x) = \sqrt{\frac{1}{A}\sum_{a=1}^{A}\sigma^2{}_{s,a}(x)}. \tag{5.28}$$

The total random error is also calculated in the same way.

The coefficient α of the 3D SD vector $\boldsymbol{\sigma}_s$ of the systematic error determines the margin to tolerate the systematic error with a confidence level of C. Let a 3D density probability function of a CTV location be $p(x, y, z; \sigma_s)$, which is given by

$$p(x, y, z; \sigma_s) = \frac{1}{\left(\sqrt{2\pi\sigma^2{}_s}\right)^3}\exp\left(-\frac{x^2 + y^2 + z^2}{2\sigma^2{}_s}\right). \tag{5.29}$$

It is assumed that the SDs are equal in the x, y, and z directions. The probability is considered the confidence level. Therefore, the probability that an error with the density probability function occurs between $-w$ and w can be computed by an integration of the density probability function from $-w$ to w with respect to x, y, z. $2w$ corresponds to the margin for the systematic error.

By integrating the density probability function $p(x, y, z; \sigma_s)$ in a polar coordinate system, the probability (confidence level of C) of the error occurrence is reduced to (van Herk et al. 2000):

$$C = -\sqrt{\frac{2}{\pi}\alpha \cdot e^{-\frac{\alpha^2}{2}} + erf\left(\frac{\alpha}{\sqrt{2}}\right)} \quad \left(\alpha = \frac{w}{\sigma_s}\right), \tag{5.30}$$

where erf(·) represents an error function. Readers can calculate the coefficients α for the confidence levels required by using a root-finding algorithm such as a bisection method or Newton method. For instance, a coefficient α of 2.5 is obtained for a confidence level of 0.9 (Table 2 in van Herk et al. 2000).

The coefficient β of the 3D SD vector $\boldsymbol{\sigma_r}$ of the random error controls the margin to allow the random error with a dose level of D. The blurred dose distribution of a step function affected by the random error is expressed by

$$D(x, y, z) = D_{nominal} \cdot p(x, y, z; \sigma_r) * S(x, y, z, w), \tag{5.31}$$

where D_{nominal} is the nominal total dose (prescribed dose), $S(x, y, z, w)$ is the 3D step function (a solid sphere), and w is the radius of the dose distribution at the 50 % dose level. According to van Herk et al. (2000), the coefficient β is given by

$$\beta = \sqrt{2} \cdot erf^{-1}(2D - 1), \tag{5.32}$$

where $\text{erf}^{-1}(\cdot)$ is the inverse error function and D is the dose level which is desired. For example, a coefficient β of 1.64 is obtained for a dose level of 0.95 (second column of Table 3 in van Herk et al. 2000). The term including the SDs of the random error and penumbra is approximated by using a linear function within small random errors as follows:

$$\beta\{\sigma(x) - \sigma_p(x)\} = \beta\{\sqrt{\sigma^2{}_r(x) + \sigma^2{}_p(x)} - \sigma_p(x)\} \tag{5.33}$$

$$\beta\{\sigma(x) - \sigma_p(x)\} \approx \gamma \sigma_r(x), \tag{5.34}$$

where γ is the coefficient of the SD of the random error. For instance, if $\sigma_p(x) =$ 3.2 mm at a dose level of 0.95, γ is around 0.7 within the range of the random error of 0–5 mm (third column of Table 3 in van Herk et al. 2000). Readers can verify this approximation using a curve-fitting algorithm. When having more than 5 mm random errors, we may need to use an exact equation as shown above for determination of the additional PTV margins. In general, such random errors do not happen in clinical practice.

5.4 Computational Approaches for Determination of CTV-to-PTV Margins

Computational anatomies are useful for developing mathematical models to predict uncertainties related to anatomy in radiation therapy such as organ motions and/or organ deformations by patient and/or fraction (Okada et al. 2008; van der Wielen et al. 2008; Söhn et al. 2005, 2007, 2012; Thörnqvist et al. 2013; Xu et al. 2014, 2015). Computational anatomy includes mathematical models of anatomical structures using statistical shape models, which is a novel field between medical anatomy and statistical computational image analysis. The authors believe that computational anatomy may be feasible for radiation therapy, because many parameters (e.g., CTV-to-PTV margin) should be determined based on statistical data by taking into account uncertainties (e.g., setup errors, intra-fractional organ motion) in the radiation therapy steps (diagnosis, treatment planning, patient positioning, and treatment execution).

5.4.1 Analysis of Target Deformation Using Point Distribution Models

Computational anatomical approaches based on point distribution models (PDMs) (Okada et al. 2008) are promising tools for the determination of CTV-to-PTV margins, because we can analyze the motion of each point (displacement) on an objective surface, such as CTV surfaces, for a population of patients at a number of treatment fractions.

Let $\boldsymbol{p}_{i,j}(k) = (p_{i,j,x}(k), p_{i,j,y}(k), p_{i,j,z}(k))^T$ be a 3D position vector of the kth vertex ($k = 1$ to M) on the objective (CTV) surface $S_{i,j}$ for the ith patient ($i = 1$ *to* N) at the jth fraction ($j = 1$ *to* F ; $j = 1$: reference fraction), where x, y, and z correspond to right-left (LR), anterior-posterior (AP), and superior-inferior (SI) directions, respectively. Figure 5.5 illustrates a point distribution model of an object. The surface (shape) of an object is defined as a matrix (a set of vertex vectors) as follows:

$$\boldsymbol{S}_{i,j} = \left(\boldsymbol{p}_{i,j}(1)\ \boldsymbol{p}_{i,j}(2) \ldots \boldsymbol{p}_{i,j}(k) \ldots \boldsymbol{p}_{i,j}(M)\right). \tag{5.35}$$

The systematic and random displacements at the vertices of surfaces can be calculated using the PDMs (van der Wielen et al. 2008). Let a displacement matrix of the transformed surface $\boldsymbol{D}_{i,j}^{(1)} = (\boldsymbol{d}_{i,j}(1)\ \boldsymbol{d}_{i,j}(2) \ldots \boldsymbol{d}_{i,j}(k) \ldots \boldsymbol{d}_{i,j}(M))$ be for the jth fraction of the ith patient from the surface $\boldsymbol{S}_{i,1}$ for the first fraction (reference fraction) of the ith patient. The displacement matrix is derived from

$$\boldsymbol{D}_{i,j}^{(1)} = \boldsymbol{T}_{i,j}^{(1)} \boldsymbol{S}_{i,j} - \boldsymbol{S}_{i,1}, \tag{5.36}$$

where $\boldsymbol{T}_{i,j}^{(1)}$ is the nonrigid transformation matrix (e.g., a thin plate spline robust point matching (TPS-RPM) algorithm (Chui and Rangarajan 2003)) to register each surface $\boldsymbol{S}_{i,j}$ with a reference surface $\boldsymbol{S}_{i,1}$.Therefore, the average surface $\overline{\boldsymbol{S}_i}$ for all fractions of the ith patient is obtained from

$$\bar{\boldsymbol{S}}_i = \boldsymbol{S}_{i,1} + \overline{\boldsymbol{D}_i}, \tag{5.37}$$

where

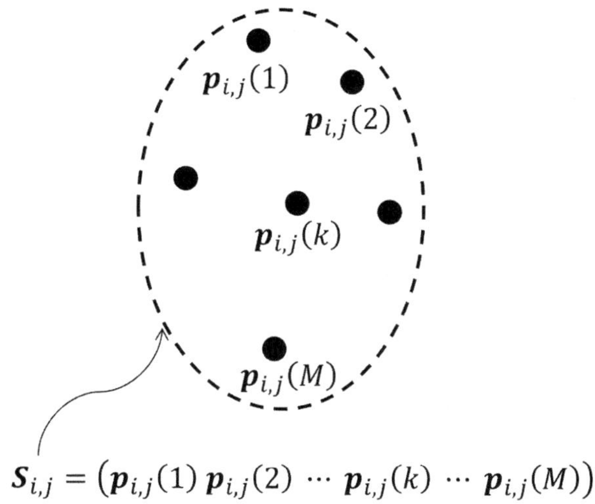

Fig. 5.5 A point distribution model of an object

$$\overline{\boldsymbol{D}_i} = \frac{1}{F}\sum_{j=1}^{F}\boldsymbol{D}_{i,j} \tag{5.38}$$

and

$$\bar{\boldsymbol{D}}_i = \left(\bar{\boldsymbol{d}}_i(1)\ \ \bar{\boldsymbol{d}}_i(2)\ldots\bar{\boldsymbol{d}}_i(k)\ldots\bar{\boldsymbol{d}}_i(M)\right). \tag{5.39}$$

The displacement matrix $\boldsymbol{D}_i^{(a)}$ of the transformed average surface $\boldsymbol{T}_i^{(a)}\bar{\boldsymbol{S}}_i$ of the ith patient from the average surface for all fractions of the first patient $\bar{\boldsymbol{S}}_1$ is given by

$$\boldsymbol{D}_i^{(a)} = \boldsymbol{T}_i^{(a)}\bar{\boldsymbol{S}}_i - \bar{\boldsymbol{S}}_1, \tag{5.40}$$

Therefore, the average surface $\bar{\boldsymbol{S}}$ for all fractions of all patients is obtained from

$$\bar{\boldsymbol{S}} = \bar{\boldsymbol{S}}_1 + \boldsymbol{D}^{(a)} \tag{5.41}$$

where

$$\boldsymbol{D}^{(a)} = \frac{1}{N}\sum_{i=1}^{N}\boldsymbol{D}_i^{(a)}. \tag{5.42}$$

Finally, the systematic displacement $\varepsilon_i(k)$ along the surface normal vector $\boldsymbol{n}_i(k)$ at the kth vertex, which is distributed on the average surface $\overline{\boldsymbol{S}_i}$ of the ith patient, can be defined as (van der Wielen et al. 2008):

$$\varepsilon_i(k) = \frac{1}{F-1}\sum_{j=1}^{F}\left(\boldsymbol{d}_{i,j}^{(1)}(k), \boldsymbol{n}_i(k)\right), \tag{5.43}$$

where $(\cdot,\cdot)$ denotes the inner product. Then, the corresponding SDs of the random displacement along the surface normal vector are calculated by

$$\delta_i(k) = \frac{1}{F-1}\sum_{j=1}^{F}\left(\boldsymbol{d}_{i,j}^{(1)}(k) - \bar{\boldsymbol{d}}_i(k), \boldsymbol{n}_i(k)\right)^2. \tag{5.44}$$

5.4.2 Statistical Shape Models of Targets

Statistical shape models of targets with statistical shape analysis are utilized for prediction of CTV day-by-day deformations or variations for a population of patients, which is useful in radiation treatment planning (van der Wielen et al. 2008; Söhn et al. 2005, 2007, 2012; Thörnqvist et al. 2013; Xu et al. 2014, 2015). van der Wielen et al. (2008) analyzed the deformation of the prostate and, in particular, the seminal vesicles relative to intraprostatic fiducial markers. Söhn et al. (2005, 2007, 2012) applied principal component analysis (PCA) to rectal DVHs of prostate cancer patients and investigated the correlation of the PCA parameters with late bleeding, because the variability of dose-volume histogram (DVH) shapes in a patient population can be quantified using PCA. Thörnqvist et al. (2013) introduced a statistical deformable motion model for multiple targets based on PCA. They applied the model to treatment simulations for dosimetric evaluation of margins for the multiple targets in radiation therapy of locally advanced prostate cancer. Xu et al. (2014, 2015) compared a standard fixed margin-based planning technique with two coverage-based planning techniques with a consideration of the dosimetric impact of interfraction deformable organ motion exclusively for high-risk prostate treatments. The coverage-based plans were made by using the PCA for reconstruction of the model of patient-specific inter-fractional deformable organ changes. The PCA was used to predict patient geometries for virtual treatment course simulation. Figure 5.6 describes a big picture of a computational anatomy in a coordinate system reconstructed by eigenvectors ($\boldsymbol{e}_1, \boldsymbol{e}_2, \ldots, \boldsymbol{e}_r$) obtained from principal component analysis.

In general, the statistical shape analysis is based on PCA. PCA is a statistical technique, which uses a principal axis transform (one of orthogonal transforms) to find a new coordinate system based on eigenvectors called "principal components." Figure 5.7 illustrates an original coordinate system and a new coordinate system obtained by a principal axis transform. A Fourier series expansion is one of orthogonal transforms, in which sine and cosine waves are employed as orthogonal functions, which are mathematically orthogonal to each other like a set of

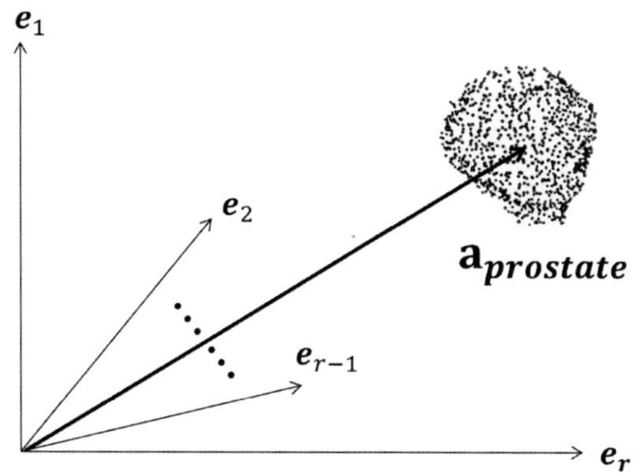

Fig. 5.6 A big picture of a computational anatomy in a coordinate system reconstructed by eigenvectors ($\boldsymbol{e}_1, \boldsymbol{e}_2, \ldots, \boldsymbol{e}_r$) obtained from principal component analysis. The vector $\boldsymbol{a}_{prostate}$ represents a computational anatomy (e.g., a computational prostate)

orthogonal vectors. Arbitrary waves can be expressed as a linear combination of a direct current, sine, and/or cosine waves as shown in Fig. 5.8, which means decomposition of arbitrary waves by sine and/or cosine waves. Similarly, PCA can produce a linear combination of a mean vector and eigenvectors, which are orthogonal to each other, for arbitrary data. Figure 5.9 shows a linear combination of a mean vector ($\bar{\boldsymbol{q}}_i$) and eigenvectors ($\boldsymbol{e}_{i,1}, \boldsymbol{e}_{i,2}, \boldsymbol{e}_{i,3} \ldots$) for an arbitrary PDM-based shape, which were computed by PCA. The advantage of PCA is that the readers can visualize the eigenvectors, which is generally quite a boring linear algebra subject.

The problem of the application of PCA to PDMs is how to determine the coefficients and eigenvectors. The procedure of PCA is described below:

1. Calculation of a covariance matrix
2. Applying a singular value decomposition (SVD) for covariance matrix
3. Analysis of eigenvectors and eigenvalues for your purposes

We now consider the case where we want to reconstruct a computational anatomy for the jth fraction ($j = 1$ *to* F) of the ith patient ($i = 1$ *to* N). Let a surface or shape vector including all vertex position vectors ($k = 1$ to M) be $\boldsymbol{q}_{i,j} = (p_{i,j,x}(1), \ldots, p_{i,j,x}(M), p_{i,j,y}(1), \ldots, p_{i,j,y}(M), p_{i,j,z}(1), \ldots, p_{i,j,z}(M))$ for the jth fraction of ith patient. Furthermore, the patient matrix can be defined as

$$\boldsymbol{P}_i = \left(\widehat{\boldsymbol{q}}_{i,1} - \bar{\boldsymbol{q}}_i \;\; \widehat{\boldsymbol{q}}_{i,2} - \bar{\boldsymbol{q}}_i \;\; \ldots \widehat{\boldsymbol{q}}_{i,F} - \bar{\boldsymbol{q}}_i\right), \tag{5.45}$$

where

$$\bar{\boldsymbol{q}}_i = \frac{1}{F} \sum_{j=1}^{F} \widehat{\boldsymbol{q}}_{i,j}, \tag{5.46}$$

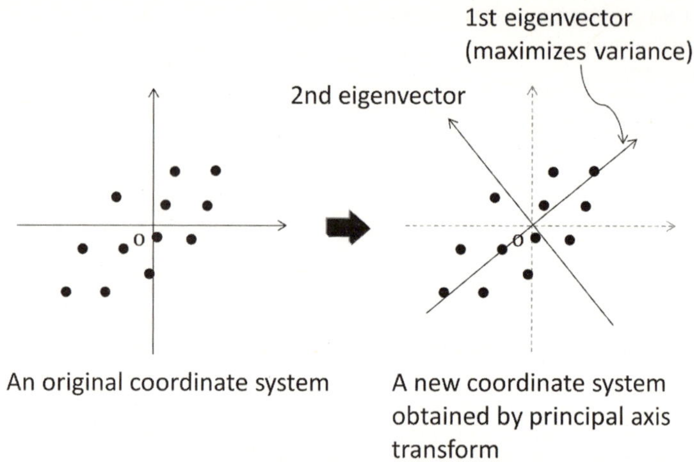

Fig. 5.7 An illustration of an original coordinate system and a new coordinate system obtained by a principal axis transform

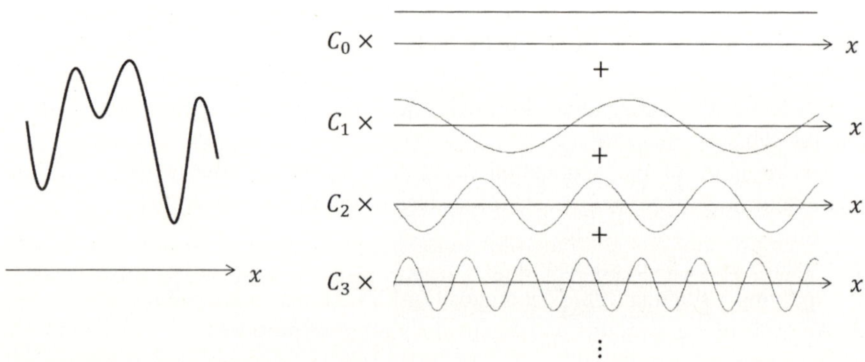

Fig. 5.8 A linear combination of a direct current, sine, and/or cosine waves for an arbitrary wave, whose coefficients were calculated by the Fourier series expansion

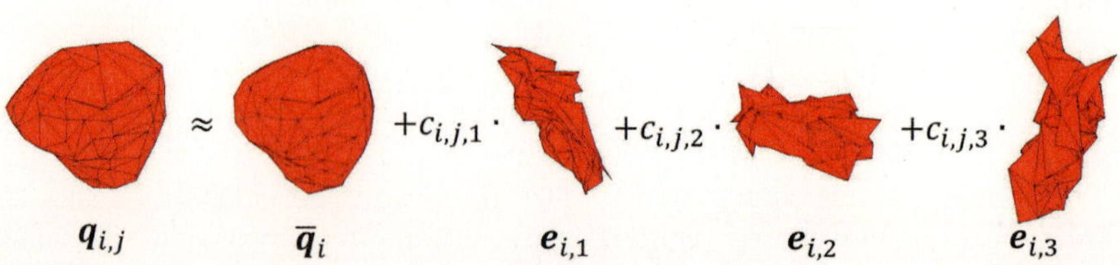

Fig. 5.9 A linear combination of a mean vector ($\bar{q}_i$) and eigenvectors ($\boldsymbol{e}_{i,1}, \boldsymbol{e}_{i,2}, \boldsymbol{e}_{i,3} \ldots$) for an arbitrary PDM-based shape, which were computed by PCA

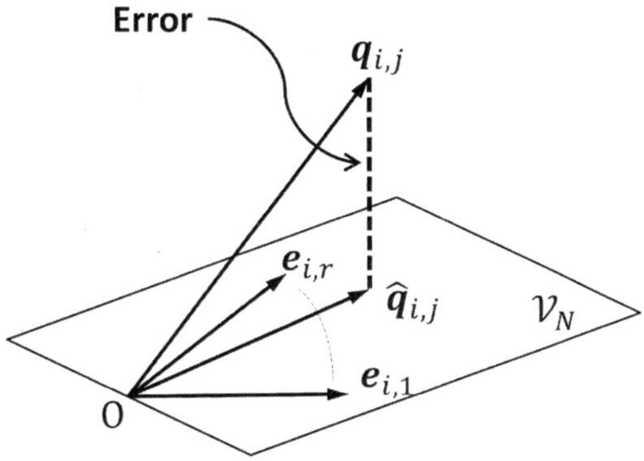

Fig. 5.10 A projection of original data $\boldsymbol{q}_{i,j}$ to a low-dimensional space $\mathcal{V}_N$

$\widehat{\boldsymbol{q}}_{i,j}$ is the transformed shape vector $\boldsymbol{q}_{i,j}$ to a reference shape vector, and $\bar{\boldsymbol{q}}_i$ was a mean vector of $\widehat{\boldsymbol{q}}_{i,j}$. The covariance matrix for all fractions of ith patient is given by

$$\boldsymbol{V}_i = \frac{1}{F}\boldsymbol{P}_i^T\boldsymbol{P}_i. \tag{5.47}$$

This matrix size is N × N, which is much smaller than a $\boldsymbol{P}_i\boldsymbol{P}_i^T$ matrix size of 3M × 3M. Singular values and eigenvectors $(\boldsymbol{e}_{i,1}, \boldsymbol{e}_{i,2}, \ldots, \boldsymbol{e}_{i,r}; r \leq N)$ are obtained by applying SVD for the covariance matrix. Eigenvectors and nonnegative eigenvalues for the matrices $\frac{1}{F}\boldsymbol{P}_i\boldsymbol{P}_i^T$ and $\frac{1}{F}\boldsymbol{P}_i^T\boldsymbol{P}_i$ are identical to each other (Trefethen LN and Bau III D 1997). The eigenvectors correspond to nonnegative eigenvalues, which are ranked in descending order. Finally, the shape vector for the jth fraction of ith patient is approximated by

$$\boldsymbol{q}_{i,j} \approx \bar{\boldsymbol{q}}_i + c_{i,j,1}\boldsymbol{e}_{i,1} + c_{i,j,2}\boldsymbol{e}_{i,2} + \cdots + c_{i,j,r}\boldsymbol{e}_{i,r} \quad (r \leq N), \tag{5.48}$$

where

$$\boldsymbol{c}_{i,j} = \boldsymbol{U}_i^T\left(\boldsymbol{q}_{i,j} - \bar{\boldsymbol{q}}_i\right) \ \left\{\boldsymbol{c}_{i,j} = \left(c_{i,j,1}\ c_{i,j,2} \ldots c_{i,j,r}\right)^T\right\}, \tag{5.49}$$

$$\boldsymbol{U}_i = \left(\boldsymbol{e}_{i,1}\ \boldsymbol{e}_{i,2} \ldots \boldsymbol{e}_{i,r}\right). \tag{5.50}$$

The coefficient vector is an optimum solution to approximate the original data using a linear combination of eigenvectors. The coefficient vector can be obtained by minimizing the following cost function:

$$J = \frac{1}{2}\left\|\boldsymbol{q}_{i,j} - \left(\bar{\boldsymbol{q}}_i + c_{i,j,1}\boldsymbol{e}_{i,1} + c_{i,j,2}\boldsymbol{e}_{i,2} + \cdots + c_{i,j,r}\boldsymbol{e}_{i,r}\right)\right\|^2 \rightarrow \text{min}. \tag{5.51}$$

Readers can solve this minimization problem by using a least squares method. Figure 5.10 shows a projection of original data $\boldsymbol{q}_{i,j}$ to a low-dimensional space $\mathcal{V}_N$. The error represents the difference between the original data and an approximated data in a cost function J.

References

Aristophanous M, Penney BC, Martel MK, Pelizzari CA (2007) A Gaussian mixture model for definition of lung tumor volumes in positron emission tomography. Med Phys 34:4223–4235

Belhassen S, Zaidi H (2010) A novel fuzzy C-means algorithm for unsupervised heterogeneous tumor quantification in PET. Med Phys 37:1309–1324

Biehl KJ, Kong FM, Dehdashti F et al (2006) ^{18}F-FDG PET definition of gross tumor volume for radiotherapy of non-small cell lung cancer: is a single standardized uptake value threshold approach appropriate? J Nucl Med 47:1808–1812

Boellaard R (2009) Standards for PET image acquisition and quantitative data analysis. J Nucl Med 50(Suppl 1):11S–20S

Bradley JD, Perez CA, Dehdashti F, Siegel BA (2004) Implementing biologic target volumes in radiation treatment planning for non-small cell lung cancer. J Nucl Med 45:96S–101S

Chan TF, Sandberg BY, Vese LA (2000) Active contours without edges for vector-valued images. J Vis Commun Image Represent 11:130–141

Chao KS, Bhide S, Chen H et al (2007) Reduce in variation and improve efficiency of target volume delineation by a computer-assisted system using a deformable image registration approach. Int J Radiat Oncol Biol Phys 68:1512–1521

Chui H, Rangarajan A (2003) A new point matching algorithm for non-rigid registration. Comput Vis Image Underst 89:114–141

Crum WR, Camara O, Hill DLG (2006) Generalized overlap measures for evaluation and validation in medical image analysis. IEEE Trans Med Imaging 25:1451–1461

Day E, Betler J, Parda D, Reitz B, Kirichenko A, Mohammadi S, Miften M (2009) A region growing method for tumor volume segmentation on PET images for rectal and anal cancer patients. Med Phys 36:4349–4358

El Naqa I, Yang D, Apte A et al (2007) Concurrent multimodality image segmentation by active contours for radiotherapy treatment planning. Med Phys 34:4738–4749

Gardner SJ, Wen N, Kim J, Liu C, Pradhan D, Aref I, Elshaikh MA (2015) Contouring variability of human-and deformable-generated contours in radiotherapy for prostate cancer. Phys Med Biol 60:4429–4447

Geets X, Lee JA, Bol A, Lonneux M, Gregoire V (2007) A gradient-based method for segmenting FDG-PET images: methodology and validation. Eur J Nucl Med Mol Imaging 34:1427–1438

Hatt M, Cheze Le Rest C, Albarghach N et al (2011) PET functional volume delineation: a robustness and repeatability study. Eur J Nucl Med Mol Imaging 38:3663–3672

Ikushima K, Arimura H, Jin Z, Yabu-uchi H, Kuwazuru J, Shioyama Y, Sasaki T, Honda H, Sasaki M (2016) Computer-assisted framework for machine-learning-based delineation of GTV regions on datasets of planning CT and PET/CT images. J Radiat Res:57. doi:10.1093/jrr/rrw082

International Commission on Radiation Units and Measurements, (ICRU) (1993) Prescribing, recording, and reporting photon beam therapy, ICRU Report 50. ICRU, Bethesda

International Commission on Radiation Units and Measurements, (ICRU) (1999) Prescribing, Recording and Reporting Photon Beam Therapy. (Supplement to ICRU Report 50), ICRU Report 62. ICRU, Bethesda

Jin Z, Arimura H, Shioyama Y et al (2014) Computer-assisted delineation of lung tumor regions in treatment planning CT images with PET/CT image sets based on an optimum contour selection method. J Radiat Res 55(6):1153–1162

Kerhet A, Small C, Quon H et al (2010) Application of machine learning methodology for PET-based definition of lung cancer. Curr Oncol 17(1):41–47

Leunens G, Menten J, Weltens C et al (1993) Quality assessment of medical decision making in radiation oncology: variability in target volume delineation for brain tumours. Radiother Oncol 29(2):169–175

Niyazi M, Landrock S, Elsner A et al (2013) Automated biological target volume delineation for radiotherapy treatment planning using FDG-PET/CT. Radiat Oncol 8:180. doi:10.1186/1748-717X-8-180

Okada T, Shimada R, Hori M et al (2008) Automated segmentation of the liver from 3D CT images using probabilistic atlas and multilevel statistical shape model. Acad Radiol 15:1390–1403

Rousson M, Khamene A, Diallo M, Carlos Celi J, Sauer F (2005) Constrained surface evolutions for prostate and bladder segmentation in CT images. Lect Notes Comput Sci (LNCS) 3765:251–260

Sethian JA (1999) Level set methods and fast marching methods: evolving interfaces in computational geometry, fluid mechanics, computer vision, and materials science. Cambridge University Press, Cambridge, UK

Söhn M, Birkner M, Yan D et al (2005) Modelling individual geometric variation based on dominant eigenmodes of organ deformation: implementation and evaluation. Phys Med Biol 50:5893–5908

Söhn M, Alber M, Yan D (2007) Principal component analysis-based pattern analysis of dose-volume histograms and influence on rectal toxicity. Int J Radiat Oncol Biol Phys 69 (1):230–239

Söhn M, Sobotta B, Alber M (2012) Dosimetric treatment course simulation based on a statistical model of deformable organ motion. Phys Med Biol 57:3693–3709

Stroom JC, Heijmen BJ (2002) Geometrical uncertainties, radiotherapy planning margins, and the ICRU-62 report. Radiother Oncol 64:75–83

Thörnqvist S, Hysing LB, Zolnay AG et al (2013) Treatment simulations with a statistical deformable motion model to evaluate margins for multiple targets in radiotherapy for high-risk prostate cancer. Radiother Oncol 109(3):344–349

Trefethen LN, Bau D III (1997) Numerical linear algebra. Society for Industrial and Applied Mathematics, Philadelphia

van de Steene J, Linthout N, de Mey J, Vinh-Hung V, Claassens C, Noppen M, Bel A, Storme G (2002) Definition of gross tumor volume in lung cancer: inter-observer variability. Radiother Oncol 62:37–49

van der Wielen GJ, Mutanga TF, Incrocci L et al (2008) Deformation of prostate and seminal vesicles relative to intraprostatic fiducial markers. Int J Radiat Oncol Biol Phys 72:1604–1611

van Herk M (2004) Errors and margins in radiotherapy. Semin Radiat Oncol 14(1):52–64

van Herk M, Remeijer P, Rasch C et al (2000) The probability of correct target dosage: dose-population histograms for deriving treatment margins in radiotherapy. Int J Radiat Oncol Biol Phys 47:1121–1135

Vapnik VN (1999) The nature of statistical learning theory, 2nd edn. Springer, New York

Weiss E, Hess CF (2003) The impact of gross tumor volume (GTV) and clinical target volume (CTV) definition on the total accuracy in radiotherapy theoretical aspects and practical experiences. Strahlenther Onkol 179:21–30

Xu H, Vile DJ, Sharma M et al (2014) Coverage-based treatment planning to accommodate deformable organ variations in prostate cancer treatment. Med Phys 41(10):101705. doi:10.1118/1.4894701

Xu H, Gordon JJ, Siebers JV (2015) Coverage-based treatment planning to accommodate delineation uncertainties in prostate cancer treatment. Med Phys 42(9):5435–5443

Zhang T, Tachiya Y, Sakaguchi Y et al (2010) Phantom study on three-dimensional target volume delineation by PET/CT-based auto-contouring. Fukuoka Acta Med 101:238–246

Chapter 6
Computer-Assisted Treatment Planning Approaches for SBRT

Taiki Magome

Abstract This chapter describes computer-assisted treatment planning approaches for stereotactic body radiation therapy (SBRT), focusing especially on beam angle optimization and similar-case-based treatment planning. The determination of appropriate treatment plans for SBRT is a substantial and demanding task for inexperienced treatment planners. A computer-aided treatment planning system for SBRT could help treatment planners by capitalizing on the knowledge and skills that are stored in radiotherapy treatment planning databases. First, the chapter describes a computer-aided method of determining beam arrangements based on similar cases in a radiotherapy treatment planning database. Second, the chapter discusses a similar-case-based optimization method for beam arrangements that was designed to assist treatment planners. The methods introduced herein could be employed as computer-aided tools that assist treatment planners. The quality of radiotherapy could thus be normalized across treatment planners with different levels of experience in SBRT.

Keywords Treatment planning • Similar case • Knowledge based • Computer aided • Stereotactic body radiation therapy

6.1 Introduction

Stereotactic body radiation therapy (SBRT) can be used to deliver highly conformal doses to tumors while minimizing doses to surrounding organs at risk (OARs) and normal tissues with steep dose gradients (Nagata et al. 2005, Takayama et al. 2005; Timmerman et al. 2006a, 2007; Glide-Hurst and Chetty 2014). In general, hypofractionated regimens (10–20 Gy in five or fewer fractions) have been used. Numerous phase I/II studies of early-stage lung and liver cancers have shown high local control rates and good tolerability (Nagata et al. 2005, 2011; Timmerman et al. 2006b, 2010; Onishi et al. 2011; Taremi et al. 2012; Shioyama et al. 2013).

T. Magome (✉)
Department of Radiological Sciences, Faculty of Health Sciences, Komazawa University, 1-23-1, Komazawa, Setagaya-ku, Tokyo 154-8525, Japan
e-mail: magome@komazawa-u.ac.jp

H. Arimura (ed.), *Image-Based Computer-Assisted Radiation Therapy*,
DOI 10.1007/978-981-10-2945-5_6

Recently, this technique has made substantial progress with intensity-modulated radiation therapy (IMRT), volumetric modulated arc therapy (VMAT), and flattening filter-free (FFF) beams (Videtic et al. 2010; Holt et al. 2011; Zhang et al. 2011; Takahashi et al. 2013; Hrbacek et al. 2014; Nakagawa et al. 2014; Yamashita et al. 2014a).

Radiotherapy treatment planning (RTP), which is one of the most important procedures for SBRT, is determined by treatment planners in a time-consuming iterative manner. In particular, it is essential to determine an appropriate beam arrangement, which generally consists of a large number of coplanar and noncoplanar static beams or rotational beams (Takayama et al. 2005; Liu et al. 2006; Lim et al. 2010).

In general, the choice of an appropriate beam arrangement for lung SBRT has varied across institutions, depending on their individual circumstances. Regarding the number of beams, Takayama et al. (2005) reported routine use of five to ten beams with coplanar and noncoplanar directions in order to deliver homogeneous target dose distributions during lung SBRT, while avoiding high doses to normal tissues. Liu et al. (2006) found that the optimal number of beams for lung SBRT was 13–15 with coplanar and noncoplanar directions. A large number of beams increase the required treatment time, which should be as short as possible to reduce intra-fractional patient motion. Moreover, the available beam direction space is restricted by the size of the gantry and the immobilizer. The beam arrangement plans are not limited to the beam directions; planning also includes nominal beam energies, collimator angles, beam weights, and other parameters.

One of the most difficult problems in RTP is the patient-specific trade-off between the benefit of irradiating the tumor and the risk to surrounding normal tissues. Therefore, treatment planners should select a plan that is most suitable for the individual patient who is in their care. In the rest of this chapter, several methods of overcoming the abovementioned problems are discussed.

6.2 Target and Organ Determination in SBRT

The majority of treatment planning procedures for SBRT are the same as those used for conventional treatment planning: (1) contouring of a target and OARs, (2) determination of the beam arrangements, and (3) optimization of the dose distribution (via a trial-and-error approach or inverse planning, such as in IMRT and VMAT). The four-dimensional motions of the target and OARs should be considered in SBRT. Report 62 of the International Commission on Radiation Units & Measurements (ICRU 1999) introduced the concept of the internal target volume (ITV), in which the internal margin due to physiological motion (e.g., respiration) is added to clinical target volume (CTV). The ITV can be created individually according to the internal respiratory motion of the patient, which can be measured with an X-ray simulator or four-dimensional computed tomography (4DCT) (Underberg et al. 2004; Rietzel et al. 2005; Yamashita et al. 2014b). When 4DCT is used for this purpose, the motions of the target and organ are visualized in different phases of the respiratory cycle. CTVs can be delineated on all 4DCT phases, and a union can be defined as the ITV.

6.3 Beam Angle Optimization

Many researchers have investigated automated methods for beam angle optimization (BAO) (Rowbottom et al. 1999; Pugachev and Xing 2002; Djajaputra et al. 2003; Gaede et al. 2004; Wang et al. 2004; Meyer et al. 2005; de Pooter et al. 2006, 2008; Liu et al. 2006; Aleman et al. 2008; Potrebko et al. 2008; Li and Lei 2010; Vaitheeswaran et al. 2010; Breedveld et al. 2012; Bertsimas et al. 2013). Rowbottom et al. (1999) suggested a method in which the coplanar beam orientation was determined using an artificial neural network. Li et al. (Li and Lei 2010) developed a DNA-based genetic algorithm to solve the BAO problem in coplanar directions for IMRT planning. De Pooter et al. (2006, 2008) investigated an optimization method for noncoplanar beams based on the cycle algorithm for SBRT of liver tumors. Meyer et al. (2005) developed an automated method for the selection of noncoplanar beams by using a cost function based on radiation absorption in normal tissue and OARs for three-dimensional conformal radiotherapy. The majority of the abovementioned methods maximize or minimize a cost function, which is often defined without information on the dose distribution in order to reduce computational costs. Treatment planning time could be reduced by using these BAO algorithms, as compared with trial-and-error approaches.

6.4 Similar-Case-Based Treatment Planning

In the field of diagnostic radiology, the presentation of similar cases as a diagnostic aid has been suggested when making diagnoses based on chest images (Aisen et al. 2003), lung computed tomography images (Kumazawa et al. 2008), and mammography images (Kumazawa et al. 2008, Muramatsu et al. 2005, 2009, 2010). These studies have indicated that it is feasible to use similar cases as a diagnostic aid. To date, the usefulness of similar cases in the field of radiation oncology has been shown in several studies. Commowick and Malandain (2007) used a similar image in a database for the segmentation of critical structures. Chanyavanich et al. (2011) developed new prostate IMRT plans based on similar cases. Mishra et al. (2011) investigated the case-based reasoning approach to determine the most appropriate dose plans for prostate cancer patients. Schlaefer and Dieterich (2011) showed the feasibility of case-based beam generation for robotic radiosurgery. Therefore, the clinically usable beam arrangements for SBRT might also be determinable based on past similar cases.

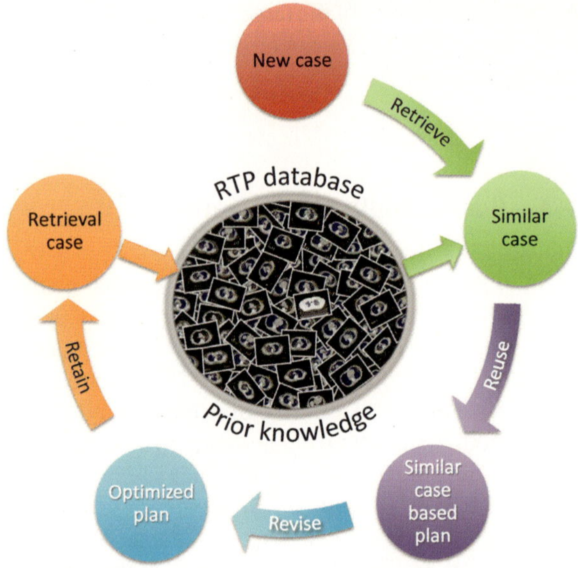

Fig. 6.1 Conceptual scheme of similar-case-based radiotherapy treatment planning

RTP is a time-consuming task, especially for less experienced treatment planners. Treatment planning skills are developed by repeated planning experiences in clinical practice, often under the guidance of experienced planners or appropriate textbooks. As they gain experience, treatment planners should memorize many planning patterns and construct an evolving "database" in their memory, which can then be searched for past cases that are similar to the case under consideration. Therefore, a similar-case-based treatment planning tool (Fig. 6.1) may reduce both the workload for treatment planners and the inter-planner variability of treatment plans. Moreover, the similar-case-based approach to RTP could be adjusted to the specific circumstances and contexts of different institutions by replacing the RTP database.

6.5 Similar-Case-Based Beam Angle Optimization

The accuracy and efficiency of beam arrangement determinations could potentially be improved by combining similar-case-based treatment planning and BAO algorithms (Magome et al. 2013a, b). Figure 6.2 shows the overall scheme of the similar-case-based beam angle optimization method, which consisted of three main steps. First, cases that were similar to an objective case were automatically selected from the RTP database based on geometrical features related to structures, such as the location, size, and shape of the target and OARs. Second, the initial beam arrangements of the objective case were determined by registering similar cases to the objective case, using a linear registration technique (Burger and Burge

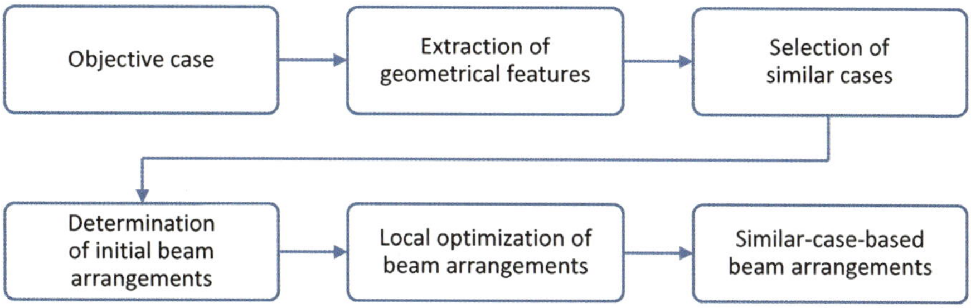

Fig. 6.2 Overall scheme of similar-case-based beam angle optimization

2007). Finally, the beam directions of the objective case were locally optimized based on the cost function, which took the radiation absorption in normal tissues and OARs into account.

6.5.1 Feature Extraction for Searching Similar Cases

It is very important to consider the exact meaning of "similarity" in the radiation oncology field. "Similarity" could be defined in many different ways, for example, based on the similarity of the tumor type (histological type or staging), the patient (gender, age, height, weight, etc.), or other characteristics. However, similar cases should be defined from the viewpoint of treatment planning because they are intended to be useful for the treatment planner. It should be assumed that the geometrical similarity with respect to tumor and OAR among clinical cases may be a key in the similar-case-based treatment planning. Therefore, four types of features (comprising 10 features in total) were defined for lung SBRT: the planning target volume (PTV) shape, the PTV size, the lung dimensions, and the geometrical relationship between the PTV and the spinal cord (Fig. 6.3), as assessed using the DICOM-RT structure set (Magome et al. 2013a).

The ten defined geometrical features were described as follows: PTV centroid in left-right (*LR*), anterior-posterior (*AP*), and superior-inferior (*SI)* directions; effective diameter of the PTV; sphericity of the PTV; lung dimension in *LR*, *AP*, and SI directions; distance between the PTV and the spinal cord in the isocenter plane; and angle from the spinal cord to the PTV in the isocenter plane. The PTV centroid was determined by registering the lung structure image of each case in the RTP database with that of a reference case, using a linear registration technique (Burger and Burge 2007). The effective diameter was defined as the diameter of a sphere with the same volume as the PTV. The sphericity was defined as the roundness of the PTV without directional dependence, and given by the ratio of the number of logical AND voxels between the PTV and its equivalent sphere with the same centroid and volume as the PTV to the number of PTV voxels. The lung dimensions were defined as the three side lengths of the circumscribed parallelepiped of the

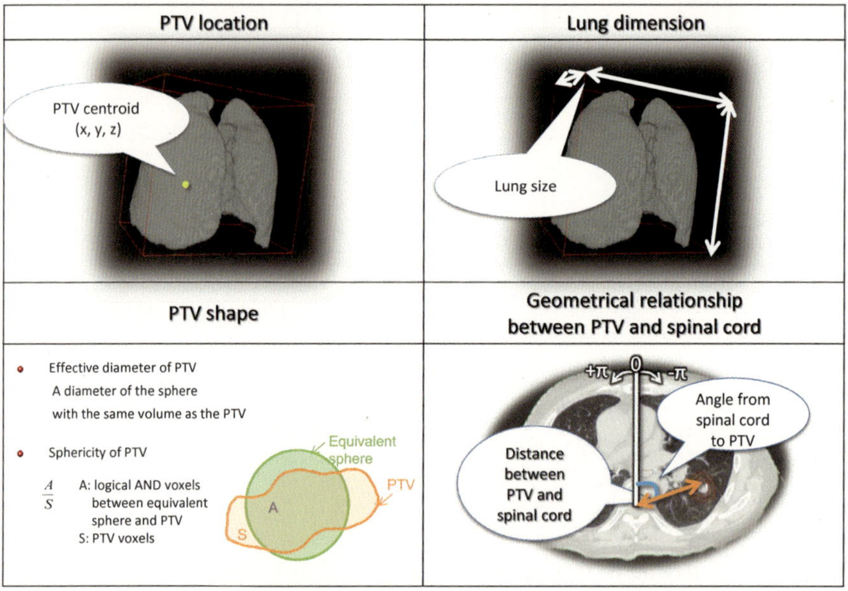

Fig. 6.3 Geometrical features, which were used to search for similar cases in a lung SBRT database (Magome et al. 2013a)

lung regions in the *LR*, *AP*, and *SI* directions. The distance between the PTV and spinal cord was measured between the centroid of the PTV and that of the spinal cord in the isocenter plane. The angle from the spinal cord to the PTV was defined in the two-dimensional coordinate system with the origin at the centroid of the spinal cord in the isocenter plane, and ranged from $-\pi$ (clockwise) to π (counter-clockwise) for a baseline of the posterior-anterior direction. Although only the PTV centroid was determined in a fixed reference coordinate system by registering the lung regions of each case in the RTP database with those of a reference case, the other features were calculated with respect to each of their original coordinate systems. The calculations were performed in this way in order to consider both the relative similarity of the tumor in the lung regions and absolute similarities, such as of the lung dimensions and spinal cord position.

6.5.2 Selection of Similar Planning Cases Using Geometrical Features

The RTP database was searched for the cases that resembled the objective case by considering the weighted Euclidean distances between the geometrical feature vector of the objective case and the geometrical feature vectors of all other cases in the RTP database (Fig. 6.4). The weighted Euclidean distance was thus regarded

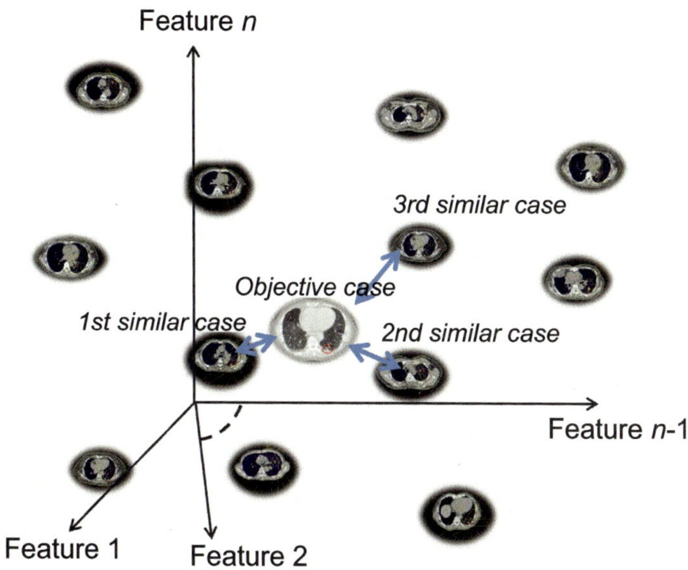

Fig. 6.4 Conceptual illustration of an objective case and similar cases in a *n*-dimensional feature space. Most similar case was defined as the case that was closest to the objective case in the feature space, as measured with a weighted Euclidean distance

as a similarity measure. The weighted Euclidean distance d_{image} was calculated using the following equation:

$$d_{\text{image}} = \sqrt{\sum_{i=1}^{G} w_i (A_i - B_i)^2}, \tag{6.1}$$

where G is the number of geometrical features, w_i is the weight of the i-th geometrical feature, A_i is the i-th geometrical feature for the objective case, and B_i is the i-th geometrical feature for another case in the RTP database. Note that each geometrical feature was normalized by subtraction of a mean of the feature and dividing it by the standard deviation of its value for all cases in the RTP database.

Weights were needed for the geometrical features in order to incorporate their relative importance from the viewpoint of treatment planning. Therefore, when applying the proposed method to their own databases, each institute should determine the appropriate weights for the geometrical features based on their own philosophy or policy of treatment planning. In our investigation, the weights for geometrical features were empirically set as follows: PTV centroid (three-dimension) = 0.3, effective diameter of PTV = 0.1, sphericity of PTV = 0.1, lung dimension (three-dimension) = 0.3, distance between PTV and spinal cord = 1.0, and angle from spinal cord to PTV = 1.0.

6.5.3 Determination of Initial Beam Arrangements Based on the Linear Registration Technique

In the second step, beam arrangements for the objective case were automatically determined (Magome et al. 2013a) based on the registration of similar cases with the objective case in terms of lung regions, using a linear registration technique (i.e., affine transformation) (Burger and Burge 2007). The beam arrangement of the similar case was modified to fit the objective case with respect to the lung regions.

First, a beam angle (i.e., a beam direction with a gantry angle θ and couch angle φ) was described as a point in a Cartesian coordinate system. As shown in Fig. 6.5, the beam direction with gantry angle θ and couch angle φ can be considered as a line in a spherical polar coordinate system, with the origin as the isocenter. An arbitrary point $(x_{\theta,\varphi}, y_{\theta,\varphi}, z_{\theta,\varphi})$ on the line is described in a Cartesian coordinate system as follows:

$$\begin{pmatrix} x_{\theta,\phi} \\ y_{\theta,\phi} \\ z_{\theta,\phi} \end{pmatrix} = \begin{pmatrix} x_{\text{iso}} + r\sin\theta\cos\phi \\ y_{\text{iso}} - r\cos\theta \\ z_{\text{iso}} + r\sin\theta\sin\phi \end{pmatrix}. \tag{6.2}$$

where r is distance from the isocenter $(x_{\text{iso}}, y_{\text{iso}}, z_{\text{iso}})$. In this study, r has no meaning ($r = 1$ for simplicity) because the purpose of the analysis is registration of the beam angle.

Second, each beam point of the similar case in the Cartesian coordinate system was modified based on a linear registration technique (i.e., an affine transformation) (Burger and Burge 2007). Please note that the linear registration maps straight lines to straight lines, and thus the beam directions—which can be considered as points—are uniquely and automatically determined by the registration. The beam point $(x_{\theta,\varphi}, y_{\theta,\varphi}, z_{\theta,\varphi})$ was modified to the point $(x'_{\theta,\varphi}, y'_{\theta,\varphi}, z'_{\theta,\varphi})$ by using the affine transformation matrix to register the lung regions of each similar case with those of the objective case, as follows:

$$\begin{pmatrix} x'_{\theta,\phi} \\ y'_{\theta,\phi} \\ z'_{\theta,\phi} \\ 1 \end{pmatrix} = \begin{pmatrix} u_{11} & u_{12} & u_{13} & u_{14} \\ u_{21} & u_{22} & u_{23} & u_{24} \\ u_{31} & u_{32} & u_{33} & u_{34} \\ 0 & 0 & 0 & 1 \end{pmatrix} \begin{pmatrix} x_{\theta,\phi} \\ y_{\theta,\phi} \\ z_{\theta,\phi} \\ 1 \end{pmatrix}, \tag{6.3}$$

where $u_{11} \ldots u_{34}$ are the transformation parameters. The isocenter point $(x_{\text{iso}}, y_{\text{iso}}, z_{\text{iso}})$ was also modified to the point $(x'_{\text{iso}}, y'_{\text{iso}}, z'_{\text{iso}})$ in the same manner. The affine transformation can apply a linear combination of translation, scaling, rotation, and/or shear mapping. Further details can be found in the literature (Burger and Burge 2007). The vertices of a circumscribed parallelepiped of a lung (including the left and right lung regions) were automatically obtained as feature points to calculate the parameters of the affine transformation matrix. In this study, the

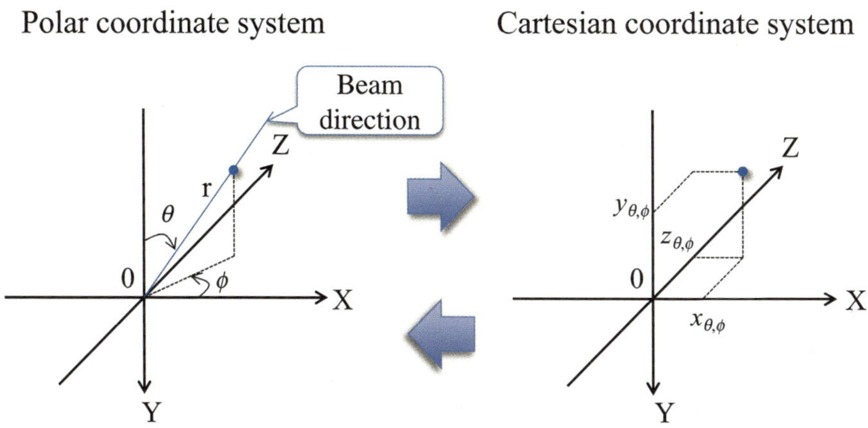

Fig. 6.5 Illustration of a beam direction with gantry angle θ and couch angle φ in a spherical polar coordinate system and a Cartesian coordinate system. Here, the origin indicates an isocenter and couch angle φ is defined with respect to the patient-fixed coordinate system

circumscribed parallelepiped was chosen to reduce the calculation time that was necessary to find the feature points of the lung.

Finally, the resulting direction vector ($x'_{\theta,\varphi} - x'_{\mathrm{iso}}$, $y'_{\theta,\varphi} - y'_{\mathrm{iso}}$, $z'_{\theta,\varphi} - z'_{\mathrm{iso}}$) in the Cartesian coordinate system was converted into the spherical polar coordinate system as gantry angle θ' and couch angle φ', as follows:

$$\theta' = \tan^{-1}\left(\frac{\sqrt{\left(x'_{\theta,\phi} - x'_{\mathrm{iso}}\right)^2 + \left(z'_{\theta,\phi} - z'_{\mathrm{iso}}\right)^2}}{-\left(y'_{\theta,\phi} - y'_{\mathrm{iso}}\right)}\right), \tag{6.4}$$

$$\phi' = \tan^{-1}\left(\frac{\left(z'_{\theta,\phi} - z'_{\mathrm{iso}}\right)}{\left(x'_{\theta,\phi} - x'_{\mathrm{iso}}\right)}\right). \tag{6.5}$$

6.5.4 Local Optimization of Beam Arrangements

The beam directions of the objective case were locally optimized based on the cost function, which took into account the radiation absorption in normal tissues and OARs (Magome et al. 2013b). Although Meyer et al. (2005) developed the cost function for a global optimization of beam arrangements, the cost function was used for the local optimization of each beam direction in this study. The cost function $C_{\theta,\varphi}$ of a beam with gantry angle θ and couch angle φ was defined as follows:

$$C_{\theta,\varphi} = C_{\theta,\varphi}(\mathrm{PTV}) + \sum_k w_k C_{\theta,\varphi}(\mathrm{OAR}_k), \tag{6.6}$$

where $C_{\theta,\varphi}$(PTV) represents the dose absorption in normal tissue until the X-ray beams reach the PTV surface, $C_{\theta,\varphi}(\mathrm{OAR}_k)$ is a term for the irradiation of k-th OAR, and w_k is a weight for the k-th OAR. The first term $C_{\theta,\varphi}$(PTV) was determined by the following equation:

$$C_{\theta,\varphi}(\mathrm{PTV}) = 1 - \exp\left(-\mu d_{\theta,\varphi}(\mathrm{PTV})\right), \tag{6.7}$$

where μ is a linear attenuation coefficient in water, and $d_{\theta,\varphi}$(PTV) is the mean distance in centimeters from the body surface to the PTV surface. The second term for the k-th OAR $C_{\theta,\varphi}(\mathrm{OAR}_k)$ was defined as follows:

$$C_{\theta,\phi}(\mathrm{OAR}_k) = \lambda v_{\theta,\phi}(\mathrm{OAR}_k) + (1-\lambda)\exp\left(-\mu d_{\theta,\phi}(\mathrm{OAR}_k)\right), \tag{6.8}$$

where $v_{\theta,\varphi}(\mathrm{OAR}_k)$ is an irradiated fractional volume of the k-th OAR, $d_{\theta,\varphi}(\mathrm{OAR}_k)$ is the mean depth from the body surface to the k-th OAR surface, and λ is a parameter for controlling the relative significance of the first and second terms. The term exp $(-\mu d_{\theta,\varphi}(\mathrm{OAR}_k))$ represents the number of incident photons in the k-th OAR. Figure 6.6 presents a conceptual illustration of the cost function.

Each beam direction was locally optimized in the range of $\pm\, p$ degrees at an interval of q degrees. The lung and spinal cord were incorporated as OARs in the cost function, and both weights (for the lung and the spinal cord) were set to 5.0. The parameters for the local optimization of the beam arrangement λ, p, and q, were set to 0.6, 4°, and 2°, respectively. Although the parameters for the local optimization of beam arrangements were set empirically based on the preferences of our institution, each institute could determine the appropriate parameters based on their own philosophy or policy of treatment planning, in resemblance with the geometrical feature weights. Each optimal beam direction was defined as the direction of the beam which had the lowest cost value among the beam directions of the local range.

6.5.5 *Evaluation of Beam Arrangements Using Planning Evaluation Indices*

The similar-case-based beam arrangements were evaluated by manually preparing plans based on both the beam arrangements and other planning parameters (such as nominal beam energies, collimator angles, and beam weight) derived from the treatment plans of similar cases in a radiation treatment planning system. The following 11 planning evaluation indices were used for validation.

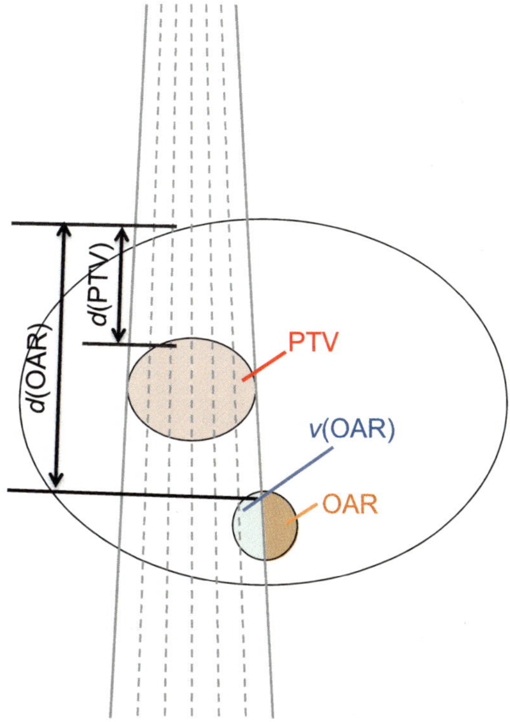

Fig. 6.6 Conceptual diagram of the cost function for local optimization of beam angles

The planning evaluation indices for the PTVs calculated in this study were the D95, homogeneity index (HI), conformity index (CI), and tumor control probability (TCP). The D95 was defined as the minimum dose in the PTV that encompassed at least 95 % of the PTV. The HI was calculated as the ratio of the maximum dose to the minimum dose in the PTV. The CI was the ratio of the treated volume to the PTV. The treated volume was defined as the tissue volume that was receiving the minimum PTV dose. The TCP was estimated based on a linear-quadratic (LQ) model according to a Poisson distribution by considering the radiosensitivity variation and nonuniform dose distribution (Sanchez-Nieto and Nahum 1999, 2000). The TCP was averaged over a population with variability in radiosensitivity, which was simulated as a Gaussian distribution of α_k values with mean $\overline{\alpha}$ and standard deviation σ_α in K groups of patients (Webb and Nahum 1993; Kanai et al. 2006). Specifically, TCP was given by

$$\mathrm{TCP} = \sum_{k=1}^{K}\left(\frac{1}{\sqrt{2\pi}\sigma_{\alpha}}\right)\exp\left\{-\frac{(\alpha_k-\overline{\alpha})^2}{2\sigma_{\alpha}^2}\right\}$$
$$\times\prod_{l=1}^{L}\exp\left[-\rho_c v_l\cdot\exp\left\{-\alpha_k D_l\left(1+\frac{d_l}{\alpha_k/\beta_k}\right)\right\}\right], \tag{6.9}$$

where ρ_c is the number of initial clonogenic cells per volume cm^3, L is the number of dose bins of the differential dose-volume histogram (DVH) in the PTV, v_l is the volume (cm^3) irradiated by a dose d_l (Gy) per fraction in the PTV, and D_l is the total dose (Gy) at v_l. The α_k ranged $\alpha_k \pm \gamma\sigma_\alpha$, and increased in certain intervals divided by K. The parameters for the TCP calculation were obtained from Kanai et al.'s (2006) study of patients with lung cancers.

The planning evaluation indices for normal tissues (i.e., the lung and spinal cord) were calculated as described below. For the lung volume, which was defined as the total lung volume minus the PTV, a $V5$, $V10$, $V20$, and mean dose were calculated. Each Vk was defined as the percentage of the total lung minus PTV receiving $\geq k$ Gy. The maximum dose for the spinal cord was also calculated. Moreover, the normal tissue complication probability (NTCP) values for the lung and spinal cord were calculated using the Lyman-Kutcher-Burman model (Lyman 1985; Kutcher and Burman 1989; Burman et al. 1991). For the calculation of the NTCP, the dose scale of a DVH was rescaled as a linear-quadratic equivalent dose (LQED) for 2 Gy fractions, as follows:

$$\mathrm{LQED}_s = D_s\frac{\alpha/\beta+d_s}{\alpha/\beta+2}, \tag{6.10}$$

where D_s is the total dose (Gy), α/β is a parameter for a linear-quadratic model (Wheldon et al. 1998; Thames et al. 1990), and d_s is the dose per fraction (Gy) at D_s in the differential DVH. Then, the NTCP was calculated as

$$\mathrm{NTCP} = \frac{1}{\sqrt{2\pi}}\int_{-\infty}^{t}\exp\left(-\frac{x^2}{2}\right)dx = \frac{1}{2}\left\{1+\mathrm{erf}\left(\frac{t}{\sqrt{2}}\right)\right\}, \tag{6.11}$$

$$t = \frac{\mathrm{LQED}_{\max} - TD_{50}(v)}{mTD_{50}(v)}, \tag{6.12}$$

$$v = \frac{v_{\mathrm{eff}}}{v_{\mathrm{ref}}}, \tag{6.13}$$

$$v_{\mathrm{eff}} = \sum_{s=1}^{S}\left(\frac{\mathrm{LQED}_s}{\mathrm{LQED}_{\max}}\right)^{1/n} v_s, \tag{6.14}$$

$$TD_{50}(v) = TD_{50}(v_{\mathrm{ref}})\cdot v^{-n}, \tag{6.15}$$

where erf(·) is an error function, $TD_{50}(v)$ and $TD_{50}(v_{\mathrm{ref}})$ are the tolerance doses in Gy that cause 50 % complication rates within 5 years after treatment for uniform irradiation of the partial volume v according to Eqs. (6.13) and (6.15), and reference volume v_{ref}, respectively. The parameters n and m control the volume effect and the slope of the dose-response curve, respectively. By using an effective volume method (Kutcher and Burman 1989), a nonuniform dose distribution, which has a volume bin v_s with a dose of $\mathrm{LQED_s}$ in the differential DVH, was transformed into a uniform dose distribution with an effective volume v_{eff} at the maximum dose of $\mathrm{LQED_{max}}$ in Eq. (6.14). The fitting parameter values for the NTCP calculation were obtained from Burman et al. (1991).

6.5.6 Assessment of Usable Beam Arrangements

In practice, treatment planners could manually select the best plan for each patient from among the treatment plans that are based on similar cases, according to the planner's own policies and the patient's performance. However, some indices that are representative of the treatment plan's usefulness could be helpful during decision making. The usefulness of each treatment plan can be estimated by the following Euclidean distance, d_{plan}, of the plan evaluation vector between an ideal treatment plan and each treatment plan that has been determined based on a similar case. This quantity is designated as the RTP evaluation measure:

$$d_{\mathrm{plan}} = \sqrt{\sum_{j=1}^{J} \left(E(\mathrm{ideal})_j - E(\mathrm{plan})_j\right)^2}, \tag{6.16}$$

where J is the number of plan evaluation indices, $E(\mathrm{ideal})_j$ is the j-th plan evaluation index for the ideal treatment plan, and $E(\mathrm{plan})_j$ is the j-th plan evaluation index for the treatment plan based on a similar case. The ideal treatment plan was created under the assumption that it produces perfect, uniform irradiation with a prescription dose in the PTV and no irradiation in the surrounding OARs or normal tissues. Although equal weights for were set for all of the indices in this study, the weights for each index could be determined based on each patient's condition or the treatment planners' policies.

6.5.7 Experimental Results

The proposed method was assessed using an RTP database that included 81 cases of lung cancer (right lung: 46 cases, left lung: 35 cases), as well as 10 test cases (right lung: 3 cases, left lung: 7 cases) that were chosen at random from all 91 available

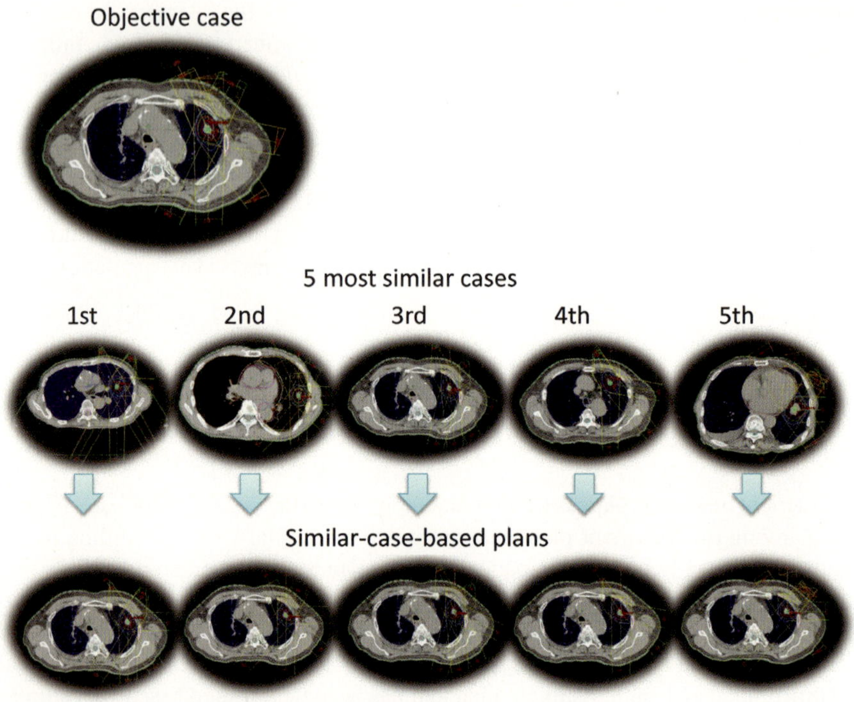

Fig. 6.7 An objective case, the first to fifth most similar cases to the objective case, and similar-case-based treatment plans

cases. The 10 test cases were not included in the RTP database of 81 cases (Magome et al. 2013a, b). The five most similar cases were selected from among the cases of lung cancers that were ipsilateral to the test case. The effectiveness of the combination method of determining the initial beam arrangement based on similar cases and the local optimization of the beam arrangement was evaluated by comparing the planning evaluation indices of 50 plans (5 plans × 10 test cases) with and without the local optimization of the beam arrangement. The same beam weights and wedges from the similar case were used for the plan, with the beam arrangement determined by our method.

Figure 6.7 shows an objective case, the first to fifth most similar cases to this objective case, and the similar-case-based treatment plans. In practice, a treatment planner could select one of the suitable plans for the patient from among several similar-case-based plans.

Figure 6.8 illustrates dose distributions of the original plan and one of the similar-case-based plan (specifically, the most usable plan). Although the lateral beam passed the spinal cord in the beam arrangement, the optimized beam arrangement avoided the spinal cord. Figure 6.9 provides DVHs for the case shown in Fig. 6.8. Regarding the PTV, the similar-case-based plan had a DVH curve that was almost the same as that of the original plan. However, the similar-case-based plan

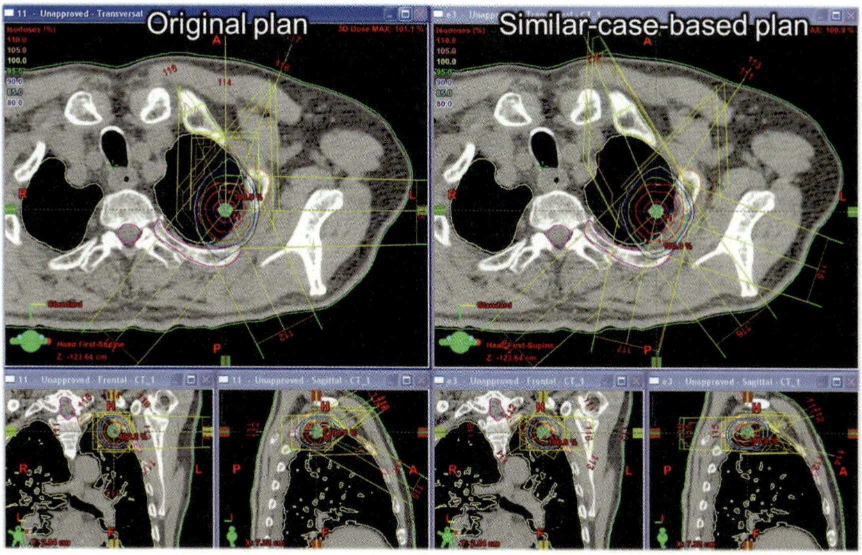

Fig. 6.8 Dose distributions of the original plan and one of the similar-case-based plans

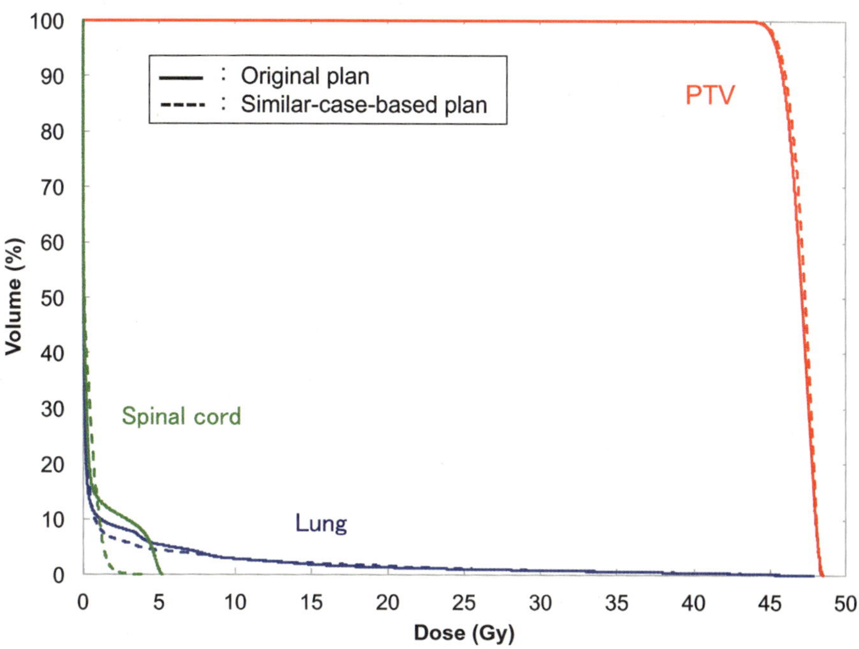

Fig. 6.9 Dose-volume histograms of the original plan and the similar-case-based plan for the case shown in Fig. 6.8

also resulted in better sparing of spinal cord and lung regions, as compared with the original plan. Magome et al. (2013b) have reported detailed results indicating that the local BAO algorithm improved the quality of treatment plans with significant differences ($P < 0.05$) in the homogeneity index and conformity index for the PTV, $V10$, $V20$, mean dose, and NTCP for the lung. Moreover, the proposed method may provide usable beam arrangements that are not significantly different from the original beam arrangements ($P > 0.05$) in terms of the ten planning evaluation indices. The mean value of D95 was significantly improved based on the proposed method, as compared with the D95 of the original beam arrangements ($P = 0.029$).

6.6 Estimation of Available Beam Direction Space

Because collision of the gantry and the patient must be avoided, the available beam direction space is limited by the gantry head, immobilizer, and patient's size. Magome et al. (2013b) constrained the available beam space, and these constraints were used in past cases included in the RTP database. Takayama et al. (2005) determined the applicable areas of beam arrangement at different isocenter heights. Ideally, however, the space should be determined separately for individual patients. Recently, several researchers have developed a collision prediction methodology for the patient and gantry by reconstructing the patient's surface on a treatment couch (Padilla et al. 2015; Yu et al. 2015). These studies allow more extensive use of noncoplanar beam directions, which can provide a better dose distribution.

6.7 Summary and Future Direction

In this chapter, computer-assisted treatment planning approaches for SBRT have been discussed, especially focusing on beam angle optimization and similar-case-based treatment planning. In general, the RTP database at each hospital has been generated by experienced planners after many trials and incorporates substantial amount of their knowledge and skills. The aim of the discussed studies was to use these records of knowledge and skill. The similar-case-based RTP was able to provide several usable beam arrangements based on similar cases in the RTP database. These methods could be useful for treatment planners, thereby improving the quality and efficiency of radiotherapy. Although the plan evaluation indices were calculated to evaluate the treatment plans, they may not cover all aspects of the dose distribution. Regarding the future direction of research, it will be important to incorporate clinical outcomes in order to improve the quality of the RTP database.

Acknowledgments The author would like to thank the radiation oncology group at the University of Tokyo Hospital for their support. This work was supported by a Grant-in-Aid for the Japan Society for the Promotion of Science (JSPS) Fellows (13J02944), as well as by a Grant-in-Aid for Young Scientists (B) (26860397).

References

Aisen AM, Broderick LS, Winer-Muram H, Brodley CE, Kak AC, Pavlopoulou C, Dy J, Shyu CR, Marchiori A (2003) Automated storage and retrieval of thin-section CT images to assist diagnosis: system description and preliminary assessment. Radiology 228(1):265–270

Aleman DM, Kumar A, Ahuja RK, Romeijn HE, Dempsey JF (2008) Neighborhood search approaches to beam orientation optimization in intensity modulated radiation therapy treatment planning. J Glob Optim 42:587–607

Bertsimas D, Cacchiani V, Craft D, Nohadani O (2013) A hybrid approach to beam angle optimization in intensity-modulated radiation therapy. Comput Oper Res 40:2187–2197

Breedveld S, Storchi PRM, Voet PWJ, Heijmen BJM (2012) iCycle: integrated, multicriterial beam angle, and profile optimization for generation of coplanar and noncoplanar IMRT plans. Med Phys 39:951–963

Burger W, Burge MJ (2007) Digital image processing an algorithmic introduction using Java. Springer, New York

Burman C, Kutcher GJ, Emami B, Goitein M (1991) Fitting of normal tissue tolerance data to an analytic function. Int J Radiat Oncol Biol Phys 21:123–135

Chanyavanich V, Das SK, Lee WR, Lo JY (2011) Knowledge-based IMRT treatment planning for prostate cancer. Med Phys 38:2515–2522

Commowick O, Malandain G (2007) Efficient selection of the most similar image in a database for critical structures segmentation. Med Image Comput Comput Assist Interv 10(Pt 2):203–210

de Pooter JA, Romero AM, Jansen WPA, Storchi PRM, Woudstra E, Levendag PC, Heijmen BJM (2006) Computer optimization of noncoplanar beam setups improves stereotactic treatment of liver tumors. Int J Radiat Oncol Biol Phys 66:913–922

de Pooter JA, Romero AM, Wunderink W, Storchi PRM, Heijmen BJM (2008) Automated non-coplanar beam direction optimization improves IMRT in SBRT of liver metastasis. Radiother Oncol 88:376–381

Djajaputra D, Wu Q, Wu Y, Mohan R (2003) Algorithm and performance of a clinical IMRT beam-angle optimization system. Phys Med Biol 48:3191–3212

Gaede S, Wong E, Rasmussen H (2004) An algorithm for systematic selection of beam directions for IMRT. Med Phys 31:376–388

Glide-Hurst CK, Chetty IJ (2014) Improving radiotherapy planning, delivery accuracy, and normal tissue sparing using cutting edge technologies. J Thorac Dis 6:303–318

Holt A, van Vliet-Vroegindeweij C, Mans A, Belderbos JS, Damen EMF (2011) Volumetric-modulated arc therapy for stereotactic body radiation therapy of lung tumors: a comparison with intensity-modulated radiotherapy techniques. Int J Radiat Oncol Biol Phys 81:1560–1567

Hrbacek J, Lang S, Graydon SN, Klöck S, Riesterer O (2014) Dosimetric comparison of flattened and unflattened beams for stereotactic ablative radiotherapy of stage I non-small cell lung cancer. Med Phys 41:031709

ICRU (1999) Prescribing, recording and reporting photon beam therapy (supplement to ICRU report 50). Interna-tional Commission on Radiation Units and Measurements, Bethesda

Kanai T, Matsufuji N, Miyamoto T, Mizoe J, Kamada T, Tsuji H, Kato H, Baba M, Tsujii H (2006) Examination of GyE system for HIMAC carbon therapy. Int J Radiat Oncol Biol Phys 64:650–656

Kumazawa S, Muramatsu C, Li Q, Li F, Shiraishi J, Caligiuri P, Schmidt RA, MacMahon H, Doi K (2008) An investigation of radiologists' perception of lesion similarity: observations with paired breast masses on mammograms and paired lung nodules on CT images. Acad Radiol 15(7):887–894

Kutcher GJ, Burman C (1989) Calculation of complication probability factors for non-uniform normal tissue irradiation: the effective volume method. Int J Radiat Oncol Biol Phys 16:1623–1630

Li Y, Lei J (2010) A feasible solution to the beam-angle-optimization problem in radiotherapy planning with a DNA-based genetic algorithm. IEEE Trans Biomed Eng 57:499–508

Lim DH, Yi BY, Mirmiran A, Dhople A, Suntharalingam M, D'Souza WD (2010) Optimal beam arrangement for stereotactic body radiation therapy delivery in lung tumors. Acta Oncol (Stockh) 49:219–224
Liu R, Buatti JM, Howes TL, Dill J, Modrick JM, Meeks SL (2006) Optimal number of beams for stereotactic body radiation therapy of lung and liver lesions. Int J Radiat Oncol Biol Phys 66:906–912
Lyman JT (1985) Complication probability as assessed from dose-volume histograms. Radiat Res Suppl 8:S13–S19
Magome T, Arimura H, Shioyama Y, Mizoguchi A, Tokunaga C, Nakamura K, Honda H, Ohki M, Toyofuku F, Hirata H (2013a) Computer-aided beam arrangement based on similar cases in radiation treatment-planning databases for stereotactic lung radiation therapy. J Radiat Res 54:569–577
Magome T, Arimura H, Shioyama Y, Nakamura K, Honda H, Hirata H (2013b) Similar-case-based optimization of beam arrangements in stereotactic body radiation therapy for assisting treatment planners. BioMed Res Int 6:1–10
Meyer J, Hummel SM, Cho PS, Austin-Seymour MM, Phillips MH (2005) Automatic selection of non-coplanar beam directions for three-dimensional conformal radiotherapy. Br J Radiol 78:316–327
Mishra N, Petrovic S, Sundar S (2011) A self-adaptive case-based reasoning system for dose planning in prostate cancer radiotherapy. Med Phys 38:6528
Muramatsu C, Li Q, Suzuki K, Schmidt RA, Shiraishi J, Newstead GM, Doi K (2005) Investigation of psychophysical measure for evaluation of similar images for mammographic masses: preliminary results. Med Phys 32(7):2295–2304
Muramatsu C, Li Q, Schmidt RA, Shiraishi J, Doi K (2009) Determination of similarity measures for pairs of mass lesions on mammograms by use of BI-RADS lesion descriptors and image features. Acad Radiol 16(4):443–449
Muramatsu C, Schmidt RA, Shiraishi J, Li Q, Doi K (2010) Presentation of similar images as a reference for distinction between benign and malignant masses on mammograms: analysis of initial observer study. J Digit Imaging 23(5):592–602
Nagata Y, Takayama K, Matsuo Y, Norihisa Y, Mizowaki T, Sakamoto T, Sakamoto M, Mitsumori M, Shibuya K, Araki N, Yano S, Hiraoka M (2005) Clinical outcomes of a phase I/II study of 48 Gy of stereotactic body radiation therapy in 4 fractions for primary lung cancer using a stereotactic body frame. Int J Radiat Oncol Biol Phys 63:1427–1431
Nagata Y, Wulf J, Lax I, Timmerman R, Zimmermann F, Stojkovski I, Jeremic B (2011) Stereotactic Radiotherapy of Primary Lung Cancer and Other Targets: Results of Consultant Meeting of the International Atomic Energy Agency. Int J Radiat Oncol Biol Phys 79:660–669
Nakagawa K, Haga A, Sakumi A, Yamashita H, Igaki H, Shiraki T, Ohtomo K, Iwai Y, Yoda K (2014) Impact of flattening-filter-free techniques on delivery time for lung stereotactic volumetric modulated arc therapy and image quality of concurrent kilovoltage cone-beam computed tomography: a preliminary phantom study. J Radiat Res 55:200–202
Onishi H, Shirato H, Nagata Y, Hiraoka M, Fujino M, Gomi K, Karasawa K, Hayakawa K, Niibe Y, Takai Y, Kimura T, Takeda A, Ouchi A, Hareyama M, Kokubo M, Kozuka T, Arimoto T, Hara R, Itami J, Araki T (2011) Stereotactic body radiotherapy (SBRT) for operable stage I non-small-cell lung cancer: can SBRT be comparable to surgery? Int J Radiat Oncol Biol Phys 81:1352–1358
Padilla L, Pearson EA, Pelizzari CA (2015) Collision prediction software for radiotherapy treatments. Med Phys 42:6448–6456
Potrebko PS, McCurdy BMC, Butler JB, El-Gubtan AS (2008) Improving intensity-modulated radiation therapy using the anatomic beam orientation optimization algorithm. Med Phys 35:2170–2179
Pugachev A, Xing L (2002) Incorporating prior knowledge into beam orientaton optimization in IMRT. Int J Radiat Oncol Biol Phys 54:1565–1574

Rietzel E, Pan T, Chen GTY (2005) Four-dimensional computed tomography: image formation and clinical protocol. Med Phys 32:874–889

Rowbottom CG, Webb S, Oldham M (1999) Beam-orientation customization using an artificial neural network. Phys Med Biol 44:2251

Sanchez-Nieto B, Nahum AE (1999) The delta-TCP concept: A clinically useful measure of tumor control probability. Int J Radiat Oncol Biol Phys 44:369–380

Sanchez-Nieto B, Nahum AE (2000) BIOPLAN: software for the biological evaluation of. Radiotherapy treatment plans. Med Dosim 25:71–76

Schlaefer A, Dieterich S (2011) Feasibility of case-based beam generation for robotic radiosurgery. Artif Intell Med 52:67–75

Shioyama Y, Nakamura K, Sasaki T, Ohga S, Yoshitake T, Nonoshita T, Asai K, Terashima K, Matsumoto K, Hirata H, Honda H (2013) Clinical results of stereotactic body radiotherapy for Stage I small-cell lung cancer: a single institutional experience. J Radiat Res 54:108–112

Takahashi W, Yamashita H, Kida S, Masutani Y, Sakumi A, Ohtomo K, Nakagawa K, Haga A (2013) Verification of Planning Target Volume Settings in Volumetric Modulated Arc Therapy for Stereotactic Body Radiation Therapy by Using In-Treatment 4-Dimensional Cone Beam Computed Tomography. Int J Radiat Oncol Biol Phys 86:426–431

Takayama K, Nagata Y, Negoro Y, Mizowaki T, Sakamoto T, Sakamoto M, Aoki T, Yano S, Koga S, Hiraoka M (2005) Treatment planning of stereotactic radiotherapy for solitary lung tumor. Int J Radiat Oncol Biol Phys 61:1565–1571

Taremi M, Hope A, Dahele M, Pearson S, Fung S, Purdie T, Brade A, Cho J, Sun A, Bissonnette J-P, Bezjak A (2012) Stereotactic Body Radiotherapy for Medically Inoperable Lung Cancer: Prospective, Single-Center Study of 108 Consecutive Patients. Int J Radiat Oncol Biol Phys 82:967–973

Thames HD, Bentzen SM, Turesson I, Overgaard M, Van den Bogaert W (1990) Time-dose factors in radiotherapy: a review of the human data. Radiother Oncol 19:219–235

Timmerman R, Galvin J, Michalski J, Straube W, Ibbott G, Martin E, Abdulrahman R, Swann S, Fowler J, Choy H (2006a) Accreditation and quality assurance for Radiation Therapy Oncology Group: Multicenter clinical trials using Stereotactic Body Radiation Therapy in lung cancer. Acta Oncol (Stockh) 45:779–786

Timmerman R, McGarry R, Yiannoutsos C, Papiez L, Tudor K, DeLuca J, Ewing M, Abdulrahman R, DesRosiers C, Williams M, Fletcher J (2006b) Excessive toxicity when treating central tumors in a phase ii study of stereotactic body radiation therapy for medically inoperable early-stage lung cancer. J Clin Oncol 24:4833–4839

Timmerman RD, Kavanagh BD, Cho LC, Papiez L, Xing L (2007) Stereotactic body radiation therapy in multiple organ sites. J Clin Oncol 25:947–952

Timmerman R, Paulus R, Galvin J, Michalski J, Straube W, Bradley J, Fakiris A, Bezjak A, Videtic G, Johnstone D, Fowler J, Gore E, Choy H (2010) Stereotactic body radiation therapy for inoperable early stage lung cancer. JAMA 303:1070–1076

Underberg RWM, Lagerwaard FJ, Cuijpers JP, Slotman BJ, Van Sörnsen De Koste JR, Senan S (2004) Four-dimensional CT scans for treatment planning in stereotactic radiotherapy for stage I lung cancer. Int J Radiat Oncol Biol Phys 60:1283–1290

Vaitheeswaran R, Narayanan VKS, Bhangle JR, Nirhali A, Kumar N, Basu S, Maiya V (2010) An algorithm for fast beam angle selection in intensity modulated radiotherapy. Med Phys 37:6443–6452

Videtic GMM, Stephans K, Reddy C, Gajdos S, Kolar M, Clouser E, Djemil T (2010) Intensity-modulated radiotherapy-based stereotactic body radiotherapy for medically inoperable early-stage lung cancer: excellent local control. Int J Radiat Oncol Biol Phys 77:344–349

Wang X, Zhang X, Dong L, Liu H, Wu Q, Mohan R (2004) Development of methods for beam angle optimization for IMRT using an accelerated exhaustive search strategy. Int J Radiat Oncol Biol Phys 60:1325–1337

Webb S, Nahum AE (1993) A model for calculating tumour control probability in radiotherapy including the effects of inhomogeneous distributions of dose and clonogenic cell density. Phys Med Biol 38(6):653–666

Wheldon TE, Deehan C, Wheldon EG, Barrett A (1998) The linear-quadratic transformation of dose-volume histograms in fractionated radiotherapy. Radiother Oncol 46:285–295

Yamashita H, Haga A, Takahashi W, Takenaka R, Imae T, Takenaka S, Nakagawa K (2014a) Volumetric modulated arc therapy for lung stereotactic radiation therapy can achieve high local control rates. Radiat Oncol 9:243

Yamashita H, Takahashi W, Haga A, Kida S, Saotome N, Nakagawa K (2014b) Stereotactic body radiotherapy for small lung tumors in the university of Tokyo hospital. BioMed Res Int 2014:1–13

Yu VY, Tran A, Nguyen D, Cao M, Ruan D, Low DA, Sheng K (2015) The development and verification of a highly accurate collision prediction model for automated noncoplanar plan delivery. Med Phys 42:6457–6467

Zhang GG, Ku L, Dilling TJ, Stevens CW, Zhang RR, Li W, Feygelman V (2011) Volumetric modulated arc planning for lung stereotactic body radiotherapy using conventional and unflattened photon beams: a dosimetric comparison with 3D technique. Radiat Oncol (Lond) 6:152

Chapter 7
Computer-Assisted Treatment Planning Approaches for Carbon-Ion Beam Therapy

Shinichiro Mori

Abstract In this chapter, we introduced the basic concept of the charged particle beam therapy from a physics point of view. Although treatment procedures for particle beam therapy are closely similar to those for the photon beam therapy, beam range (penetration depth) should be taken into account carefully in the particle beam therapy due to different characteristics of them. Moreover, heavy charged particle beam leads to complex biological effect compared to proton beam. For readers not familiar with charged particle beam therapy, therefore, we provide the sufficient information of the particle therapy physics and its clinical application.

Keywords Image guidance • Motion management • Particle beam • Treatment planning

7.1 Introduction

State-of-the-art radiotherapy techniques improve dose conformation to the target and dose sparing to normal tissues compared to conventional methods. These precise delivery techniques, which include intensity-modulated radiotherapy (IMRT) and volumetric modulated arc therapy (VMAT) in the photon world and intensity-modulated particle therapy (IMPT) in the particle world, allow much steeper dose gradients between the target region and surrounding healthy tissue. The physics of interactions differ between charged particle and photon beams, one result of which is that particle beam therapy reduces excessive dose to healthy tissues and maintains a high target dose, leading to good tumor control rates with less toxicity and improved patient quality of life (Fig. 7.1). Those unfamiliar with particle beam treatment might feel that charged particle beam treatment planning is both difficult and markedly different from photon beam treatment planning. But as

S. Mori (✉)
Research Center for Charged Particle Therapy, National Institute of Radiological Sciences, 4-9-1 Anagawa, Inage-ku, Chiba-city, Chiba 263-8555, Japan
e-mail: mori.shinichiro@qst.go.jp

H. Arimura (ed.), *Image-Based Computer-Assisted Radiation Therapy*,
DOI 10.1007/978-981-10-2945-5_7

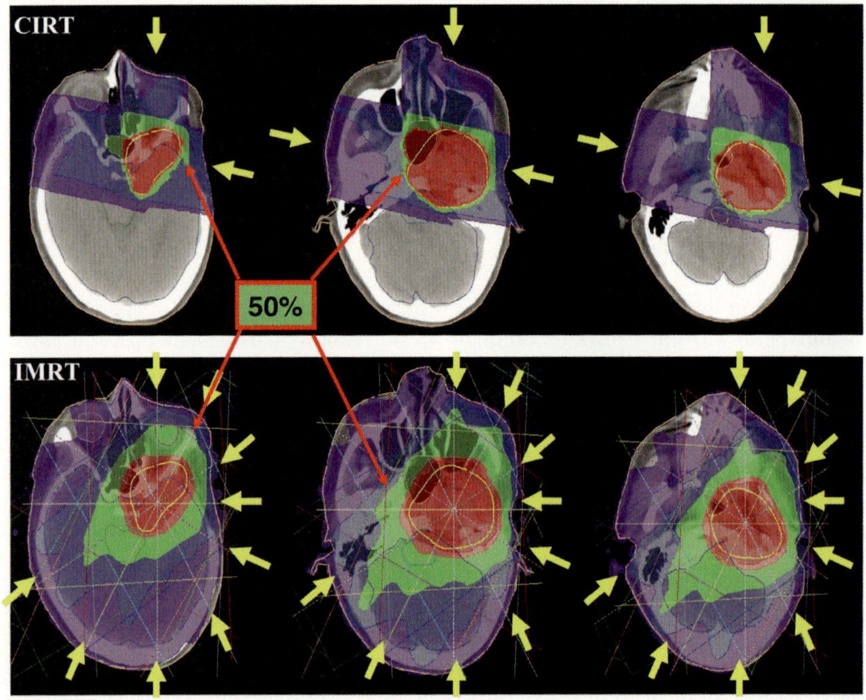

Fig. 7.1 Dose distribution with passive scattering carbon-ion radiotherapy (CIRT) (*upper panel*) and IMRT (*lower panel*). *Yellow arrows* show beam fields (With permission from Tsujii et al. 2014)

noted by Dr. Goitein at the Particle Therapy Co-Operative Group (PTCOG) meeting in 2006 (Goitein 2006), they share most of the same treatment planning procedures and primarily differ only in particle beam's finite penetration and sensitivity to tissue density variation along a given ray. Moreover, treatment planning for heavy charged particle beams (commonly used to characterize ions heavier than protons) should take account of the nonlinear additivity of the biologically weighted dose. The more precise beam delivery and treatment planning techniques developed recently require image guidance, which provides visualization and quantification of patient geometrical information from medical images and improves treatment workflow.

In this chapter, we introduce basic concepts of carbon-ion beam treatment planning with image guidance/image processing (in a sense, image-guided particle therapy, IGPT) and emphasize the differences between particle beam therapy and photon beam therapy. Several recent articles on particle beam therapy provide important additional skill-building information (Jakel et al. 2008; Tsujii and Kamada 2012; Chen et al. 2009, 2006).

7.2 Why Choose Carbon Ions?

It is well known that the high energy of a therapeutic photon beam decreases in a steep exponential curve with penetration depth and that the dose close to the entrance surface shows "buildup" caused by forward-scattered Compton electrons. In contrast, charged particle beams provide superior dose conformation to photon beams and minimize excessive dose to normal tissues. These strengths owe to the characteristic increase in energy deposition of particle beams with penetration depth (proton and carbon-ion beams) up to a sharp maximum at the end of the beam range (Bragg peak) (Fig. 7.2) (Bragg and Kleeman 1904). Explained simply, accelerated particle beam interactions lose kinetic energy along the ray line due to the interaction of Coulomb forces with the target electrons (stopping power). This is expressed by the Bethe-Bloch formula. Stopping power is approximately proportional to $(Z/v)^2$:

$$\frac{dE}{dx} \sim \frac{KnZ^2}{v^2}\left[\ln\left(\frac{2m_e v^2}{I}\right)\right] \propto \left(\frac{Z}{v}\right)^2, \tag{7.1}$$

where K, n, and m_e are the constant, electron density of the target material, and mass of electrons, respectively. Z is the charge of the projectile particle, v is the projectile velocity, and I is the mean ionization energy of the target atoms.

Accordingly, projectile velocity slows down as material penetration deepens, and stopping power is increased. Projectile velocity at the end of range is close to zero, and a high dose is deposited there.

In 1975–1992, neon ions and helium ions were used to treat 433 cancer patients and 2054 patients, respectively, at the Lawrence Berkeley National Laboratory (Alonso 2000), while in 1994, the heavy ion medical accelerator (HIMAC) at the National Institute of Radiological Sciences (NIRS) began providing carbon-ion radiotherapy (CIRT). From clinical experience gained at Berkeley, most heavy charged particle beam centers have selected carbon ions, mainly for the following reasons:

1. *Ions heavier than carbon have an increased nuclear fragmentation tail dose.* Protons did not deposit dose beyond the Bragg peak (Fig. 7.2a). In contrast, ions heavier than protons still had low projectile energy nuclear interactions (elastic collisions with target nuclei), providing a small dose (fragment particles with lower atomic number) beyond the Bragg peak (Fig. 7.2b).
2. *Ions heavier than carbon increase LET and relative biological effectiveness (RBE).*
   Conceptually, RBE represents the particle beam dose which provides the same biological effect as would be provided by the reference dose (typically X-rays or γ-rays). The RBE of light ions (proton, helium, etc.) does not significantly change between the entrance region and distal spread-out Bragg peak (SOBP) (Fig. 7.3). In contrast, the RBE of carbon ions is similar to that of light ions at the

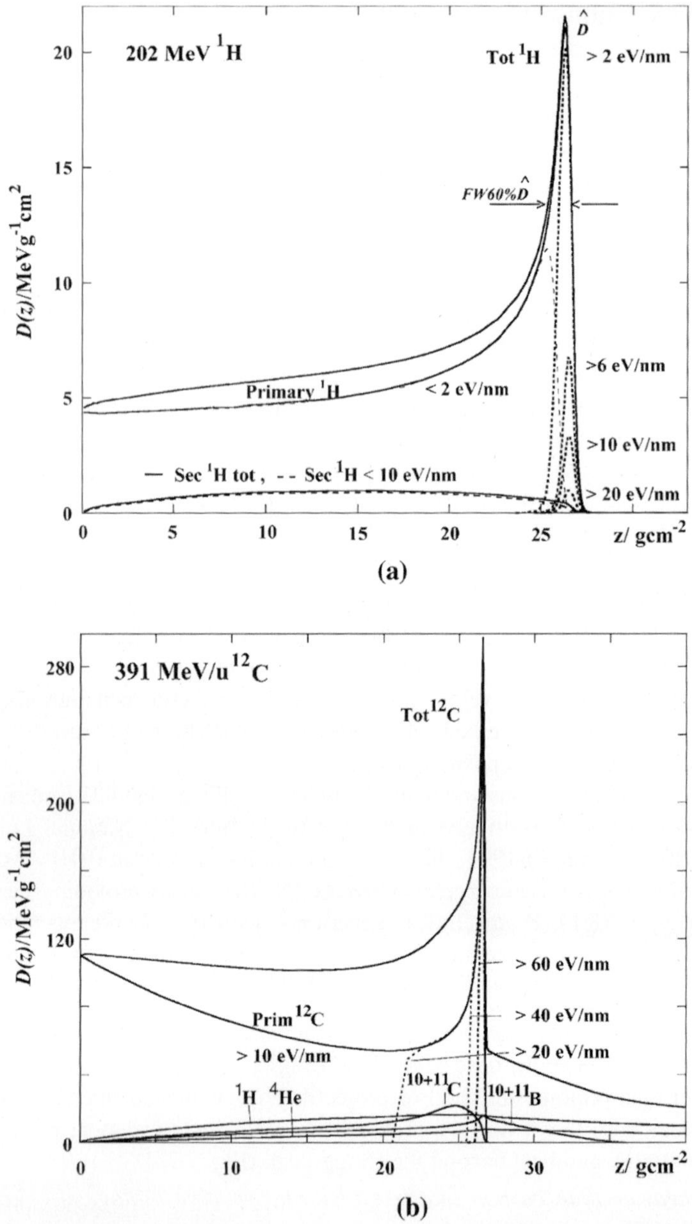

Fig. 7.2 Depth absorbed dose distributions of (**a**) a primary proton beam and its secondary particles and (**b**) a carbon-ion beam and its secondary particles (Reproduced from Kempe et al. 2007)

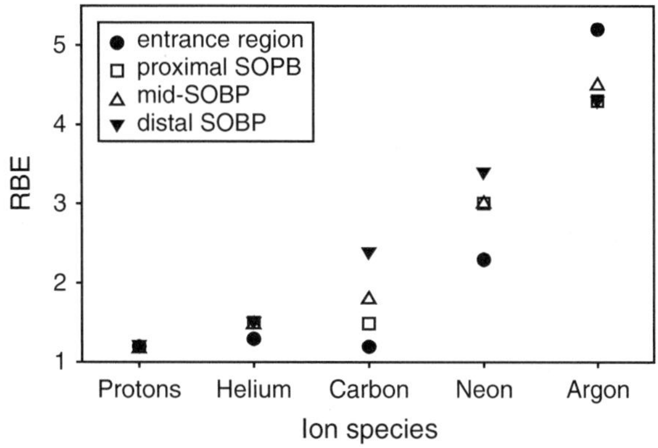

Fig. 7.3 Relative biological effectiveness (RBE) of different ions in fractionated irradiation of jejunal crypt cells of mice (With permission from Jakel 2009)

proximal SOBP but increased at the distal SOBP. The light-ion relative biological dose at the plateau region is therefore higher than the carbon-ion relative biological dose (Fig. 7.4). In contrast, the RBE of heavier ions (neon, argon, etc.) at the proximal and distal SOBPs is higher than that of carbon ions (although the RBE of neon at the entrance region is smaller than that of carbon ions at the distal SOBP). Although the relative biological dose of heavier ions at the SOBP is the same as that of carbon ions, the relative biological dose at the entrance region and proximal and distal SOBPs is higher than that of carbon ions. As a result, the peak to plateau ratio for carbon ions is higher and therefore improved, over that of other particle beams, including protons.

3. *Heavier ions minimize the magnitude of range straggling and lateral scattering.* These factors blur out the sharp ionization peak. Range straggling causes smearing out of the depth of penetration of the stopping particle beam due to statistical fluctuations in the ionization process. The variance of the range straggling is expressed from Bohr's theory as follows:

$$\varphi(x) = \frac{1}{\sigma_x\sqrt{2\pi}}\exp\left(\frac{-(x-R(E))^2}{2\sigma_x^2}\right), \tag{7.2}$$

$$R(E) = \int_0^E \left(\frac{\mathrm{d}E'}{\mathrm{d}x}\right)^{-1}\mathrm{d}E', \tag{7.3}$$

where x is the penetration depth, σ_x is almost proportional to range R and inverse to the square root of the particle mass, and range straggling for helium and neon are about 50 and 20 % of that for protons, respectively. Lateral scattering is mainly caused by elastic Coulomb interactions with the target nuclei and can be approximated by Gaussian functions as follows (Highland 1975):

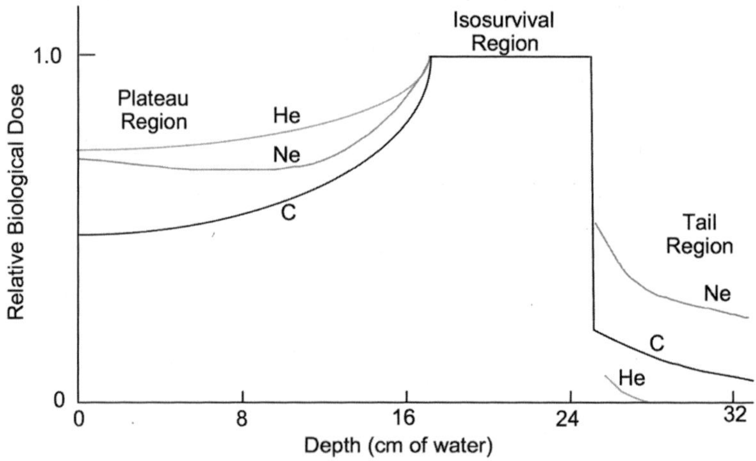

Fig. 7.4 Relative biological dose of the SOBP of ion beams. Doses are normalized at the SOBP region (With permission by the IAEA 2007)

$$\sigma_\theta = \frac{14.1\text{MeV}}{\beta pc} Z_p \sqrt{\frac{d}{L}\left[1 + \frac{1}{9}\log_{10}\left(\frac{d}{L}\right)\right]}, \tag{7.4}$$

where L and d are the radiation length and penetration length, respectively, β is particle beam velocity, and p and c are the momentum of the incident particle and the speed of light, respectively. The magnitude of the lateral scattering of photons and protons is larger than that for carbon ions at the same depth (Fig. 7.5).

4. *Heavier ions require a large accelerator.*
   Due to differences in their mass-to-charge ratio, it is two times more difficult to bend a carbon-ion beam with an accelerator than protons under same magnetic field, and the range of carbon ions is three time shorter than that of protons under the same velocity. Carbon-ion beams therefore require higher energy than protons to obtain the same range by enlarging accelerator size. Current particle beam center construction costs are dominated by size of the accelerator, which requires a large housing size. Progress in accelerator technology over the last 20 years has contributed to cost reductions by reducing accelerator size. For example, the cost of the synchrotron ring at Gunma University, which was constructed in 2009, was 63 m, approximately half that of the NIRS, constructed in 1993.

Given the above, it appears that carbon ions represent a well-balanced particle in both physical and biological aspects (Table 7.1). In 2015, more than ten treatment centers were operating CIRT, as shown on the website of the PTCOG. The NIRS

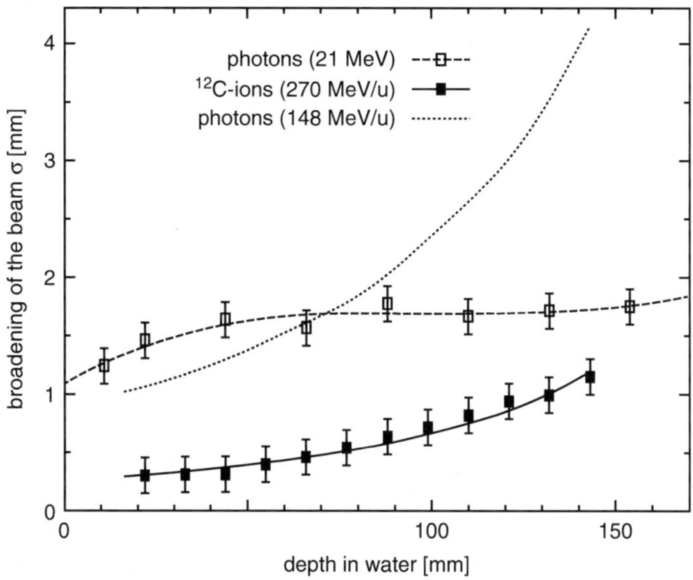

Fig. 7.5 Lateral scattering of photon, proton, and carbon-ion beams as a function of penetration depth (With permission from Kraft 2000)

Table 7.1 Summary of the characteristics of particle beams

	Biological dose distribution	Range straggling and lateral scattering	Construction cost
Proton	Good	Poor	Excellent
Carbon ion	Excellent	Good	Good
Neon	Good	Excellent	Poor

has treated over 8000 patients using carbon ions, and their clinical experience is reported here (Tsujii and Kamada 2012).

7.3 Particle Beam Treatment Planning

7.3.1 Planning CT

CT imaging provides both patient 3D anatomical information and effective density information, making it an essential part of treatment planning. This 3D information is markedly helpful in deciding treatment parameters, especially beam angle and dose distribution. An immobilization device is typically used in the planning CT acquisition and treatment stages to improve patient positional reproducibility throughout the treatment course. Several treatment centers have installed a large bore CT (over 80 cm diameter) to avoid the conflict between positioning of the raised arm and immobilization which occurs with a standard bore CT (about 72 cm diameter).

Recent commercial CT scanners are equipped with a 4D mode to capture respiratory-induced organ motion. 4DCT is a breakthrough technique which allows the quantification of intrafractional uncertainties. This technique is applied in cardiac CT imaging and has already become practical for identifying patients with significant coronary artery stenosis by ECG-correlated preprocessing. Given the heartbeat (~ 1 s) is faster than respiratory motion (~ 4 s) and coronary arteries (~ a few mm) are smaller than lung tumors (~ a few cm), it should therefore be feasible to visualize intrafractional motion. Although the respiratory pattern shows variations (e.g., phase shift/drift), 4DCT scans provide information of a single exemplary respiratory cycle only. Thus, serial CT/4DCT image acquisition is performed over a certain time axis (daily, weekly, etc.) to obtain potential anatomical changes. This information can be helpful in considering replanning during the treatment course.

In photon beam therapy, megavoltage X-ray interaction in material is dominated by Compton scattering, and effective density is calibrated using relative electron density. Typically, HU (Hounsfield unit) values within the patient are measured by the planning CT image and converted to linear attenuation coefficients (μ):

$$\mu = (HU - HU_{\text{air}})(HU_{\text{water}} - HU_{\text{air}})^{-1}, \tag{7.5}$$

The linear attenuation coefficient is derived from the formula or photon attenuation (Rutherford et al. 1976):

$$\mu = \rho_e\left(K^{\text{ph}}Z^{3.62} + K^{\text{coh}}Z^{1.86} + K^{\text{KN}}\right), \tag{7.6}$$

where K^{ph}, K^{coh}, and K^{KN} are constants for the contribution of the photoelectric effect, coherent scattering, and Compton scattering, respectively.

Particle beam ranges in materials are scaled by the stopping-power ratio relative to water based on measurement in water during beam commissioning. Accordingly, effective density in charged particle beams should be defined as the stopping power relative to water (ρ_s):

$$\rho_s = \rho_e\left[\ln\left(\frac{2m_ec^2}{I_{\text{material}}}\frac{\beta^2}{1-\beta^2}\right) - \beta^2\right]\left[\ln\left(\frac{2m_ec^2}{I_{\text{water}}}\frac{\beta^2}{1-\beta^2}\right) - \beta^2\right]^{-1}, \tag{7.7}$$

where ρ_e and m_e are relative electron density and the electron mass, respectively, and I_{material} and I_{water} are the mean ionization energies in material and water, respectively. Several carbon-ion beam treatment centers in Japan use CT calibration using the polybinary tissue model (muscle (water), air, fat (ethanol), and bone (40 % K_2HPO_4 water)) due to the good balance it provides between quality and cost (Kanematsu et al. 2003). By doing this, dose distribution can be calculated by converting all CT image sets to the effective density in the treatment planning system (TPS).

7.3.2 Contouring

7.3.2.1 Volume of Interest (VOI)

Since the planning CT image contains patient anatomical information that the TPS does not recognize, the volume of interest (VOI) on the CT image should be input into the TPS to conform the prescribed dose to the tumor and to minimize dose to normal tissues. The International Commission on Radiation Units and Measurement (ICRU) first defined the VOI in ICRU report 50 (1993) and refined it further in ICRU reports 62 (1999), 71 (2005), and 78 (2007). These VOI terms are illustrated in Fig. 7.6, in which the target-related terms are gross tumor volume (GTV), clinical target volume (CTV), internal target volume (ITV), and planning target volume (PTV). The term "target volume" is often used for both target and healthy tissues but is more specific to the tumor. We therefore use VOI here to describe both tumor and normal tissues. Although the VOI is fully defined in these ICRU reports, I introduce it briefly here as follows.

The GTV consists of a primary/metastatic tumor and demonstrable visible tumor region on planning images. It is generally delineated by the oncologist and may not be present following irradiation treatment. The CTV contains the GTV and subclinical malignant disease region (microscopic tumor spread region), which in some cases is difficult to observe in the planning CT image. To compensate for expected internal uncertainties such as physiologic movement and temporal size/shape/positional variations, the ITV is defined by adding an internal margin to the CTV. This internal margin technique is often used in thoracoabdominal treatment. The PTV is designed by adding a setup margin to the ITV. This setup margin accounts for the inaccuracy and low reproducibility of patient positioning to the treatment beam. The PTV in photon beam therapy generally uses the geometrical-based margins of the beam field to compensate for organ motion and setup errors. Since particle beam therapy considers uncertainties in beam penetration, the PTV should include the range-based proximal and distal margins of the beam field as well as the lateral margins. The PTV is therefore designed for each beam direction. The margin for respiratory-induced range uncertainties is described in Sect. 7.4.

In addition, critical normal structures (organs at risk, OARs) are also delineated on the TPS. Because OARs are likely affected by intra-/interfractional movement, patient setup error, etc., planning organ at risk volume (PRV) is delineated in addition to the ITV and PTV concepts by adding an internal margin and setup margin to OARs (Fig. 7.6). In some cases, the PTV overlaps another PTV, OAR, or PRV; however, ICRU reports 78 and 83 recommend that delineating the VOIs should not be compromised because recent TPS can optimize sufficient dose

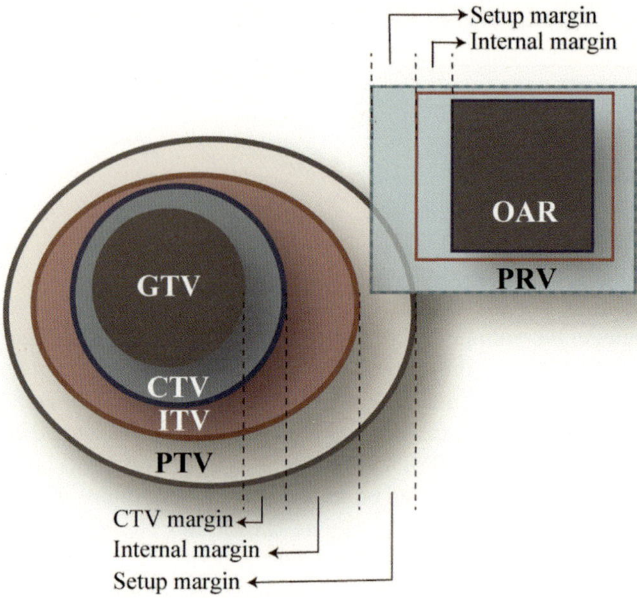

Fig. 7.6 Schematic drawing of the volumes of interest relating to the definition of target and organs at risk

sparing of the OAR. As described here, GTV, CTV, and OAR are oncological or anatomical concepts, while ITV, PTV, and PRV are physical constructions.

7.3.2.2 Image Registration/Segmentation

The image registration/segmentation technique is mandatory in current radiotherapy procedures, particularly in treatment planning. Generally, image registration is used for contouring and 4D dose calculation. The latter is described in Sect. 7.4. Image segmentation supports the inputting of target and normal organ contours automatically (auto-contouring) without a huge burden on the oncologist. In contrast, image registration is used to transform contours between different CT data sets for the same patient and in replanning (from original CT to new CT) and 4DCT (from a reference phase to other phases). Deformable image registration (DIR) is used in place of rigid image registration to reflect realistic human geometrical changes. In treatment planning, multiple sets of image data (CT, MRI, PET, and their combinations) are generally registered. The DIR process finds a deformation vector field (DVF) between two image data sets.

DVF is obtained by applying a transforming function (generally *B*-spline with control points) to the reference image and calculating similarity measure between the two images. This process is repeated until the similarity measure reaches the criterion value. When the same imaging modality data set is used, image voxel values for each image data set are similar; therefore, to avoid the time-consuming in user input of further information, the intensity-based DIR method is more suitable than the landmark-based or segmentation-based methods, because it operates on image voxel values directly. Voxel similarity measure generally uses sum of squared differences and cross correlation etc.; these contours are transferred to the next image data set by applying DVF to the contours on the reference image (warping). As an example of auto-contouring in 4DCT, an oncologist manually contours one reference CT phase (generally peak exhalation), and then DIR calculates the DVF based on the 4DCT data. These are then applied to the manual contours to transform them from the reference phase to the other respiratory phases. All contours at other respiratory phases are then automatically calculated.

DIR-related auto-contouring and 4D dose calculation (described later) can have a significant impact on treatment accuracy. It is therefore important to assess registration accuracy, which is strongly dependent on patient shape. Accordingly, it is not sufficient to evaluate the registration accuracy using a phantom only.

A simple evaluation method for the registrations is visual assessment. Point landmark-based registration is performed to obtain a quantitative result, but it is substantially time-consuming and not practical in clinical settings. It is necessary to check DIR accuracy from the CT image at exhale ($\mathrm{IM}_{\mathrm{exhale}}$) to that at inhale ($\mathrm{IM}_{\mathrm{inhale}}$):

$$\mathrm{IM}_{\mathrm{exhale}} : \boldsymbol{x}_{\mathrm{exhale}} \in \Omega_{\mathrm{exhale}},\ \ \mathrm{IM}_{\mathrm{inhale}} : \boldsymbol{x}_{\mathrm{inhale}} \in \Omega_{\mathrm{inhale}}, \tag{7.8}$$

where Ω_{exhale} and Ω_{inhale} are discrete domains of CT images at exhale and inhale and $\mathrm{x}_{\mathrm{exhale}}$ and $\mathrm{x}_{\mathrm{inhale}}$ are position vectors on CT images at exhale and inhale, respectively. Subtracted CT images at inhale and exhale show large differences in voxel values due to geometrical differences (Fig. 7.7a). DVF is calculated using CT images at exhale and inhale:

$$\mathrm{DVF} : \Omega_{\mathrm{exhale}} \rightarrow \Omega_{\mathrm{inhale}}, \tag{7.9}$$

A warped CT image at inhale is calculated by applying DVF to the CT image at exhale. If the registration error is zero, the warped CT image and CT image at inhale are the same:

$$\boldsymbol{x}_{\mathrm{inhale}} = \mathrm{DVF}(x_{\mathrm{exhale}}), \tag{7.10}$$

Geometrical differences between the warped CT image and CT image at inhale are improved (Fig. 7.7b), but the registration error is not completely zero when using patient images:

$$\boldsymbol{x}_{\mathrm{inhale}} \neq \mathrm{DVF}(x_{\mathrm{exhale}}), \tag{7.11}$$

We then calculated another DVF (DVF') by using the warped CT image at exhale and CT image at inhale and applied DVF' to the warped CT image ($\tilde{IM}_{exhale}$):

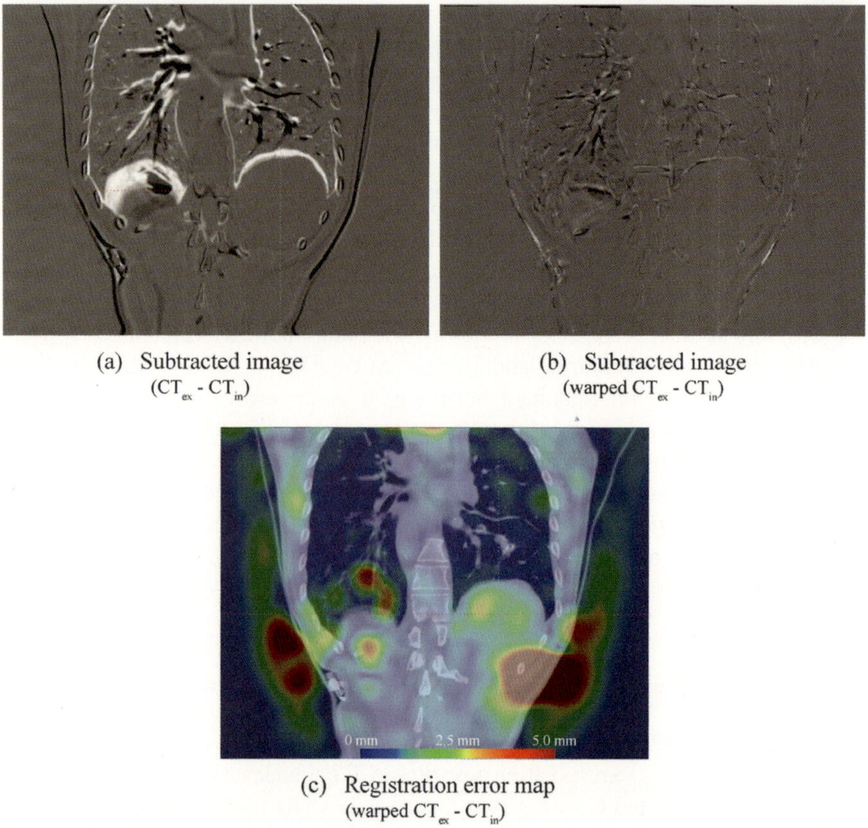

Fig. 7.7 (**a**) Subtraction CT image at inhale from that at exhale. (**b**) Subtraction CT image at inhale from warped CT at inhale. (**c**) Magnitude of the DVF color map between CT image at inhale and warped CT image at inhale

$$\widetilde{\mathrm{DVF}} : \Omega^{\mathrm{DVF}}_{\mathrm{exhale}} \rightarrow \Omega_{\mathrm{inhale}}, \tag{7.12}$$

$$\widetilde{\mathrm{IM}}_{\mathrm{exhale}} : \widetilde{\boldsymbol{x}}_{\mathrm{exhale}} \in \Omega^{\widetilde{\mathrm{DVF}}}_{\mathrm{exhale}}, \tag{7.13}$$

$$\widetilde{\boldsymbol{x}}_{\mathrm{exhale}} = \widetilde{\mathrm{DVF}}\left[\mathrm{DVF}(x_{\mathrm{exhale}})\right], \tag{7.14}$$

DIR accuracy is quantitatively visualized by the following calculation (Fig. 7.7c):

$$\left\| \widetilde{\mathrm{DVF}}(\widetilde{\boldsymbol{x}}_{\mathrm{exhale}}) - \boldsymbol{x}_{\mathrm{inhale}} \right\|_2, \tag{7.15}$$

where $\|\cdot\|$ represents a norm.

Image registration which utilizes DIR cannot remove registration error completely, and users should therefore check the contours and modify manually if necessary. In particular, a lung DIR close to the chest wall could degrade registration accuracy, because intrafractional chest wall movement is smaller than lung motion. Biomechanical intensity-based DIR considers physical properties and in one study improved target registration error, from 1.5 ± 1.4 mm (mean ± SD) compared with conventional DIR (2.6 ± 1.4 mm) (Samavati et al. 2015). The author does not provide details of the biomechanical DIR technique here, but note that it is strongly dependent on the DIR algorithm (Brock 2010). Details about image registration can be found elsewhere (Hill et al. 2001).

7.3.3 Beam Angle Configuration

Conformal photon beam treatment planning such as IMRT generally uses more than six beam fields to reduce the doses to normal tissues, while VMAT delivers the treatment beam using a rotating gantry. The use of multiple beam fields might minimize dose errors. While a few beam fields provide good target dose conformity in particle beam therapy, dose error in respective fields should not be neglected. Given that current TPS are unable to select all beam angles automatically, treatment planners should select beam angles with consideration to the following:

1. *Avoid beam angles along the target and OAR direction to spare OARs.*
   This is easy to understand in the case of OARs located proximal to the target but should also be considered for OARs at the distal side. Ideally the particle beam stops at the distal edge of the target, but range uncertainty might change particle beam stopping position; an extended particle beam position might increase harmful dose to OARs located close behind the target.
2. *Opposing beam angles achieve a good biologically effective dose.*
   Since RBE values vary as a function of depth, opposing beam angles are not good for OAR sparing; except for tumors located around the body center, beam angles should be separated within the approximate range of 25° to 70° or something similar.
3. *Avoid inhomogeneous tissue and consider patient positional variation to minimize range uncertainty.*
   Small dose differences were observed between commercial TPS and Monte Carlo (MC)-derived planning, particularly for the skull and thoracic regions, which include inhomogeneous tissues (Fig. 7.8). This is because most TPSs use empirical models for dose calculation, despite the fact that the MC algorithm is much more accurate for dose calculation. Patient anatomical intra-/interfractional positional variation is a major factor in range uncertainty. An example of intrafractional beam range variation is that a single pencil beam stops at the distal edge of a tumor when passing through the heart at diastole but penetrates the tumor at systole (Fig. 7.9). Careful selection of beam angle is one solution to minimizing range uncertainties.

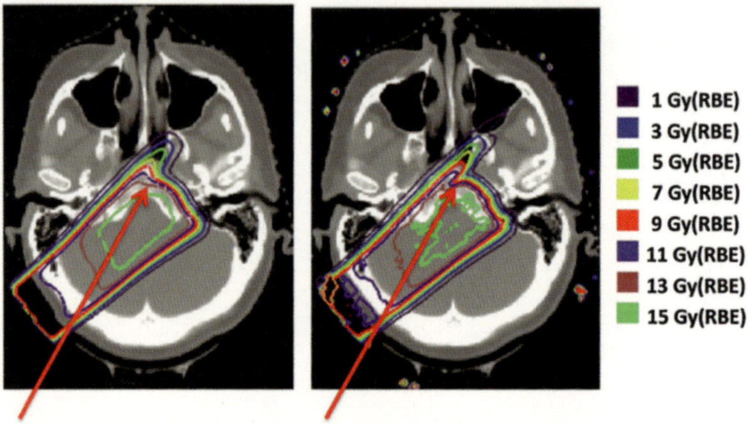

Fig. 7.8 Proton dose distribution calculated with a commercial TPS (XiO, Elekta Inc.) (*left panel*) and by Monte Carlo (MC) (*right panel*; Geant 4) (Adapted from Paganetti et.al. 2008)

Fig. 7.9 Carbon-ion pencil beam dose distribution at diastole and systole

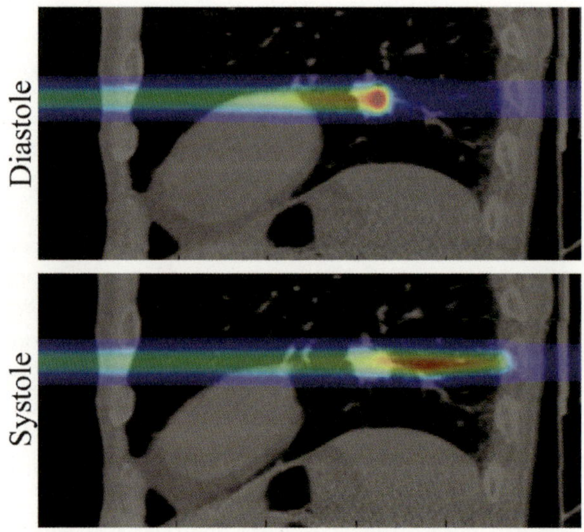

4. *Consider positioning and irradiation systems restrictions.*
   Photon beam and proton beam treatment use rotating gantry systems to irradiate from a wide range of gantry angle. However, carbon-ion beam rotating gantry systems have not been widely adopted, although a few have been constructed in Japan and Germany. These may allow the selection of beam angles which avoid the treatment couch edge. Since most CIRT centers use a fixed beam port irradiation system, extending the range of beam angles requires the treatment couch to be rotated around the patient long axis. Planners should leave this part in the tip of the corner.

7.3.4 Irradiation Method

This section provides a brief technical overview of the two most common irradiation techniques used in CIRT, passive scattering, and pencil beam scanning (PBS).

The passive scattering irradiation technique has been long and widely used in charged particle beam therapy, including proton and carbon-ion beams. A pristine beam with a narrow beam width in both lateral and depth directions is extracted from the accelerator. To cover the whole target volume, the pristine beam should be spread out in both directions. First, a wobbler magnet and scattering system are used to laterally and uniformly spread the pristine beam (Fig. 7.10a). Second, a ridge filter modulates the beam energy to obtain a uniform biological dose distribution along depth direction SOBP. Third, a patient collimator (PTC) and/or multileaf collimator (MLC) are used to adjust the beam to the target volume laterally. Finally, a compensator bolus adjusts the beam stopping position at the distal edge of the target. This method provides good dose conformity for the distal region of the target, but cannot avoid an unnecessarily high dose around the proximal side of the target.

The layer-stacking irradiation technique was developed in 1983 with the aim of maximizing dose conformation and minimizing the dose to normal tissue around the proximal side of the target with scattering beams, similar to that with PBS irradiation. It is now in clinical use at a few carbon-ion beam treatment centers (Kanai et al. 1983; Kanematsu et al. 2002). Uniform dose within the target is achieved by combining a number of small SOBPs along a depth direction. These small SOBP positions are shifted by changing range shifters (Fig. 7.10b). Beam field size is defined to fit the respective iso-energy layer regions by changing the MLC opening width.

With regard to PBS, this method was first proposed in the 1980s at NIRS, and carbon-ion PBS (C-PBS) was first implemented clinically at the Gesellschaft für Schwerionenforschung (GSI) in Darmstadt, Germany (Kanai et al. 1980; Haberer et al. 1993). Worldwide, a few treatment centers were using C-PBS as of 2015. The pencil beam is scanned in all three dimensions over the spot positions of the target to achieve a uniform dose within the target (Fig. 7.10c). Since PBS has a flexible dose distribution, OAR sparing is better than with passive scattering irradiation, and an inhomogeneous dose distribution (e.g., IMPT, additional doses to hypoxic regions) can be achieved. MLC, PTC, and a compensator bolus are not required, eliminating the treatment workflow time normally required to change these accessories and minimizing therapist entry into the treatment room. The beam energy is changed with a range shifter and/or accelerator change. A major problem with the use of a thicker range shifter is that it causes a broadening of the beam spot size with increasing depth through range shifters. By contrast, active change using an accelerator takes energy change time and requires a massively extended commissioning time for each beam energy (over a few hundred beam energies). Hybrid depth scanning with a synchrotron was developed to overcome these problems. Hybrid depth scanning provides a smaller lateral dose fall off and RBE than range shifter

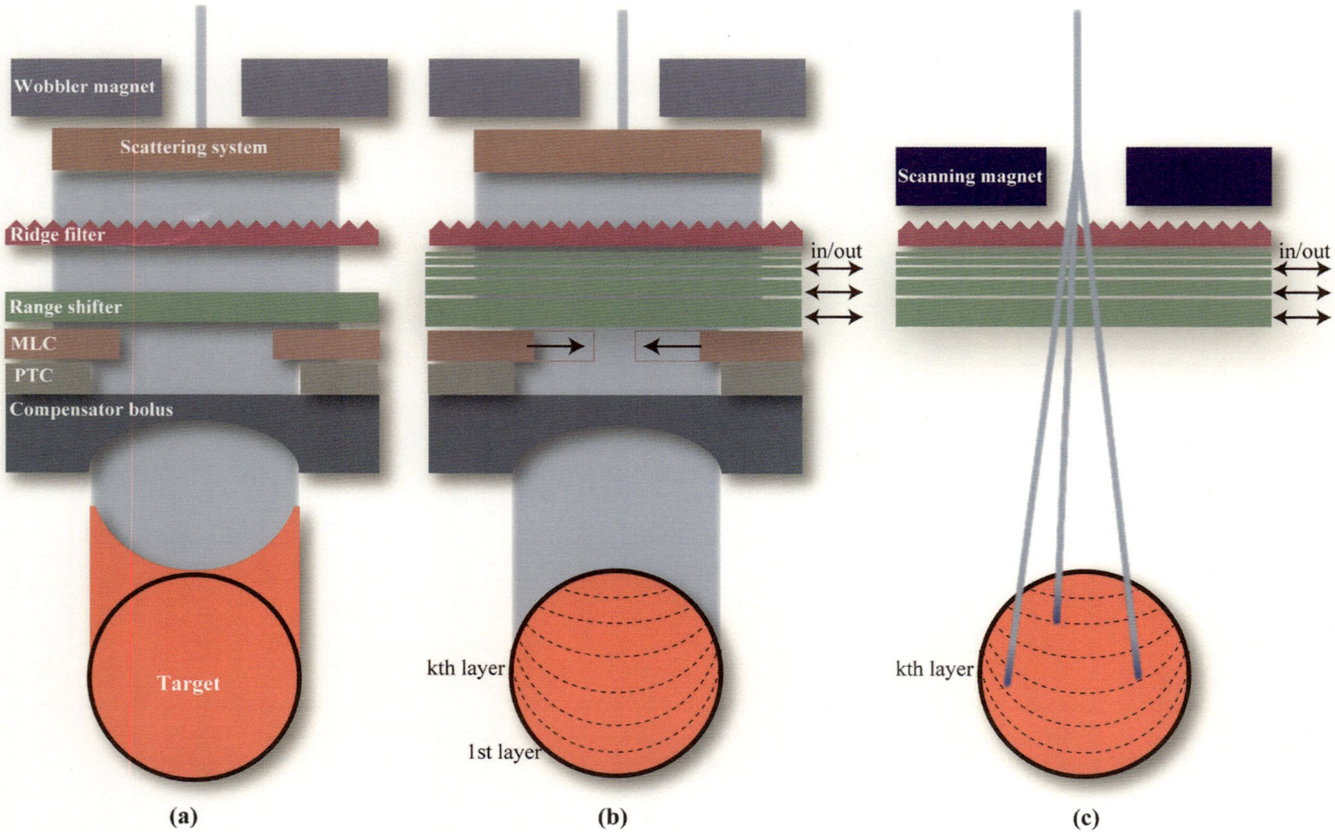

Fig. 7.10 Schematic drawing of (**a**) passive scattering, (**b**) layer-stacking, and (**c**) scanning irradiation techniques. *Dotted curved lines* show the iso-energy layers

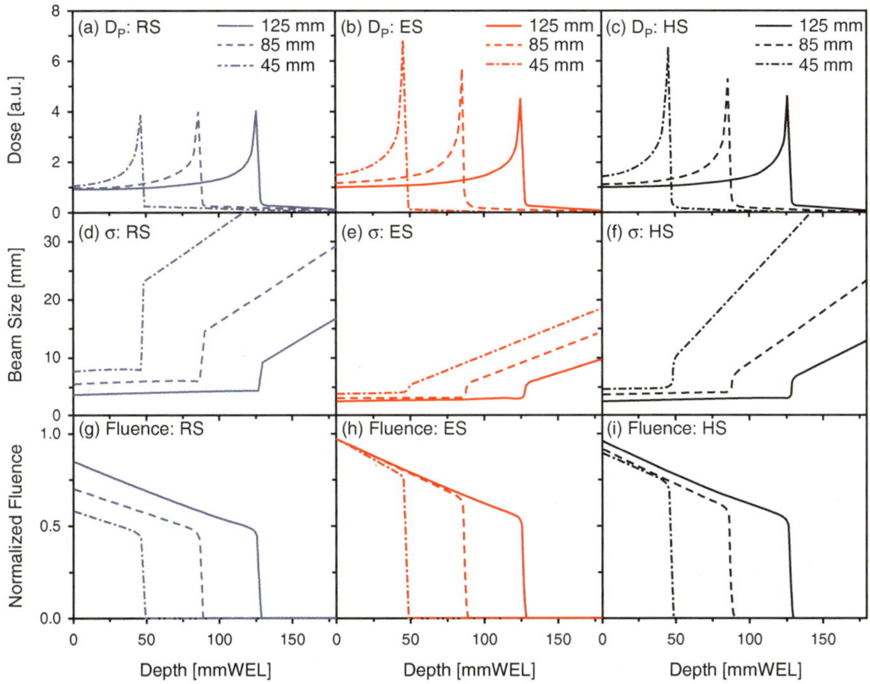

Fig. 7.11 C-PBS dose distributions in the depth direction (D_p), lateral direction (σ), and normalized fluence for RS, ES, and HS, respectively (With permission from Inaniwa et al. 2012)

scanning (Inaniwa et al. 2012) and uses the range shifter to shift the small SOBPs at a step size of 3 mm in combination with 11 distinct synchrotron energies (Fig. 7.11).

7.3.5 Dose Calculations

7.3.5.1 Beam Range Calculation

Beam spot positions are set on steps of a few millimeters (generally 2–3 mm, depending on C-PBS beam size) on CT images. Water equivalent path length (WEPL) from the irradiation system (scanning magnet) to respective spots is calculated by integrating the stopping effective density along each ray line:

$$\mathrm{WEPL}(z) = \int_0^z \rho_s(z')\mathrm{d}z', \tag{7.16}$$

where z is the total penetration depth, z' is the penetration depth, and ρ_s is the stopping power.

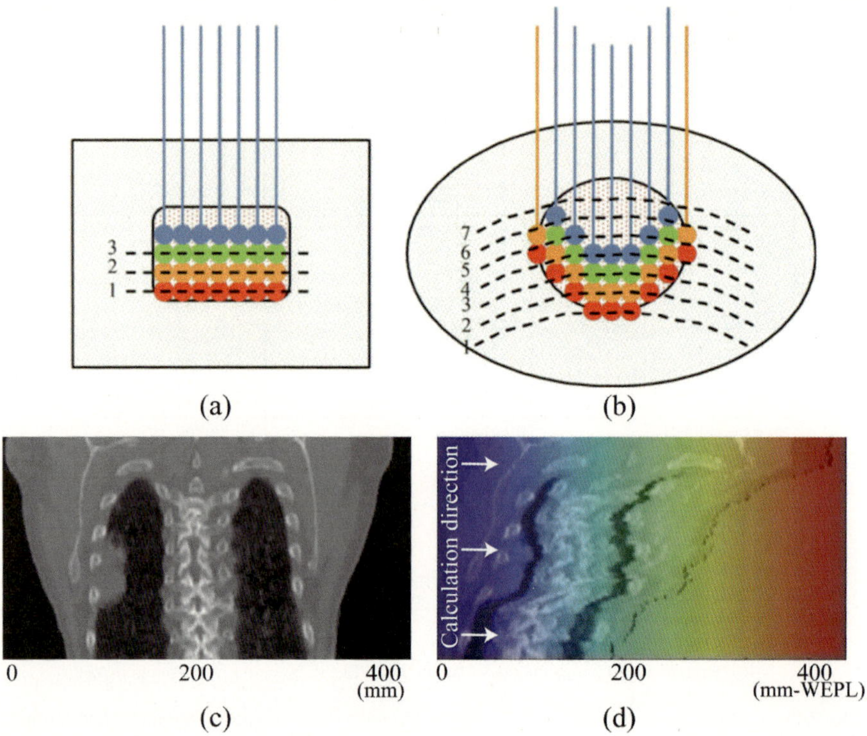

Fig. 7.12 Schematic diagram of the beam spot position in several iso-energy layers for (**a**) *rectangular shape* and (**b**) *spherical shape*. Iso-energy layer number was assigned from the distal side (With permission from ICRU-72 2007). Lung CT images in coronal section in (**c**) CT and (**d**) WEPL coordinates

For the square-shaped case in Fig. 7.12, the same WEPL position (iso-energy layer) (shown as dotted lines) is oriented in a horizontal line (Fig. 7.12a). Most distal spot positions (red circles in Fig. 7.12a) are irradiated by the same energy beam. For the spherically shaped case, in contrast, the iso-energy layer position is curved and not the same as the target shape (Fig. 7.12b). Most distal spot positions (red circles in Fig. 7.12b) are irradiated by different beam energies. In a more realistic case (lung case), the tissue density for lung may be decreased from approximately 1.0 g/cm^3 to 0.3 g/cm^3, potentially exerting a strong impact on the iso-energy layer position by making it more complex. To understand this more clearly, the lung CT image is transformed in the same WEPL value positions in Fig. 7.12d; compared to the original lung CT (Fig. 7.12c), the geometrical shape is substantially deformed, and the lung thickness is substantially shortened in the WEPL coordinate. C-PBS doses are calculated in respective beam spots.

7.3.5.2 Beam Modeling

For the C-PBS beam model, lateral dose distribution can be approximated by the Gaussian function as a function of penetration depth. Accumulated dose distribution in the PBS irradiation is superimposed on the respective pencil beam dose distributions, meaning that beam field size would be varied at the respective iso-energy layers. The dependence of photon and particle beam doses on beam field size is well known and is likely emphasized in PBS irradiation. However, a single Gaussian model does not completely compensate for the field size effect. Proton beam lateral distribution can be expressed by the sum of two Gaussians: the first and second components are the primary proton and nuclear beam halo, respectively (Pedroni et al. 2005). For carbon-ion beams, three Gaussians are used to accurately model the lateral distributions on account of nuclear fragments; the first component is primary carbon ion, the second is heavy fragments, and the third is light fragments (Inaniwa et al. 2009; Kusano et al. 2007) (Fig. 7.13), and the ith PBS dose distribution ($d_i(x,y,z)$) is expressed by the following:

$$\begin{aligned} d_i(x,y,z) = \; & d_{z,i}(z) \\ & \times \left\{ \left(1 - \sum_{j=2}^{3} f_{j,i}(z) \right) D_{1,i}(x,y,\sigma_{1,i}(z)) + \sum_{j=2}^{3} f_{j,i}(z) D_{j,i}(x,y,\sigma_{j,i}(z)) \right\}, \end{aligned} \tag{7.17}$$

where $d_{z,,i}(z)$ and $\sigma_{j,i}(z)$ are the integral dose and standard deviation at a penetration depth z, respectively; $D_{j,i}(x,y, \sigma_{j,i}(z))$ is a two-dimensional Gaussian function for the lateral distribution of the jth component; and $f_{j,i}(z)$ is the fraction of integrated dose of the jth Gaussian component. Physical dose distribution for PBS (D_{phys}) is composed by summing the respective pencil beam doses:

$$D_{\text{phys}}(x,y,z) = \sum_{i=1}^{N} d_i(x,y,z) \cdot w_i, \tag{7.18}$$

where N is the total number of spots and w_i is the ith beam spot weight.

7.3.5.3 Biological and Clinical Doses

Since biological effect in heavy charged particle therapy is strongly dependent on particle type, the primary particle and all fragment particles produced during the stopping process should be considered (Schardt et al. 2010). To discriminate the physical dose (Gy), ICRU recommends use of the term "RBE-weighted" dose (Gy (RBE)) for biological dose (ICRU-72 2007). Biological dose distribution is expressed as a typical tumor cell response, as defined by the in vitro response of human salivary gland (HSG) tumor cells. A German group adapted the local effect

Fig. 7.13 (**a**) Lateral beam spreads of the first, second, and third components for the range shifter thicknesses of 0, 50, and 100 mm WEL. (**b**) Fraction factors of the second and third components for the range shifter thicknesses of 0, 50, and 100 mm WEL (Reproduced from Inaniwa et al. 2009)

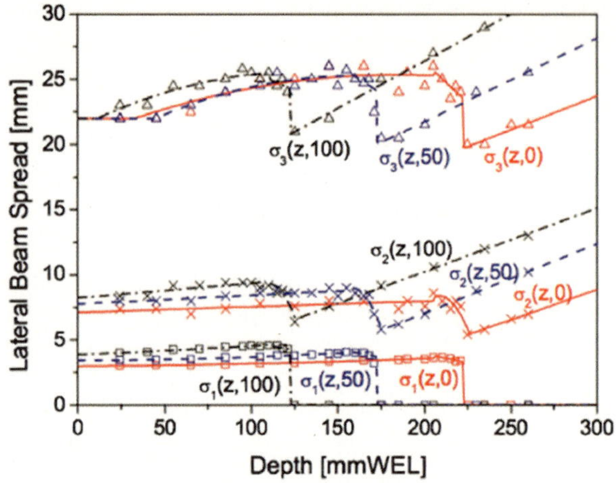

(a)

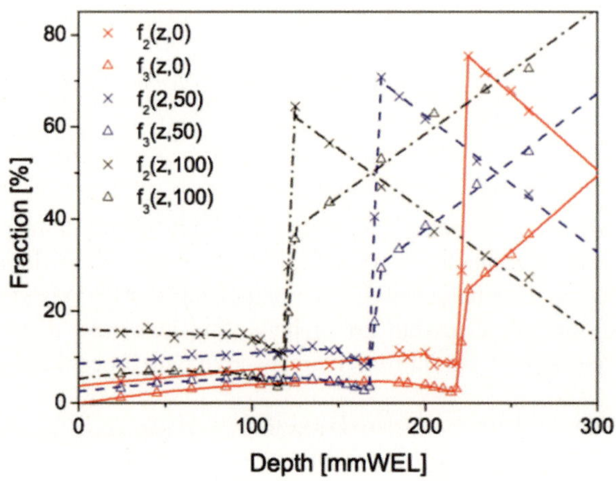

(b)

model (LEM) to CIRT (Elsasser et al. 2008). Another model was introduced as the microdosimetric kinetic model (MKM), which predicts the survival fraction of cells from the specific energy absorbed by a microscopic subcellular structure (Hawkins 1996; Hawkins 2003). However, MKM does not perfectly predict RBE due to insufficient overkill correction in high-energy regions (LET >100 keV/μm). To solve this problem, Kase et al. adapted saturation correction to express the decrease in RBE due to the overkill effect in a mixed radiation field (modified MKM) (Kase et al. 2006b). The modified MKM provides RBE values from proton to silicon using a linear quadratic (LQ) function, which simplifies the calculation of RBE under the mixed radiation field (Kase et al. 2006a) (Fig. 7.14).

Biological dose in the mixed radiation field is expressed as follows:

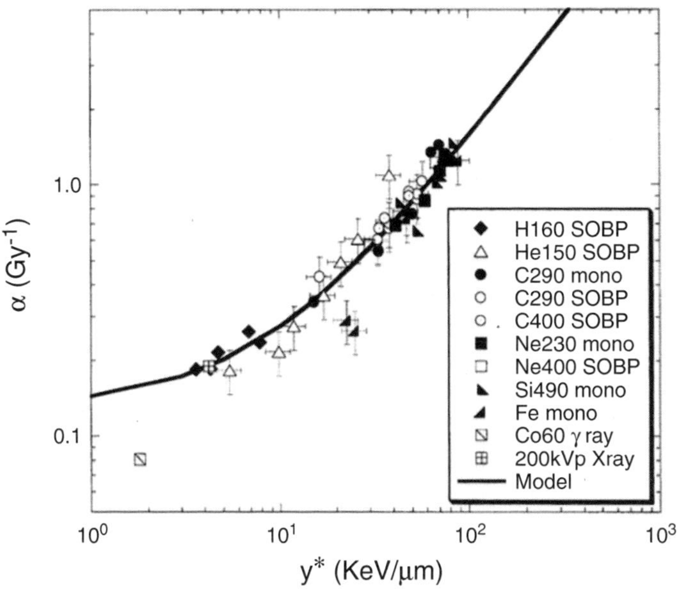

Fig. 7.14 Relationship between experimental α value and the saturation-corrected dose-mean lineal energy (With permission from Kase et al. 2006a)

$$D_{\text{biol}}(x,y,z) = D_{\text{phys}}(x,y,z)\cdot RBE_{\text{biol}}(x,y,z)$$
$$= -\frac{\alpha}{2\beta}+\sqrt{\left(\frac{\alpha}{2\beta}\right)^2-\frac{\ln S\left(D_{\text{phys}}(x,y,z)\right)}{\beta}}, \tag{7.19}$$

$$\ln\left(S\left(D_{\text{phys}}(x,y,z)\right)\right) = -\left(\alpha_0+\beta z^*_{1D\ \text{mix}}(x,y,z)\right)D_{\text{phys}}(x,y,z) - \beta D_{\text{phys}}(x,y,z)^2, \tag{7.20}$$

where α and β are the coefficients of the LQ model for the reference radiation and α_0 is the initial slope of the surviving fraction curve in the limit of LET = 0. β value is independent of radiation type and is selected as 0.0615Gy^{-2} based on the β value of HSG cells irradiated by X-ray (Furusawa et al. 2000). To predict RBE in the mixed radiation field, the saturation-corrected dose means that a single energy extended to the saturation-corrected dose-mean specific energy ($z^*_{1D\ mix}$), which can be derived by MC and the Kiefer-Chatterjee model (Kiefer and Straaten 1986), must be calculated (Fig. 7.15). Details for calculating the saturation-corrected dose-mean specific energy are described in Inaniwa et al. (2010):

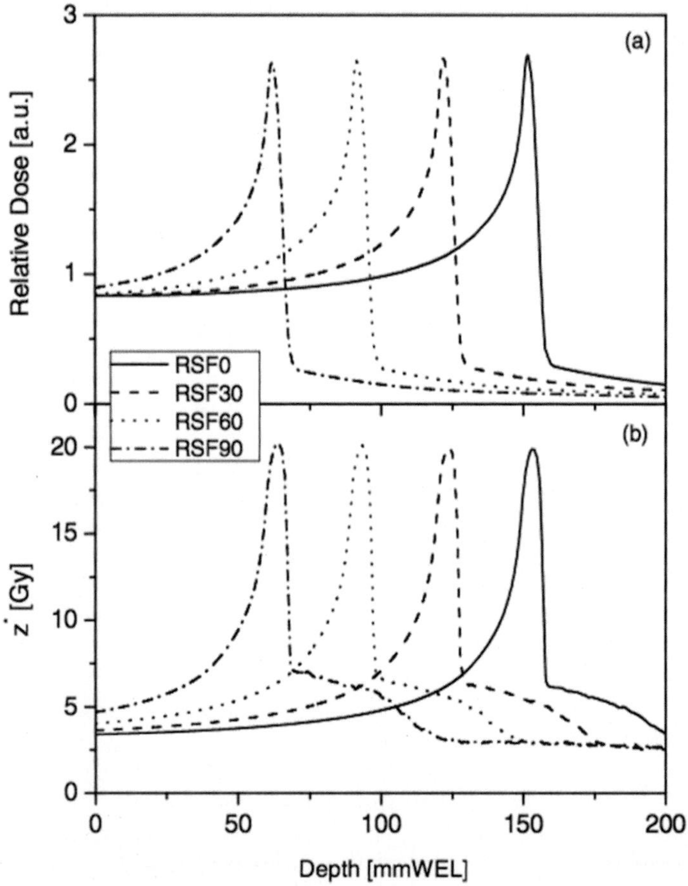

Fig. 7.15 (**a**) C-PBS depth dose distributions and (**b**) the saturation-corrected dose-mean specific energy of the domain of a 290 MeV/u for range shifter thicknesses of 0, 30, 60, and 90 mm (With permission from Inaniwa et al. 2010)

$$z^*_{1D\ \mathrm{mix}}(x, y, z) = \frac{\sum_{i=1}^{N} w_i \cdot d_i(x, y, z) \cdot \widetilde{z}^*_{1D:i}(z)}{\sum_{i=1}^{N} w_i \cdot d_i(x, y, z)}, \tag{7.21}$$

where $\widetilde{z}^*_{1D:i}(z)$ is the saturation-corrected dose-mean specific energy delivered by the *j*th beam. To adapt biological response in vitro to patient treatment (in vivo), the biological dose should be rescaled by multiplying by a clinical factor (F_{clin}). Clinical dose can be calculated by the following:

$$D_{\mathrm{clin}}(x,y,z) = D_{\mathrm{bio}}(x,y,z) \cdot F_{\mathrm{clin}}, \tag{7.22}$$

The clinical factor of 2.41 is used in our facility. Due to word count limitations, details and historical background are provided elsewhere (Kanematsu et al. 2002; Kanai et al. 1999; Inaniwa et al. 2015).

7.3.5.4 Dose Optimization

To achieve the desired target conformation and OAR sparing doses, respective beam spot weights are optimized by an iterative process (inverse planning). Generally, the objective function ($f(w)$) is defined as the errors between the current target dose and the maximum/minimum target doses (Bortfeld et al. 1990) as follows:

$$f(w) = \sum_{i \in \mathrm{target}} \left(\alpha_{\mathrm{under}}^{\mathrm{target}} \left[D_{\mathrm{min}}^{\mathrm{target}} - D_i(w) \right]^2 + \alpha_{\mathrm{over}}^{\mathrm{target}} \left[D_i(w) - D_{\mathrm{max}}^{\mathrm{target}} \right]^2 \right), \quad \underset{w>0}{\mathrm{minimum}}\ f(w) \tag{7.23}$$

where the operator [ ] is the Heaviside step function. w is the vector notation of the beam weights for all pencil beams; $D_i(w)$ is the dose at the ith spot position; $D_{\mathrm{max}}^{\mathrm{target}}$ and $D_{\mathrm{min}}^{\mathrm{target}}$ are user-defined maximum and minimum doses in the target, respectively; and $\alpha_{\mathrm{under}}^{\mathrm{target}}$ and α_{over}^{target} are the penalties for target underdosage and overdosage, respectively.

If dose constraint to the target and OAR is considered (maximum dose constraint, minimum dose constraint, dose volume constraint, etc.), these constraint mathematical expressions should be added to the objective functions. To find the optimum solutions, several types of optimization strategy have been introduced.

1. *Gradient descent*
   The gradient descent method calculates the direction (***d***) with a large magnitude of the negative gradient at the current value (series of point, ***p***) (kth iteration). A learning rate (τ) adjusts the step size to search for the next value:

$$\boldsymbol{d}_k = -\tau \nabla f(\boldsymbol{p}_k), \tag{7.24}$$

2. *Conjugate gradient*
   The conjugate gradient method finds the nearest local minimum in far fewer steps than the gradient descent method:

$$\boldsymbol{d}_k = -\nabla f(\boldsymbol{p}_k) + \beta_k \boldsymbol{d}_{k-1}, \tag{7.25}$$

The initial β value is zero, but β can be calculated thereafter using different methods:

$$\text{Fletcher \& Reeved}: \beta_k = \frac{\left(\boldsymbol{g}_k^T \cdot \boldsymbol{g}_k\right)}{\left(\boldsymbol{g}_{k-1}^T \cdot \boldsymbol{g}_{k-1}\right)}, \tag{7.26}$$

$$\text{Polak \& Ribiere}: \beta_k = \left(\boldsymbol{g}_k - \boldsymbol{g}_{k-1}\right)^T \cdot \frac{\boldsymbol{g}_k}{\left(\boldsymbol{g}_{k-1}^T \cdot \boldsymbol{g}_{k-1.}\right)}, \tag{7.27}$$

with $\boldsymbol{g}_k = \nabla f(\boldsymbol{p}_k)$,

3. *Newton*

   Newton's method finds the minimum by an iterative approach. This method provides faster convergence than the gradient descent method. However, the function $f(\boldsymbol{p}_k)$ should be differentiated:

$$\boldsymbol{d}_k = -H^{-1}(\boldsymbol{p}_k)\nabla f(\boldsymbol{p}_k), \tag{7.28}$$

   where H is the Hessian matrix as expressed by $H(\boldsymbol{p}_k) = \nabla^2 f(\boldsymbol{p}_k)$

4. *Quasi-Newton*

   To omit the calculation of Hessian and the inversed Hessian, matrix Q_k^{-1} is an approximation of the inverse of the Hessian at iteration k and is updated in every iteration. One widely used update method is the Broyden-Fletcher-Goldfarb-Shannon (BFGS):

$$\boldsymbol{d}_k = -Q_k^{-1}(\boldsymbol{p}_k)\nabla f(\boldsymbol{p}_k), \tag{7.29}$$

5. *Limited-memory BFGS*

   This method is based on the BFGS method and uses a certain number of vector corrections to estimate the inverse Hessian matrix, thereby reducing computing time and memory requirements.

For a clinical example of dose optimization, single-field uniform doses (SFUD) in which each beam delivered a homogeneous dose to the target and with optimization in a single time iteration caused large hot spots, and less than 90 % of the dose was observed within the target (left image in Fig. 7.16). However, increasing the number of iterations (up to 50 times) improved dose conformation (right image in Fig. 7.16).

As described above, while the number of beam fields in particle beam therapy is less than that in photon beam therapy, a single beam field only is not appropriate for clinical practice (see Sect. 7.3.3). Multiple beam fields are therefore overlaid to calculate final dose distributions on the CT image for treatment plan review. For photon and proton beams, the final dose can be calculated by simply summing the respective beam fields, because the RBE value is assumed to be a constant value. Where RBE value varies as a function of beam penetration depth for heavy charged particle beams, the final biological effective dose superposition from multiple beam

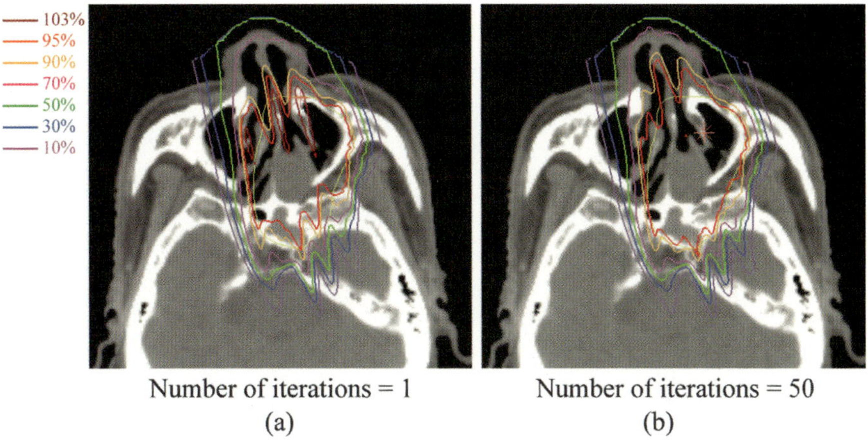

Fig. 7.16 SFUD using C-PBS (**a**) with optimization in a single iteration and (**b**) in 50 iterations. *Yellow line* shows the target volume

fields depends on the fractionation scheme (Kramer 2001). For example, when biological effective doses from multiple beam fields are superposed in the same treatment fraction (same day), the final biological effective dose is increased nonlinearly. However, since the biological repair process is mostly completed the next day, the final biological effective dose is increased linearly when a single beam field is irradiated in the same fraction. Most CIRT centers use a fixed beam port irradiation system, and most treatment cases receive a single beam field in the same day. While a limited number of carbon-ion beam rotating gantry systems are now available, a clinical request for IMPT (simultaneous dose optimization of multiple fields including all beam spots) might increase the use of a gantry to minimize OAR doses compared to SFUD.

7.3.6 Other Techniques

7.3.6.1 Hypofractionated Treatment

Owing to the unique physical and biological characteristics of heavy charged particle beams, it is theoretically possible to decrease the number of treatment fractions with dose escalation (hypofractionated treatment). A smaller number of fractions improves patient comfort and might increase the number of treated patients (improvement of treatment throughput). Hypofractionated CIRT has therefore attracted much clinical interest. Clinical doses used in our facility are based on the survival of HSG cells in vitro and on clinical experience with fast neutron beam therapy. Carbon-ion beams have the same high-LET components as fast neutrons, which tend to lower RBE for both tumor and normal tissues by increasing dose per fraction, albeit that decreasing the tumor RBE is slower than decreasing the normal

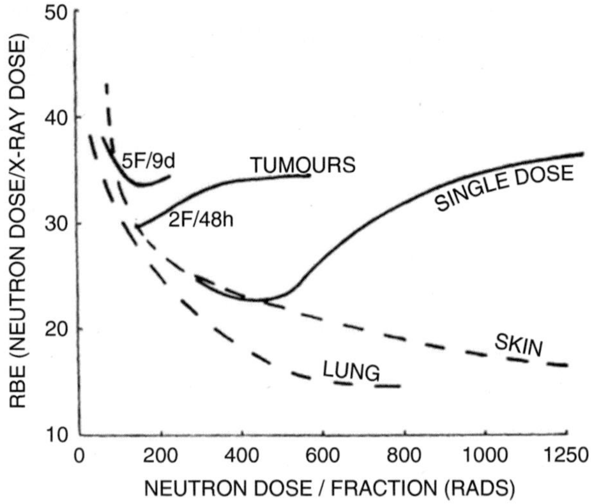

Fig. 7.17 RBE values for fast neutron beams as a function of fraction dose (With permission from Denekamp et al. 1976)

tissue RBE (Fig. 7.17) (Denekamp et al. 1976; Ando and Kase 2009). This can lead to the assumption that the therapeutic ratio can be increased by increasing the fraction dose.

Clinical dose can be expressed as equivalent dose to photon beam; in this assumption, tumor control probability (TCP) can be adopted to CIRT. We estimated TCP values in one, four, and nine treatment fractions from clinical results for non-small cell lung cancer (NSCLC) patients treated with a treatment scheme of 18 fractions (Fig. 7.18):

$$TCP=\sum_i \frac{1}{\sqrt{2\pi}\sigma}\left\{-\frac{(\alpha_i-\alpha)^2}{2\sigma^2}\right\}exp\left[-Nexp\left\{-n\alpha d\left(1+\frac{d}{(\alpha/\beta)}\right)+\frac{0.693(T-T_k)}{T_p}\right\}\right], \tag{7.30}$$

where α and β are the coefficients of the LQ model of HSG cells; σ is the standard deviation of α reflecting patient-specific variation (i) in radiosensitivity; N is the number of clonogens in a tumor (constant value of 10^9 was used); n and d are the total fraction number and dose per fraction, respectively; and T, T_k, and T_p are treatment course time, kickoff time, and average doubling time of tumor cells, respectively.

This approach is useful in determining the initially prescribed dose for hypofractionated CIRT. Because increasing the prescribed dose per fraction could cause excessive dose to OARs per fraction, however, a dose-escalation study was performed by increasing the prescribed dose steps by approximately 5 % of the initially prescribed dose to avoid the serious side effects associated with higher-dose irradiation. As a clinical example, our center has begun hypofractionated lung CIRT. In 1994, the optimum prescribed dose of 90 Gy (RBE) in 18 fractions over 6 weeks was adopted for Stage I NSCLC and achieved 95 % local control with

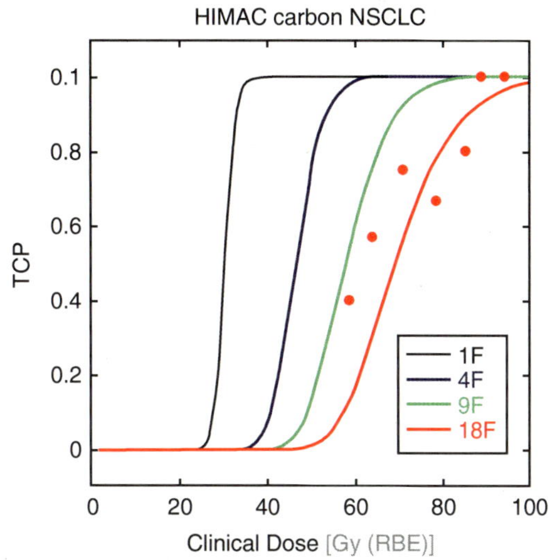

Fig. 7.18 Tumor control probability (TCP) curve of NSCLC with CIRT (Reproduced from Ref. 2012)

minimal pulmonary toxicity. Dose escalation with a small number of fractions was then continued to 72.0 Gy (RBE) in 9 fractions over 3 weeks and 52.8–60.0 Gy (RBE) in 4 fractions over 1 week. There were no severe toxic reactions, and the 5-year local control rate for 9 and 4 fractions was 95 % and 90 %, respectively (Miyamoto et al. 2003, 2007). Our center now treats NSCLC in a single fraction with dose escalation from the initially prescribed dose of 28 Gy (RBE) to 50 Gy (RBE) (Karube et al. 2015).

With regard to hepatocellular cancer (HCC), hypofractionated dose-escalation studies have been implemented in CIRT. The initial treatment fractionation scheme was 15 fractions over 5 weeks, which was then decreased to 12 fractions over 3 weeks, 8 fractions over 3 weeks, and 8 fractions over 2 weeks. The 5-year local control and survival rates for 4 fractions over 1 week (prescribed dose of 52.8 Gy (RBE)) were 81 % and 33 %, respectively (Imada et al. 2010). We have continued this fractionation scheme to 2 fractions in 2 days (prescribed dose of 45 Gy (RBE)).

7.3.6.2 Treatment Replanning

Treatment procedures are generally performed using planning CT data acquired in a single day based on the assumption that patient geometry might not change throughout the treatment course. This would be emphasized by the smaller number of treatment fractions in CIRT than in proton and photon beam therapy: the number of fractions in prostate treatment, for example, is 38 fractions for photon beam and 12 fractions for CIRT (Fowler and Ritter 1995; Tsujii and Kamada 2012). Most oncologists and physicists are likely to be anxious about both intra- and interfractional changes, however, given that the characteristics of these uncertainties can differ among individual patients. We have no quantitative information on intra-/interfractional changes if IGPT is not applied. Sources of the interfractional change, such as variations in tumor size, shape, and density, include weight loss/gain, treatment response, and setup variations. Positional changes of the tumor over a treatment course have also been reported (3, 4). In addition to range uncertainties, particle radiotherapy is also challenged by interfractional geometry changes.

One example of treatment replanning has been introduced to the treatment of locally advanced cervical cancer with CIRT. Most cervical tumors irradiated with carbon-ion beam show marked shrinkage after the start of treatment, and treatment planning is therefore routinely repeated twice during the treatment course in our hospital (Kato et al. 2006). In the first (initial) treatment plan, the CTV includes whole pelvic irradiation (gross and potentially microscopic disease, cervical tumor, uterus, parametrium, upper half of the vagina, and pelvic lymph nodes) (CTV1), and the PTV is designed by the addition of a 5-mm margin to CTV1 (PTV1). The prescribe dose of 39 Gy (RBE) in 13 fractions is given to PTV1 (Fig. 7.19a). In the first revised treatment plan, the CTV includes the gross disease at the primary site, parametrial involvement, remainder of the uterus, upper vagina, and gross lymph node involvement (CTV2). The revised PTV is CTV2 plus a 5-mm margin, and the prescribed dose of 15 Gy (RBE) in five fractions is delivered to PTV2 (Fig. 7.19b). In the second revised treatment plan, the PTV is shrunk to the GTV (PTV3), and the prescribed dose of 18 Gy (RBE) is given in two fractions (Fig. 7.19c). This procedure allows for successful delivery of the total prescribed dose of 72 Gy (RBE) to the tumor with minimal excessive dosing to normal tissues throughout the treatment course (in 20 fractions), even though tumor size is significantly changed.

7.3.6.3 LET Painting

Due to word count limitations, the author does not provide details of IMPT here. However, PBS allows the design of more flexible dose distributions and therefore has the potential to improve TCP for the hypoxia tumor region by optimizing both dose and LET distributions (LET painting) (Bassler et al. 2010; Malinen and Sovik 2015). Since CT images do not provide functional information but rather geometric information only, the effective density derived from a CT image does not provide the hypoxia region. It is well known that the hypoxia tumor region requires a higher dosage than the tumor region with a normal oxygen level to obtain the same radiation response (oxygen enhancement ratio, OER). Although heavy charged particle beams have a high-LET and low OER values, tumor control may be decreased if the hypoxia region is included in the tumor region. Functional information is obtained from positron emission tomography (PET) images used in treatment planning by combination with CT image. In an example clinical case (head and neck region), although a homogeneous C-PBS dose distribution was

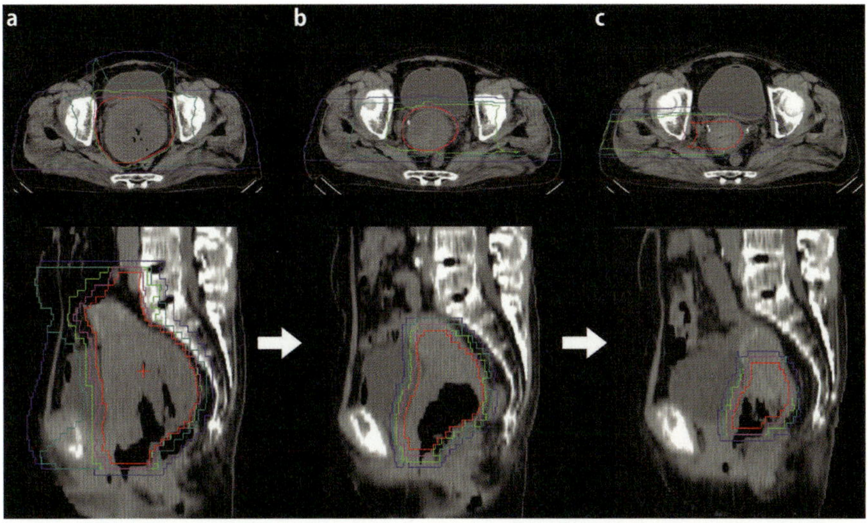

Fig. 7.19 Carbon-ion beam dose distribution using a passive scattering technique for locally advanced cervical cancer in (**a**) first (initial) treatment planning, (**b**) second (first revised) treatment planning, and (**c**) third (second revised) treatment planning. *Red* 95 %, *pink* 70 %, *green* 50 %, *blue* 30 %, *purple* 10 % (With permission from 2012)

achieved within the PTV, LET around the target edge region was higher than that around center region (upper panel in Fig. 7.20). Carbon ions were boosted to the hypoxia tumor region to increase LET, but dose distribution within the PTV was almost homogeneous (middle panel in Fig. 7.20). This group attempted to further improve LET distribution by using oxygen-ion boost irradiation instead of carbon-ion boost irradiation (lower panel in Fig. 7.20). As suggested above, the flexible dose distribution allowed by PBS provides substantial scope to increase treatment accuracy.

7.4 4D Treatment Planning

Most particle beam treatment centers using PBS currently restrict treatment to areas not affected by intrafractional organ motion. Recently, however, two treatment centers started C-PBS treatment to a moving target. In 2012, the Heidelberg Ion Therapy Center started carbon-ion treatment for liver patients, in which they apply an abdominal compression technique to significantly minimize respiratory motion (Habermehl et al. 2013), and in 2015, the NIRS started treatment under free breathing conditions with markerless tumor tracking using fluoroscopic image gating (see Sect. 7.4.5.4). Most particle beam treatment centers have already started thoracoabdominal treatment using the passive

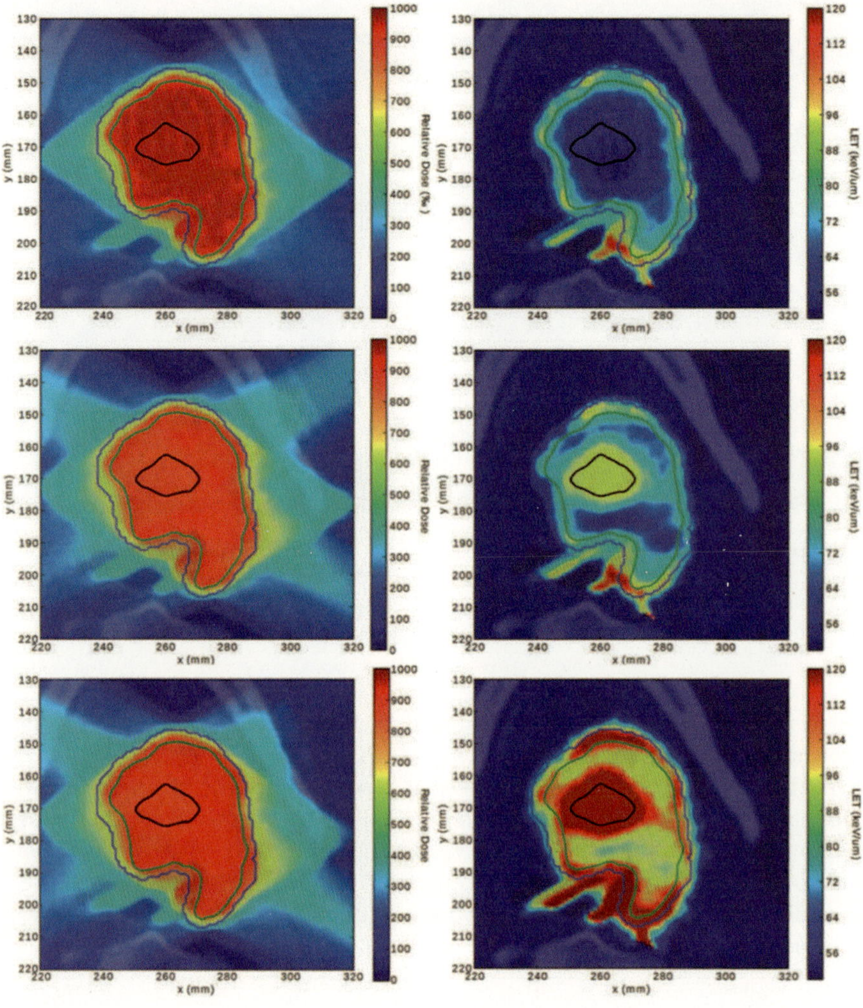

Fig. 7.20 C-PBS homogeneous dose distribution and LET distribution on irradiation by four different beam fields (*upper panel*). C-PBS dose distribution and LET distribution with boost irradiation with carbon ions (*middle panel*) or oxygen ions (*lower panel*) to the hypoxia region (marked as a *black curve*) (With permission from Bassler et al. 2014)

scattering technique. The PBS technique in these sites, however, requires additional motion mitigation techniques to improve dose conformation to the moving target. Here, we introduce the basic concept of 4D treatment planning and its motion mitigation techniques as related to C-PBS treatment. We also suggest that readers obtain more information about motion management (Bert and Durante 2011; Korreman 2012).

7.4.1 Effect of Motion

It is well known that organ geometrical changes are major problems in the degradation of dose conformation in particle beam therapy, but not in photon beam therapy. The patient is alive, and the activities required to maintain this status impact the whole body. For nearly all patients, it is impossible to stop the heartbeat, breathing, digestion, blood circulation, etc. voluntarily. Breathing can be intentionally stopped for several seconds, but not all patients can hold their breath for a long time due to decreased lung/circulation function. Respiratory and cardiac motion (intrafractional motion) is unavoidable in thoracoabdominal treatment. As of 2015, most commercially available TPS do not allow 4D dose calculation due to both patient- and machine-specific considerations. An exception is the RayStation© (RaySearch, Stockholm), whose 4D dose calculation incorporates patient-specific motion.

Independently of the use of a motion mitigation technique, particle beam stopping position is changed, and the magnitude of overdosage is increased when the solid tumor density is replaced by the lower density of the lung (left upper and middle panels in Fig. 7.21). Since a passive scattering beam provides a broadened beam field in both the lateral and depth directions to cover tumor displacement, both intrafractional motion and time axis should be considered. As a result, the temporally accumulated dose distribution to the moving target is degraded as a blurring effect (left lower panel in Fig. 7.21). PBS irradiation to the moving target also causes a blurring effect; this more severe effect results from the interplay between intrafractional tumor/organ motion and the timeline of beam spot position due to the low probability density function (PDF) between them (called the "interplay effect") (right panel in Fig. 7.21) (Furukawa et al. 2007; Bert et al. 2008, Knopf et al. 2010). Similar effects have been reported in IMRT (Bortfeld et al. 2002). PBS irradiation to a moving target should therefore consider scanned beam spot position as well as both respiratory motion and time axis.

7.4.2 4D Imaging

To achieve good treatment accuracy in the thoracoabdominal region, information on organ motion should be incorporated in planning CT imaging. The demand for time-resolved 3DCT imaging has increased in both the photon and particle beam therapeutic fields. The 4DCT technique adds time information to 3DCT data (Keall et al. 2006; Mageras et al. 2004). Two different techniques for 4DCT acquisition are commercially available and have been integrated into clinical application: cine 4D mode (Pan et al. 2004) and helical 4D mode (Keall et al. 2004). Cine 4D mode sorts reconstructed CT images into a specific respiratory phase, whereas the helical 4D mode sorts temporal scans in sinogram space before reconstruction using the respiratory signal. 4DCT is now routinely used in many treatment centers.

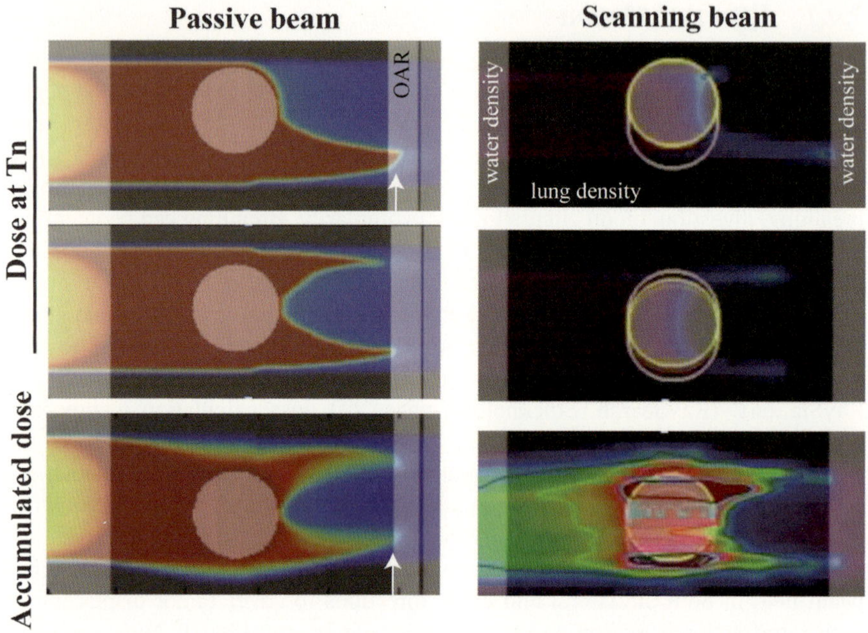

Fig. 7.21 Carbon-ion dose distributions at respective phases and accumulated dose for passive scattering and PBS. Tumor (0 HU) was placed into lung tissue (-650HU) surrounded by tissue (0HU)

However, one should be aware that 4DCT acquired with conventional multi-slice CT includes geometric errors, for example, due to resorting. The resorting process in 4DCT acquisition is based on respiratory phase, but because respiratory amplitude is not always the same during 4DCT acquisition due to the time it takes for image acquisition, resorting errors can occasionally occur. The different amplitudes apparent during the acquisition of different slices sometimes make it impossible to obtain a precise reproduction of the geometric shape (4DCT artifact) (Fig. 7.22) (Yamamoto et al. 2008). This can result in the degradation of image quality, which may in turn hamper quantitative analysis and affect the dose calculation on which the treatment planning is based.

In one example, use of 4DCT artifact-free planning CT data provided sufficient dose to the CTV (Fig. 7.23a). When planning was done using a smaller CTV shape than the actual shape due to 4DCT artifact (Fig. 7.23c), however, underdosage occurred around the diaphragm region in the treatment stage (Fig. 7.23b). To overcome these problems, state-of-the-art medical CT scanners can acquire volumetric cine CT image data with an area-detector CT, such as with 320 detector rows ("Aquilion One" by Toshiba Medical Systems) (Mori et al. 2007; Dewey et al. 2008). Because these CT scanners provide a scan region of more than 16 cm within a single rotation with a coherent absolute time in all slices, resorting of CT data at each slice position as a function of respiratory phase is not necessary. Several other

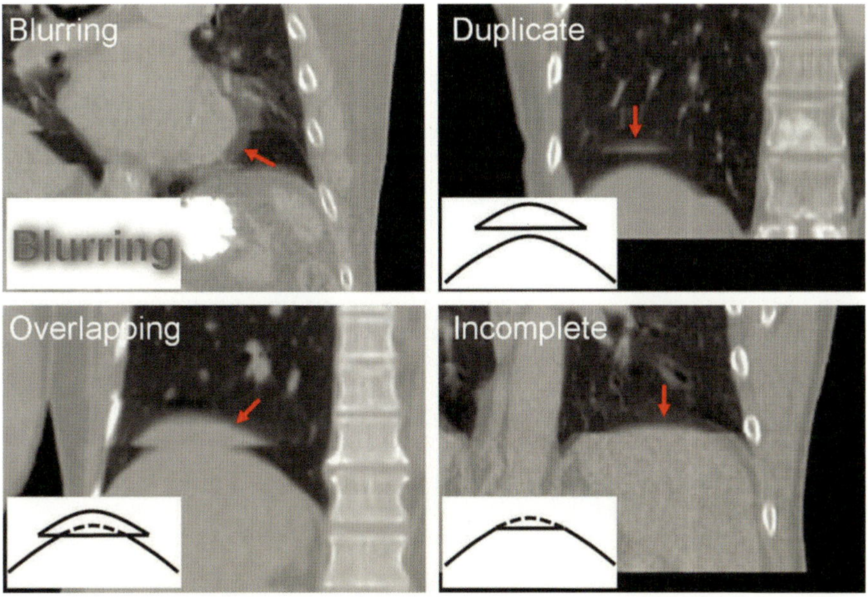

Fig. 7.22 Examples of four-dimensional CT images with schematic diagrams for the four types of artifact: blurring, duplicate structure, overlapping structure, and incomplete structure. Corresponding artifacts are indicated by *arrows* in the respective images. Note that other artifacts can also be observed in these images (With permission from Yamamoto et al. 2008)

approaches to this problem have been introduced, but medical staff generally check 4DCT image quality after acquiring 4DCT images to determine whether quality is clinically acceptable.

7.4.3 4D Dose Calculation

In a review article (Keall 2004), Dr. Paul Keall noted that "4D radiotherapy is the explicit inclusion of the temporal changes in anatomy during the imaging, planning and delivery of radiotherapy" and "4D treatment planning is designing treatment plans on CT image sets obtained for each segment of the breathing cycle." A basic approach is to convolve a static dose distribution by a probability density function, describing the probability that a volume element (voxel) is found at a particular location, on the basis that it is necessary to calculate absorbed dose at each voxel during irradiation to quantify dose assessment. As described in Sect. 7.3.5, different compositions of the mixed particle field affect each voxel, and the residual beam energy of the particles strongly affects the RBE value. Thus, although photon beam and proton beams require only simply summing of the biological dose in each voxel due to the constant RBE value, heavy charged particle beams require that the

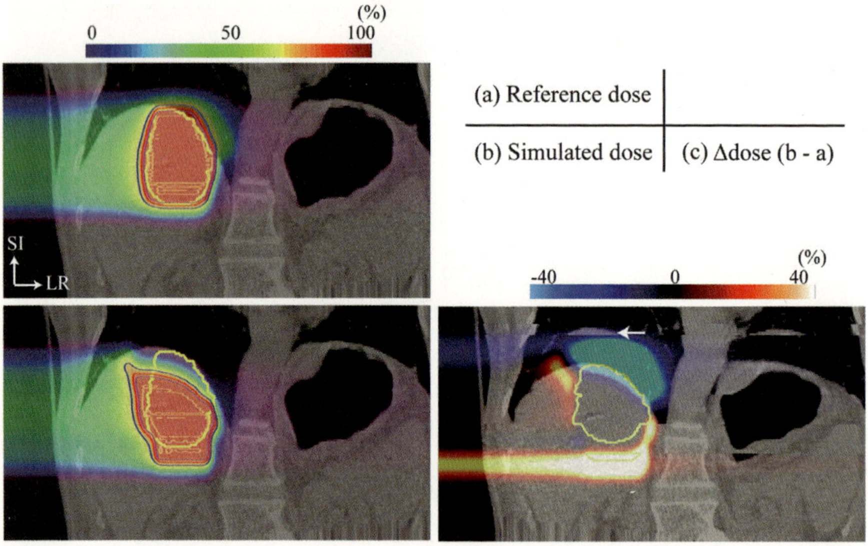

Fig. 7.23 (**a**) C-PBS dose distribution for a liver case calculated with artifact-less 4DCT and overlaid on an artifact-less 4DCT image. (**b**) C-PBS dose distribution calculated with a 4DCT artifact image and overlaid on an artifact-less 4DCT image. (**c**) C-PBS dose difference ((**b**) minus (**a**)) overlaid on the 4DCT artifact image. *Yellow line* shows the CTV

nonlinear addition of the biologically weighted dose should be accounted for in each voxel. This is more important for dose assessment with C-PBS.

Since passive scattering irradiation uses a wide beam field to sufficiently cover the target volume, if sufficient dose coverage to the moving target is achieved in respective phases even though voxel trajectories within the target are not recognized, the resultant accumulated dose will also achieve good dose coverage (left upper and left middle panels in Fig. 7.21). In this case, however, overshoot was observed over the distal side of the target region, the exact position of which changed with respiratory phase. As a result, dose to each voxel could be varied as a function of respiratory phase. Further, when hot/cold spots were caused within the target volume, the accumulated target dose was inhomogeneous. Moreover, because PBS irradiates each beam spot position as a function of time and because irradiated spot position can differ even in the same respiratory phase (right upper and middle panels in Fig. 7.21), evaluation of target dose coverage could be impossible. Therefore, calculation of dose distribution at respective phases is insufficient to evaluate dose assessment of a moving target. It is therefore necessary to calculate the accumulated dose distribution, including DIR. We have clearly defined this as "4D treatment planning."

However, because human organ structures are moved and deformed naturally by respiration, it is difficult to track each voxel in respective phases, particularly with the similar HU value voxels seen in the liver, e.g., determining which voxel (*P*2 or *P*2') at peak inhalation moved to voxel (*P*1) within the VOI at peak exhalation

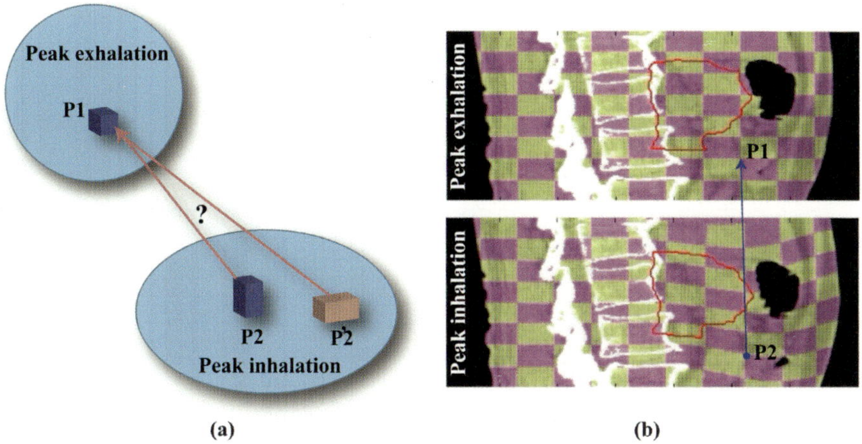

Fig. 7.24 (**a**) Schematic drawing of voxel trajectory at peak exhalation and inhalation. *Circular shapes* show VOIs at each phase. (**b**) A checkerboard image overlaid on the sagittal image in the abdominal region at peak exhalation (*upper panel*) is warped at peak inhalation by applying DVF (*lower panel*). *Red curve* shows the PTV for pancreatic treatment

(Fig. 7.24a). It is well known that human organ movement is well fitted by the B-spline curve, and this is often used in the DIR algorithm to calculate each voxel trajectory. In the abdominal region, for example, a checkerboard image overlaid on the sagittal image at peak exhalation (upper panel in Fig. 7.24b) was deformed at peak inhalation by intrafractional patient geometrical changes (lower panel in Fig. 7.24b). The same voxel at peak inhalation (*P*2 in Fig. 7.24b) can be estimated using DIR from the voxel at peak exhalation (*P*1 in Fig. 7.24b). The several DIR algorithms introduced to date have been shown to significantly affect 4D dose distribution (Castadot et al. 2008; Brock 2010; Zhang et al. 2012), and planners should therefore check DIR accuracy, as described in Sect. 7.3.2.2.

Figure 7.25 shows C-PBS dose distributions and accumulated dose distributions as a function of time for a clinical example of liver 4D dose calculation. Over 50 respiratory cycles were required to give the total prescribed dose. An ungated strategy with eight iso-energy-layered phase-controlled rescannings (PCR) (described in the next section) was applied. Dose at the distal side of the target was irradiated at T50 (T0, peak inhalation, T50, peak exhalation) in the seventh respiratory cycle; the irradiated iso-energy layer was shifted to the proximal side as treatment time proceeded (upper panel in Fig. 7.25); and the accumulated dose gradually filled the target volume (lower panel in Fig. 7.25). Almost all the total prescribed dose was given to the target at T70 by the 44th cycle.

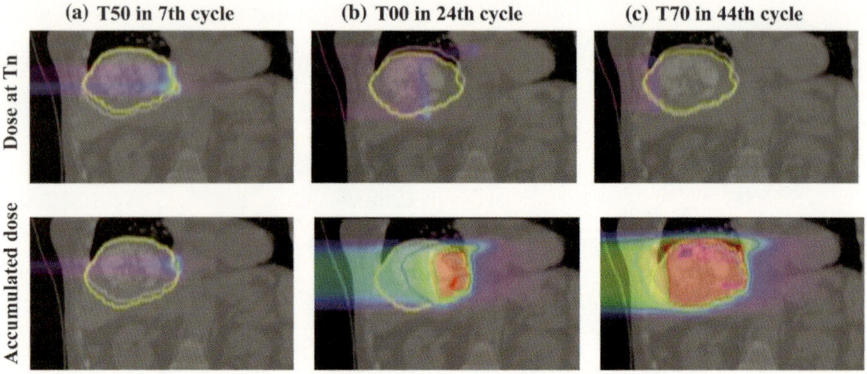

Fig. 7.25 C-PBS dose distributions for the ungated strategy at (**a**) T50 in the seventh cycle, (**b**) T00 in the 24th cycle, and (**c**) T70 in the 44th cycle. *Upper* and *lower panels* show dose distribution at the respective phases and accumulated dose. Phase control rescanning (described later) was adapted, but respiratory gating was not used

7.4.4 4D Optimization

The optimization process in treatment planning aims to find the best possible plan to satisfy user-defined criteria; clinically, this usually means that the dose is good at both sparing OARs and maintaining a good target dose. These user-defined criteria are integrated mathematically as objective functions into the TPS. Although most optimization techniques in treatment planning are 3D, state-of-the-art treatment planning now extends to 4D to allow consideration of intrafractional uncertainties (4D optimization).

Heath et al. compared two types of robust 4D optimization technique in margin-based mid-ventilation lung treatment planning (Heath et al. 2009). First, each voxel trajectory at respective phases was calculated by DIR from respective phases to the reference phase. The accumulated dose $\langle D_i \rangle$ to moving voxel i at the respective phase is calculated by summing over the contributed dose $D\left(\vec{r_{i,g}}\right)$ at the location of voxel i at the trajectory point g $\left(\vec{r_{i,g}}\right)$ and multiplying the probability distribution determined from the respiratory motion curve P_g:

$$\langle D_i \rangle = \sum_{g=1}^{n} D\left(\vec{r_{i,g}}\right) P_g, \tag{7.31}$$

where n is the number of voxel trajectory.

The first optimization technique, 4D optimization without consideration of respiratory motion uncertainties, was performed to optimize beamlet weights by using the following objective function:

$$F = F_{\text{target}} + \sum_{r}^{n\text{OAR}} F_{\text{OAR}}, \tag{7.32}$$

$$F_{\text{target}} = \sum_{i}^{N_{\text{target}}} \alpha_{\text{under}}^{\text{target}} \left[D_{\text{min}}^{\text{target}} - \langle D_i \rangle\right]^2 + \alpha_{\text{over}}^{\text{target}} \left[\langle D_i \rangle - D_{\text{max}}^{\text{target}}\right]^2, \tag{7.33}$$

$$F_{\text{OAR}} = \sum_{i}^{N_{\text{OAR}}} \alpha_{\text{over}}^{\text{OAR}} \left[\langle D_i \rangle - D_{\text{max}}^{\text{OAR}}\right]_+^2, \tag{7.34}$$

where n_{OAR} is the number of OAR and N_x is the number of voxels in object x; $\alpha^x{}_{\text{under}}$ and $\alpha^x{}_{\text{over}}$ are the penalties for the object x underdosage and overdosage, respectively; and $D^x{}_{\text{max}}$ and $D^x{}_{\text{min}}$ are user-defined maximum and minimum doses in object x, respectively. Object x is the target volume or OAR.

The second optimization technique is the probabilistic optimization technique, which was originally applied to patient setup uncertainties (Unkelbach and oelfke 2004). It has now been expanded to the temporal axis by including the variance of the dose in each voxel as follows:

$$F_{\text{target}} = \sum_{i}^{N_{\text{target}}} \alpha_{\text{under}}^{\text{target}} \left[D_{\text{min}}^{\text{target}} - \langle D_i \rangle\right]_+^2 + \alpha_{\text{over}}^{\text{target}} \left[\langle D_i \rangle - D_{\text{max}}^{\text{target}}\right]_+^2 + V_i, \tag{7.35}$$

where V_i represents the variance of the dose in each voxel within the target volume.

Another 4D optimization method involves dividing the target volume into subsections based on motion phases (Graeff et al. 2013). These subsections were consistent with the slices dividing the target volume along beam direction (Fig. 7.26a). Each slice was divided into sectors for respective motion phases (Fig. 7.26b and Fig. 7.26c), and each sector was deformed using motion function (Fig. 7.26d). The beam spots were then optimized to each target voxel in each motion phase by minimizing the error value $E(\vec{N})$ between the prescribed dose D_{pre} and particle numbers $N_{j,k}$ as follows:

$$E(\vec{N}) = \sum_{k=1}^{m} \sum_{i \in \text{CTV}(k)} \left[D_{\text{pre}}^{i} - D_{\text{act}}^{ik}(\vec{N}_k)\right]^2, \tag{7.36}$$

$$= \sum_{k=1}^{m} \sum_{i \in \text{CTV}(k)} \left[D_{\text{pre}}^{i} - \text{RBE}(\vec{N}_k) \sum_{j=1}^{r} c_{ijk} N_{j,k}\right]^2 \tag{7.37}$$

where c_{ijk} is the factor correlated to the particle number of each beam spot; i and k are the spot number and motion phase, respectively; and D_{act} is the actual dose. j is the particle number of each beam spot.

This optimization process is technically successful without introducing unpredictable respiratory variation throughout the treatment course. There are

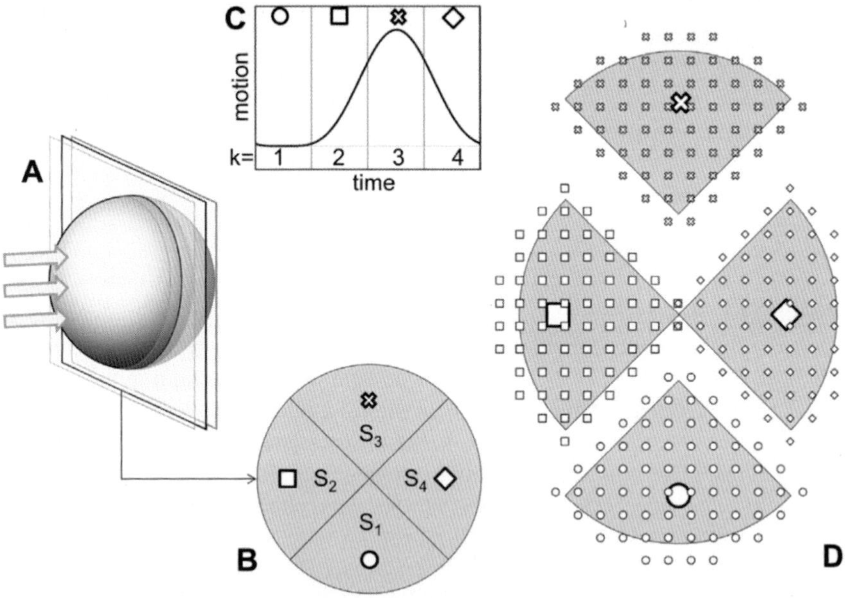

Fig. 7.26 Target volume is divided into slices along beam direction (**a**). These slices are divided into sectors (four sectors (S_1, . . ., S_4) in this example) (**b**) and assigned into motion function (**c**). Each sector is deformed according to the motion function (**d**) (With permission from Graeff et al. 2013)

fewer OARs in lung treatment than in abdominal treatment. The radiation oncologist and medical physicist should discuss any use of currently immature 4D optimization in clinical treatment planning which requires minimization of OAR dose in place of a conventional optimization technique.

7.4.5 Motion Mitigation Technique

Several approaches to motion mitigation have been introduced and some treatment centers have integrated them into clinical protocols. The major motion mitigation approaches are "margin," "rescanning," and "gating." The motion mitigation technique emphasizes clinical gain by combining these different motion mitigation approaches. The scanned beam tracking technique was introduced by a German group (Grozinger et al. 2008), but many problems required solving before it could be integrated into clinical use. Substantial additional development, simulation, and verification are required before such techniques can be used clinically.

7.4.5.1 Intrafractional Range Compensating Margins

The first approach "margin" is generally used in particle beam therapy as well as photon beam therapy. To avoid missing a moving target, internal margin has been added to the CTV to construct the internal target volume (ITV) (ICRU-62 1999, ICRU-50 1993). ITV, however, does not describe intrafractional density changes within the target volume and is "geometrically" rather than "radiologically path length oriented" (ICRU-72 2007). If ITV were used for treatment planning, 4D dose distribution would cause underdosage within the CTV, because replacing the tumor density with lower lung density produces intrafractional range variation (Fig. 7.27b). Most cases have focused on range variation around the tumor itself; however, particle beams may transit through normal tissues such as the chest wall, pulmonary vessels, esophagus, bone, heart, and other critical structures before delivering the treatment beam to the tumor. These structures could also cause range variations.

To solve this problem, we designed range-adapted ITV (called range-ITV) from respective 4DCT data by selecting maximum and minimum WEPL values at the distal and proximal sides along the same ray line at respective phases (Knopf et al. 2013). Range-ITV contours were extended along the distal direction to compensate for intrafractional range variation (Fig. 7.27a), which is the same region that had underdosage in the ITV plan (Fig. 7.27b). By applying range-ITV, sufficient dose was given to the CTV without underdosage (Fig. 7.27c).

The range-ITV contour reached the mediastinum (marked as an open arrow in Fig. 7.27a). Beam spot was set within the range-ITV region. The treatment beam reached this region around the exhalation phase due to inferior movement of the tumor, but did not reach it around the inhalation phases. Accordingly, the accumulated dose was not given to the whole range-ITV (marked as the open arrow in Fig. 7.27c) but to the whole CTV region. For this reason, even though the OAR dose was not clinically acceptable in 3D treatment planning, it might be acceptable in 4D treatment planning. This is a clinical merit of 4D treatment planning. Here, we introduce a clinical example of range-ITV for lung treatment, but this concept can be extended to OARs (range-OAR). Since range-OAR shape might also be strongly affected by density changes, especially in the lung and due to bowel gas, an overlapping problem between range-ITV and range-OAR is quite possible, more so than between PTV and PRV (see Sect. 7.3.2.1).

Range-ITV is a different shape in each beam angle (beam field-specific shape); using the example of an orthogonal beam field, the dark gray shape is required to cover intrafractional range variation for both beam fields (Fig. 7.28a). However, lateral extensions for respective beam fields would be unnecessary. These different beam-specific target volumes are not suitable for IMPT using carbon ions, which instead require the same geometrical target volumes. To perform IMPT, field-independent range-ITV was calculated using a modified geometrical and WEPL conversion table (Fig. 7.28b) (Graeff et al. 2012). This allows the same geometrical target volume to be used for both beam fields in IMPT optimization.

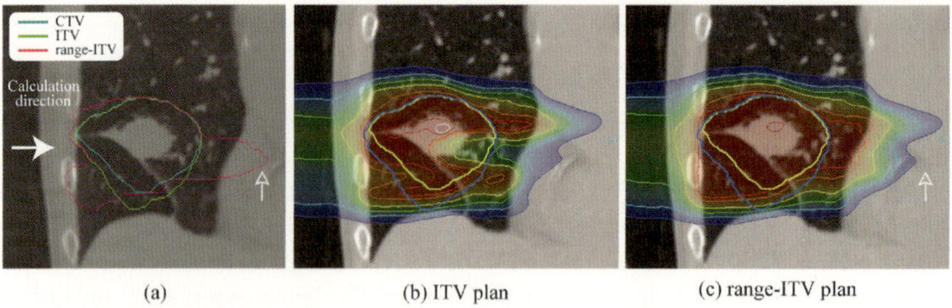

Fig. 7.27 (**a**) CTV, ITV, and range-ITV contours at the reference phase. Temporally accumulated carbon-ion beam dose distributions using (**b**) ITV and (**c**) range-ITV. Single-field uniform dose optimization was selected

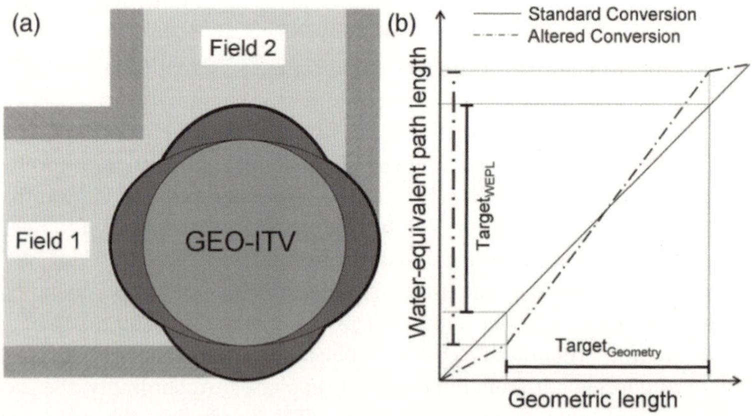

Fig. 7.28 (**a**) Schematic drawing of field-independent range-ITV for orthogonal beam fields. Geometrical ITV and field-specific range-ITV are shown as a light *gray circle* (GEO-ITV) and *dark ellipses*, respectively. (**b**) Standard and altered geometrical and WEPL conversion table (With permission from Graeff et al. 2012)

7.4.5.2 Rescanning

Rescanning, first proposed by Phillips et al. more than 20 years ago (Phillips et al. 1992), is based on the idea of averaging the positional errors of intrafractional motion and thereby smoothing associated dose errors. Rescanning minimizes the magnitude of the interplay effect and improves dose conformation within the target. A basic concept of rescanning is to irradiate the pencil beam to respective beam spots on multiple times. There are two major rescanning methods: layered and volumetric rescanning.

Layered rescanning performs repetitive scanning of the same iso-energy layer; after completing rescanning of the layer, the beam energy is changed to irradiate the next adjacent iso-energy layer. This process is repeated until all iso-energy layers are irradiated. The interplay effect is affected by the scanning speed, beam energy change time, beam spot size, number of beam fields, etc. Several researchers have reported optimum rescanning parameters to minimize the interplay effect (Dowdell et al. 2013; Grassberger et al. 2013; Knopf et al. 2011). However, multiple rescanning (e.g., 20 times) is not good for the scanning magnet system; and if raster-scanning method, which makes the spot transition without turning off the beam, were used, doses between beam spots could be increased. Rescanning is applied to a moving target, albeit that rescanning does not consider respiratory cycle and performs the rescanning as rapidly as possible in the irradiation system. A correlation of rescanning with respiratory motion techniques has been introduced, namely, breath-sampled rescanning and phase-controlled rescanning (PCR) (Seco et al. 2009; Furukawa et al. 2010). PCR deposits the dose to respective spots included in each iso-energy layer to ensure the completion of irradiation within a single respiratory cycle or within the gating window if gating is applied by changing the dose rate (Fig. 7.29a). Scanning order in the iso-energy layer is inversely switched after each rescanning by optimization to minimize total scanning path length. Adequate PCR frequency minimizes the magnitude of the interplay effect by averaging the probability density function between the target and beam spot positions.

One clinical example uses the accumulated dose distribution of a horizontal beam field with a variable number of rescannings under free breathing conditions (Fig. 7.30). Dose conformation without rescanning is severely and rapidly degraded when respiratory cycle is not considered, indeed, as rapidly as the treatment system can achieve. Although a single PCR (1 × PCR) also resulted in severe dose degradation due to the slow scanning speed resulting from irradiating a single layer for a 4-sec respiratory cycle, four or more rescannings improved dose conformity, and sufficient prescribed dose was successfully delivered to a moving target. This strategy is already implemented in the Toshiba heavy charged particle beam treatment system and was in use in treating patients in our hospital and at Kanagawa Cancer Center in Japan in 2015. A similar system is now under construction at Yamagata University.

Volumetric rescanning irradiates beam spots in the iso-energy layer; beam energy is then changed to irradiate beam spots in the next iso-energy layer. The process is repeated until the prescribed dose is delivered to the entire target volume. This method is preferred to an irradiation system with a short energy change time. Volumetric PCR irradiation is made to complete at the end of a gating window by setting the appropriate dose rate constant for all iso-energy layers (Fig. 7.29b).

These rescanning methods are strongly dependent on machine specification. In comparisons using our irradiation system, we found that volumetric PCR was not a suitable alternative to layered PCR (Mori et al. 2013).

7.4.5.3 Gating

Although gating is widely used in photon and particle beam therapies, it has a long history in proton therapy and was in fact integrated into proton therapy in Tsukuba

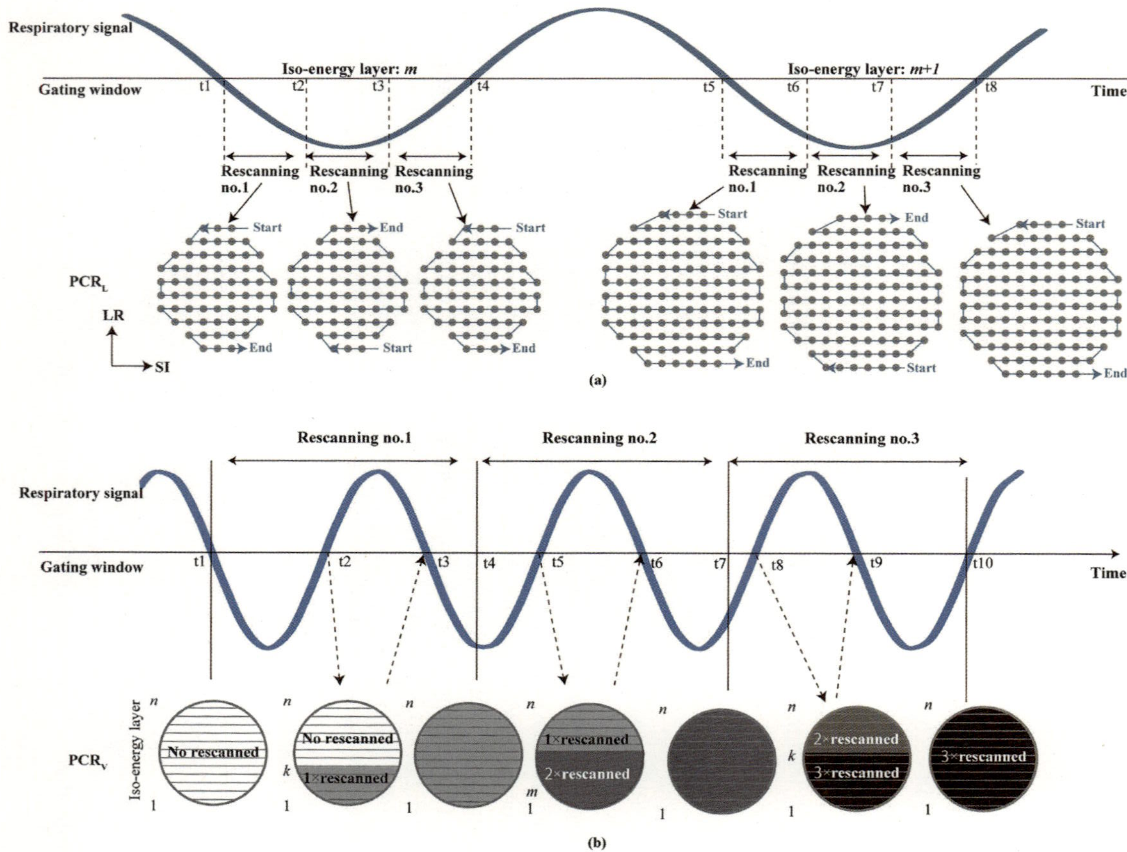

Fig. 7.29 (**a**) Layered and (**b**) volumetric PCR with three rescannings. The *curved line* shows the respiratory signal. *Gray points* are scan spots. (Lower panel) White are not yet rescanned, *light gray* area = 1× rescanned, *gray area* = 2× rescanned, *black area* = 3× rescanned (With permission from Mori et al. 2013)

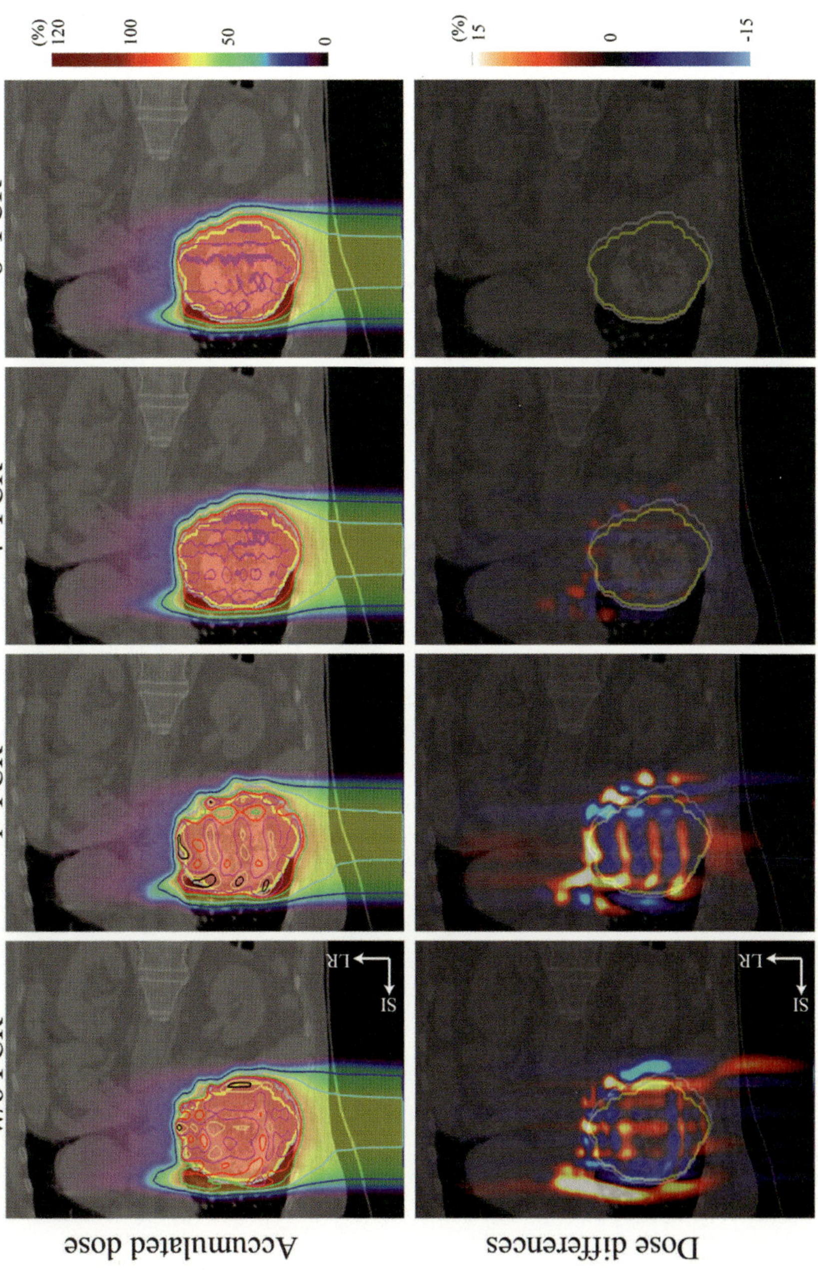

Fig. 7.30 *Upper panel:* C-PBS accumulated dose distributions for liver treatment without PCR and with 1 × PCR, 4 × PCR, and 8 × PCR. *Lower panel:* dose differences (8 × PCR − n × PCR or w/o PCR). Ungated irradiation of a single field was applied

University in the late 1980s (Ohara et al. 1989). The general concept of gating is to irradiate the treatment beam at a specific respiratory phase with a gating signal, typically obtained by observing the patient's respiration. Gating is useful in mitigating the interplay effect via the minimization of tumor displacement during irradiation; nevertheless, it is not a fundamental approach but rather adequate for PCR/breath-sampled rescanning. Here, the author would like to emphasize that the aim of "gating" is to reduce excessive dose to normal tissues by minimizing beam field size. A smaller beam field with gating requires greater accuracy to irradiate a moving tumor than a wide beam field without gating. This gating accuracy could be affected by both machine inheritance and patient inheritance factors. While technical progress in hardware and software will likely improve machine inheritance (e.g., delay time between actual motion and creation of the gating signal), patient inheritance factors described below should be approached by a reconsideration of the fundamental concepts of treatment planning.

The first patient inheritance factor is respiratory pattern variation during treatment. The second is imperfect reproducibility of the respiratory pattern and correlation between the skin surface and internal tumor motion across exhalations (Hoisak et al. 2004; Koch et al. 2004; Liu et al. 2004; Ahn et al. 2004). Together, these may result in degradation of the accuracy of gated radiotherapy and possible irradiation of the tumor beyond the gating window. This will in turn cause the position of the beam-on to be shifted relative to the actual target position (Mori et al. 2008).

Let us reconsider the basic concept of the treatment plan, which is to irradiate the treatment beam when the moving tumor is inside the PTV defined at treatment planning (called amplitude-based gating). The phase-based gating method would be insufficient to capture exact tumor position. Two commercially available amplitude-based gating systems have been recently introduced (CyberKnife® Robotic Radiosurgery System, Accuray, Inc., Sunnyvale CA, USA, and SyncTraX®, Shimadzu, Kyoto, Japan). These systems detect the position of implanted fiducial markers in real time, using paired fluoroscopic units.

Temporal dose distribution under regular breathing conditions (plan dose as a reference) was successful in delivering sufficient dose to a lung tumor (Fig. 7.31a) (Mori et al. 2014). The use of amplitude-based gating prevented dose degradation under the assumption of an irregular motion pattern, namely, motion drift in the superior direction (blue curve on Fig. 7.31b, c). Hot spots (>105 % of a prescribed dose) within the CTV were observed with the treatment dose (Fig. 7.31b), and higher and lower treatment doses not seen in the planning doses were distributed in the respective superior and inferior sides of the CTV (Fig. 7.31c). The amplitude-based gating strategy with multiple rescans preserved dose distribution to a moving target even though respiratory pattern was irregular.

7.4.5.4 Clinical Example in C-PBS Gated Treatment

In this section, the author introduces our clinical example of C-PBS treatment for the thoracic region, started in March 2015. To minimize motion effects, we applied

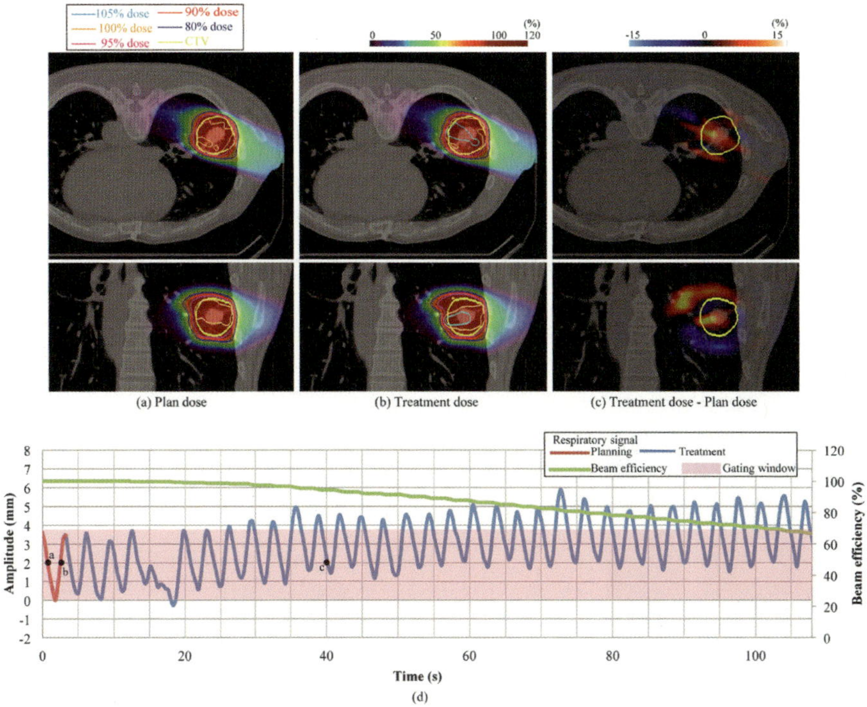

Fig. 7.31 Lung dose distributions in axial and coronal views. (**a**) Planned dose. (**b**) Delivered dose. (**c**) Dose difference. In (**d**), the respiratory wave data are displayed

motion mitigation techniques (eight times PCR and amplitude-based gating) and 4D treatment planning with range-ITV. To achieve amplitude-based gating, we use a paired fluoroscopic imaging unit to acquire real-time X-ray images to capture tumor position. However, fiducial markers are vulnerable to changes in position over the course of therapy (Imura et al. 2005), which can affect dose distribution (Newhauser et al. 2007). Further, not all patients or all tumors can be subjected to fiducial marker implantation. For these reasons, we considered that a markerless tumor tracking method would be preferable. Markerless tumor tracking uses both multi-template matching and machine-learning algorithms (Cervino et al. 2009; Cui et al. 2007, 2008). Tumor position on the fluoroscopic image was detected automatically in real time (marked as yellow lines in Fig. 7.32a) (Mori et al. 2016). When tumor position is inside the irradiation region, the treatment beam is "on" (marked as green/orange lines in Fig. 7.32a). In this case, tumor position was interfractionally changed in the 1st and 12th fractions. However, amplitude-based gating corrected the irradiated treatment beam to the moving tumor by directly capturing tumor position. External gating (monitoring surface motion) did not directly observe the tumor, so its use would degrade gating accuracy.

In this case, when external gating was used in treatment, gating accuracy was 11.1 mm (95 % confidence interval), significantly worse than the 1.1 mm achieved

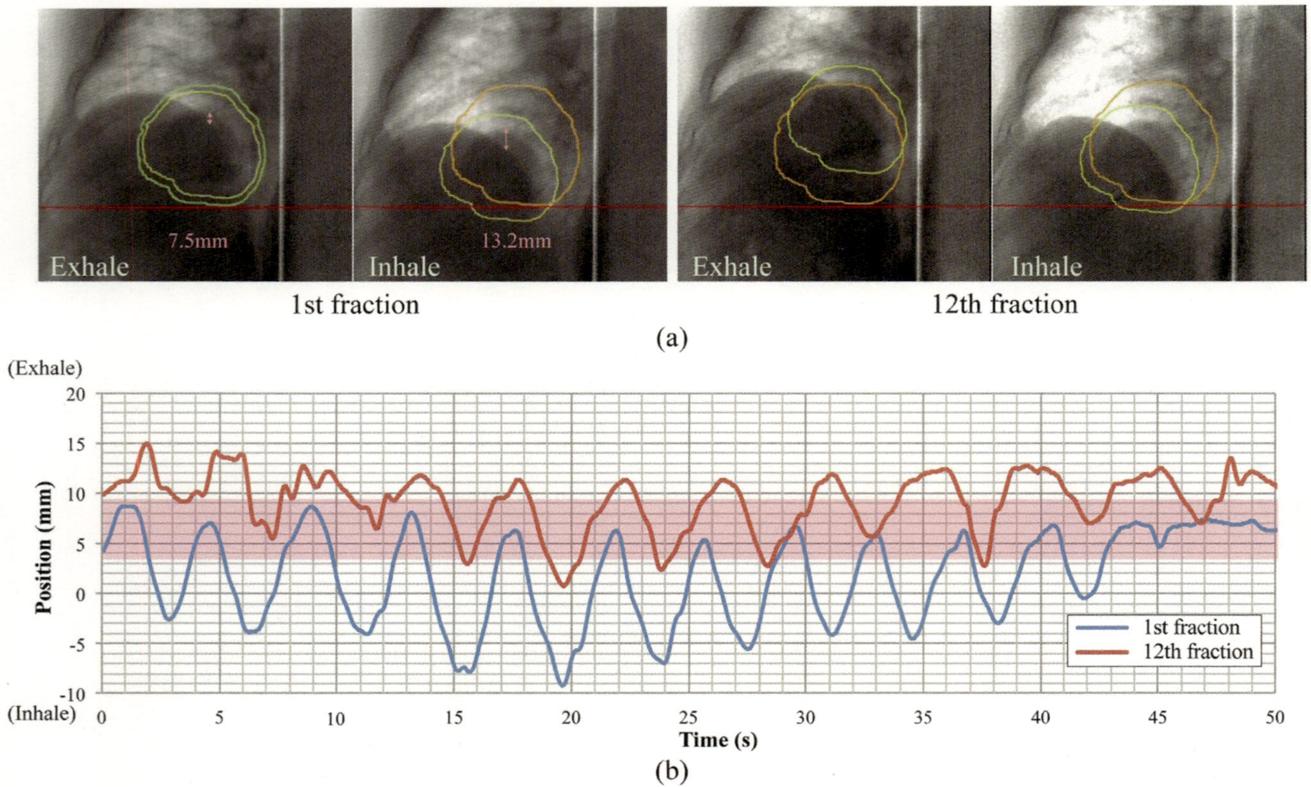

Fig. 7.32 (**a**) Fluoroscopic images for lung tumor treatment in the 1st and 12th treatment fractions. The *yellow line* shows the CTV; the *green* and *orange* borders delineate the PTV; and the *red line* shows the *bottom* position of the PTV. The *double-headed pink arrows* show tumor and diaphragm distances. (**b**) CTV position along the superior-inferior direction as a function of time at the 1st and 12th treatment fractions. The *pink* band is the treatment beam irradiation position (With permission from Mori et al. 2016)

with amplitude-based gating, due to interfractional changes. A major advantage of amplitude-based gating is its ability to target moving tumors even with large interfractional ranges. Although a large part of end-expiration in the 12th treatment fraction was out of the gating window (Fig. 7.32b), the treatment beam was "on" from end-expiration to inspiration. Despite changes in lung density and rib position during the respiratory cycle, CTV position closely corresponded to the irradiation region. Effects on dose distribution are likely smaller than the dose to the CTV using the external gating methodology, because the setup margin can compensate for these variations in density and position.

7.5 Summary and Outlook

This chapter has introduced image-guided CIRT treatment planning and emphasized differences between particle and photon beams. The basic concept of CIRT treatment planning is similar to that for photon beams. Initially, heavy charged particle therapy was used to treat rare cancers, but thanks to strong advances in medical physics and clinical research/development activities, current CIRT has been extended to treat common cancers. The CIRT treatment method and techniques have been developed to allow for safe and more robust treatment delivery.

While it is important to take account of "cost-effectiveness" in the widespread implementation of particle beam therapy around the world, this has already been achieved with photon beam therapy (Zietman 2007; Vanderstraeten et al. 2014). One solution is a reduction in constructing costs by making treatment systems more compact (accelerator and irradiation machine, etc.) and improving treatment throughput (increasing the number of patients). In this regard, our new treatment C-PBS system (Toshiba Corp., Tokyo, Japan) facility has improved treatment room occupancy time (average 10 min per patient) by integrating several technologies developed over 20 years' clinical experience and research activities. Several problems in clinical, technical, and other aspects of particle beam therapy remain, and constant collaboration efforts among medical staff and treatment system vendors are mandatory to achieve steady incremental progress over days and weeks. Higher treatment throughput via hypofractionated treatment might be one solution to hospital financing.

References

http://ptcog.web.psi.ch/ [Online]. [Accessed].

(2006) Dose reporting in ion beam therapy. In: Proceedings of a meeting organized jointly by the IAEA and the ICRU held in Ohio, USA, 18–20 March 2006

(2012) Ion beam therapy fundamentals, technology, clinical applications. Springer

Ahn S, Yi B, Suh Y, Kim J, Lee S, Shin S, Choi E (2004) A feasibility study on the prediction of tumour location in the lung from skin motion. Br J Radiol 77:588–596

Alonso JR (2000) Review of ion beam therapy: present and future

Ando K, Kase Y (2009) Biological characteristics of carbon-ion therapy. Int J Radiat Biol 85:715–728
Bassler N, Jakel O, Sondergaard CS, Petersen JB (2010) Dose- and LET-painting with particle therapy. Acta Oncol 49:1170–1176
Bassler N, Toftegaard J, Luhr A, Sorensen BS, Scifoni E, Kramer M, Jakel O, Mortensen LS, Overgaard J, Petersen JB (2014) LET-painting increases tumour control probability in hypoxic tumours. Acta Oncol 53:25–32
Bert C, Durante M (2011) Motion in radiotherapy: particle therapy. Phys Med Biol 56:R113–R144
Bert C, Grozinger SO, Rietzel E (2008) Quantification of interplay effects of scanned particle beams and moving targets. Phys Med Biol 53:2253–2265
Bortfeld T, Burkelbach J, Boesecke R, Schlegel W (1990) Methods of image reconstruction from projections applied to conformation radiotherapy. Phys Med Biol 35:1423–1434
Bortfeld T, Jokivarsi K, Goitein M, Kung J, Jiang SB (2002) Effects of intra-fraction motion on IMRT dose delivery: statistical analysis and simulation. Phys Med Biol 47:2203–2220
Bragg WH, Kleeman R (1904) On the ionisation curves of radium. Philos Mag 8:726–738
Brock KK (2010) Results of a multi-institution deformable registration accuracy study (MIDRAS). Int J Radiat Oncol Biol Phys 76:583–596
Castadot P, Lee JA, Parraga A, Geets X, Macq B, Gregoire V (2008) Comparison of 12 deformable registration strategies in adaptive radiation therapy for the treatment of head and neck tumors. Radiother Oncol 89:1–12
Cervino LI, Chao AK, Sandhu A, Jiang SB (2009) The diaphragm as an anatomic surrogate for lung tumor motion. Phys Med Biol 54:3529–3541
Chen GT, Sharp GC, Mori S (2009) A review of image-guided radiotherapy. Radiol Phys Technol 2:1–12
Cui Y, Dy JG, Sharp GC, Alexander B, Jiang SB (2007) Multiple template-based fluoroscopic tracking of lung tumor mass without implanted fiducial markers. Phys Med Biol 52:6229–6242
Cui Y, Dy JG, Alexander B, Jiang SB (2008) Fluoroscopic gating without implanted fiducial markers for lung cancer radiotherapy based on support vector machines. Phys Med Biol 53: N315–N327
Denekamp J, Harris SR, Morris C, Field SB (1976) The response of a transplantable tumor to fractionated irradiation. II Fast neutrons. Rad Res 68:93–103
Dewey M, Zimmermann E, Laule M, Rutsch W, Hamm B (2008) Three-vessel coronary artery disease examined with 320-slice computed tomography coronary angiography. Eur Heart J 29:1669
Dowdell S, Grassberger C, Sharp GC, Paganetti H (2013) Interplay effects in proton scanning for lung: a 4D Monte Carlo study assessing the impact of tumor and beam delivery parameters. Phys Med Biol 58:4137–4156
Elsasser T, Brons S, Psonka K, Scholz M, Gudowska-Nowak E, Taucher-Scholz G (2008) Biophysical modeling of fragment length distributions of DNA plasmids after X and heavy-ion irradiation analyzed by atomic force microscopy. Radiat Res 169:649–659
Fowler JF, Ritter MA (1995) A rationale for fractionation for slowly proliferating tumors such as prostatic adenocarcinoma. Int J Radiat Oncol Biol Phys 32:521–529
Furukawa T, Inaniwa T, Sato S, Tomitani T, Minohara S, Noda K, Kanai T (2007) Design study of a raster scanning system for moving target irradiation in heavy-ion radiotherapy. Med Phys 34:1085–1097
Furukawa T, Inaniwa T, Sato S, Shirai T, Mori S, Takeshita E, Mizushima K, Himukai T, Noda K (2010) Moving target irradiation with fast rescanning and gating in particle therapy. Med Phys 37:4874–4879
Furusawa Y, Fukutsu K, Aoki M, Itsukaichi H, Eguchi-Kasai K, Ohara H, Yatagai F, Kanai T, Ando K (2000) Inactivation of aerobic and hypoxic cells from three different cell lines by accelerated (3)He-, (12)C- and (20)Ne-ion beams. Radiat Res 154:485–496
Goitein M (2006) What is difference about particle treatment planning? [Abst] Prticle Therapy Co-Operative Group (PTCOG45), PTCOG45

Graeff C, Durante M, Bert C (2012) Motion mitigation in intensity modulated particle therapy by internal target volumes covering range changes. Med Phys 39:6004–6013

Graeff C, Luchtenborg R, Eley JG, Durante M, Bert C (2013) A 4D-optimization concept for scanned ion beam therapy. Radiother Oncol 109:419–424

Grassberger C, Dowdell S, Lomax A, Sharp G, Shackleford J, Choi N, Willers H, Paganetti H (2013) Motion interplay as a function of patient parameters and spot size in spot scanning proton therapy for lung cancer. Int J Radiat Oncol Biol Phys 86:380–386

Grozinger SO, Bert C, Haberer T, Kraft G, Rietzel E (2008) Motion compensation with a scanned ion beam: a technical feasibility study. Radiat Oncol 3:34

Haberer T, Becher W, Schardt D, Kraft G (1993) Magnetic scanning system for heavy-ion therapy. Nucl Instr Methods Phys Res Sect Accel Spect Detect Assoc Equip 330:296–305

Habermehl D, Debus J, Ganten T, Ganten MK, Bauer J, Brecht IC, Brons S, Haberer T, Haertig M, Jakel O, Parodi K, Welzel T, Combs SE (2013) Hypofractionated carbon ion therapy delivered with scanned ion beams for patients with hepatocellular carcinoma – feasibility and clinical response. Radiat Oncol 8:59

Hawkins RB (1996) A microdosimetric-kinetic model of cell death from exposure to ionizing radiation of any LET, with experimental and clinical applications. Int J Radiat Biol 69:739–755

Hawkins RB (2003) A microdosimetric-kinetic model for the effect of non-poisson distribution of lethal lesions on the variation of RBE with LET. Radiat Res 160:61–69

Heath E, Unkelbach J, Oelfke U (2009) Incorporating uncertainties in respiratory motion into 4D treatment plan optimization. Med Phys 36:3059

Highland VL (1975) Some practical remarks on multiple-scattering. Nucl Inst Methods 129:497–499

Hill DL, Batchelor PG, Holden M, Hawkes DJ (2001) Medical image registration. Phys Med Biol 46:R1–45

Hoisak JD, Sixel KE, Tirona R, Cheung PC, Pignol JP (2004) Correlation of lung tumor motion with external surrogate indicators of respiration. Int J Radiat Oncol Biol Phys 60:1298–1306

IAEA (2007) Dose reporting in ion beam therapy

ICRU-50 (1993) Prescribing, recording and reporting photon beam therapy. International Commission on Radiation Units and Measurements, Bethesda

ICRU-62 (1999) Prescribing, recording and eporting photon beam therapy (supplement to ICRU report 50). International Commission on Radiation Units and Measurements, Bethesda

ICRU-72 (2007) Prescribing, recording and reporting photon beam therapy (supplement to ICRU report 78). International Commission on Radiation Units and Measurements, DeLuca

Imada H, Kato H, Yasuda S, Yamada S, Yanagi T, Kishimoto R, Kandatsu S, Mizoe J-E, Kamada T, Yokosuka O, Tsujii H (2010) Comparison of efficacy and toxicity of short-course carbon ion radiotherapy for hepatocellular carcinoma depending on their proximity to the porta hepatis. Radiother Oncol 96:231–235

Imura M, Yamazaki K, Shirato H, Onimaru R, Fujino M, Shimizu S, Harada T, Ogura S, Dosaka-Akita H, Miyasaka K, Nishimura M (2005) Insertion and fixation of fiducial markers for setup and tracking of lung tumors in radiotherapy. Int J Radiat Oncol Biol Phys 63:1442–1447

Inaniwa T, Furukawa T, Nagano A, Sato S, Saotome N, Noda K, Kanai T (2009) Field-size effect of physical doses in carbon-ion scanning using range shifter plates. Med Phys 36:2889

Inaniwa T, Furukawa T, Kase Y, Matsufuji N, Toshito T, Matsumoto Y, Furusawa Y, Noda K (2010) Treatment planning for a scanned carbon beam with a modified microdosimetric kinetic model. Phys Med Biol 55:6721–6737

Inaniwa T, Furukawa T, Kanematsu N, Mori S, Mizushima K, Sato S, Toshito T, Shirai T, Noda K (2012) Evaluation of hybrid depth scanning for carbon-ion radiotherapy. Med Phys 39:2820–2825

Inaniwa T, Kanematsu N, Matsufuji N, Kanai T, Shirai T, Noda K, Tsuji H, Kamada T, Tsujii H (2015) Reformulation of a clinical-dose system for carbon-ion radiotherapy treatment planning at the National Institute of Radiological Sciences, Japan. Phys Med Biol 60:3271–3286

Jakel O (2009) Medical physics aspects of particle therapy. Radiat Prot Dosim 137:156–166

Jakel O, Karger CP, Debus J (2008) The future of heavy ion radiotherapy. Med Phys 35:5653–5663

Kanai T, Kawachi K, Kumamoto Y, ogawa H, Yamada T, Matsuzawa H, Inada T (1980) Spot scanning system for proton radiotherapy. Med Phys 7:365–369

Kanai T, Kawachi K, Matsuzawa H, Inada T (1983) Broad beam three-dimensional irradiation for proton radiotherapy. Med Phys 10:344–346

Kanai T, Endo M, Minohara S, Miyahara N, Koyama-Ito H, Tomura H, Matsufuji N, Futami Y, Fukumura A, Hiraoka T, Furusawa Y, Ando K, Suzuki M, Soga F, Kawachi K (1999) Biophysical characteristics of HIMAC clinical irradiation system for heavy-ion radiation therapy. Int J Radiat Oncol Biol Phys 44:201–210

Kanematsu N, Endo M, Futami Y, Kanai T, Asakura H, Oka H, Yusa K (2002) Treatment planning for the layer-stacking irradiation system for three-dimensional conformal heavy-ion radiotherapy. Med Phys 29:2823–2829

Kanematsu N, Matsufuji N, Kohno R, Minohara S, Kanai T (2003) A CT calibration method based on the polybinary tissue model for radiotherapy treatment planning. Phys Med Biol 48:1053–1064

Karube M, Yamamoto N, Nakajima M, Yamashita H, Nakagawa K, Miyamoto T, Tsuji H, Fujisawa T, Kamada T (2015) Single-fraction carbon-ion radiation therapy for patients 80 years of age and older with stage I non-small cell lung cancer. Int J Radiat Oncol Biol Phys

Kase Y, Kanai T, Matsumoto Y, Furusawa Y, Okamoto H, Asaba T, Sakama M, Shinoda H (2006a) Microdosimetric measurements and estimation of human cell survival for heavy-ion beams. Radiat Res 166:629–638

Kase Y, Kanematsu N, Kanai T, Matsufuji N (2006b) Biological dose calculation with Monte Carlo physics simulation for heavy-ion radiotherapy. Phys Med Biol 51:N467–N475

Kato S, Ohno T, TSUJII H, Nakano T, Mizoe JE, Kamada T, Miyamoto T, Tsuji H, Kato H, Yamada S, Kandatsu S, Yoshikawa K, Ezawa H, Suzuki M (2006) Dose escalation study of carbon ion radiotherapy for locally advanced carcinoma of the uterine cervix. Int J Radiat Oncol Biol Phys 65:388–397

Keall P (2004) 4-dimensional computed tomography imaging and treatment planning. Semin Radiat Oncol 14:81–90

Keall PJ, Starkschall G, Shukla H, Forster KM, Ortiz V, Stevens CW, Vedam SS, George R, Guerrero T, Mohan R (2004) Acquiring 4D thoracic CT scans using a multislice helical method. Phys Med Biol 49:2053–2067

Keall PJ, Mageras GS, Balter JM, Emery RS, Forster KM, Jiang SB, Kapatoes JM, Low DA, Murphy MJ, Murray BR, Ramsey CR, van Herk MB, Vedam SS, Wong JW, Yorke E (2006) The management of respiratory motion in radiation oncology report of AAPM Task Group 76. Med Phys 33:3874–3900

Kempe J, Gudowska I, Brahme A (2007) Depth absorbed dose and LET distributions of therapeutic 1H, 4He, 7Li, and 12C beams. Med Phys 34:183–192

Kiefer J, Straaten H (1986) A model of ion track structure based on classical collision dynamics. Phys Med Biol 31:1201–1209

Knopf A, Bert C, Heath E, Nill S, Kraus K, Richter D, Hug E, Pedroni E, Safai S, Albertini F, Zenklusen S, Boye D, Sohn M, Soukup M, Sobotta B, Lomax A (2010) Special report: workshop on 4D-treatment planning in actively scanned particle therapy--recommendations, technical challenges, and future research directions. Med Phys 37:4608–4614

Knopf AC, Hong TS, Lomax A (2011) Scanned proton radiotherapy for mobile targets-the effectiveness of re-scanning in the context of different treatment planning approaches and for different motion characteristics. Phys Med Biol 56:7257–7271

Knopf A-C, Boye D, Lomax A, Mori S (2013) Adequate margin definition for scanned particle therapy in the incidence of intrafractional motion. Phys Med Biol 58:6079–6094

Koch N, Liu HH, Starkschall G, Jacobson M, Forster K, Liao Z, Komaki R, Stevens CW (2004) Evaluation of internal lung motion for respiratory-gated radiotherapy using MRI: Part I–

correlating internal lung motion with skin fiducial motion. Int J Radiat Oncol Biol Phys 60:1459–1472

Korreman SS (2012) Motion in radiotherapy: photon therapy. Phys Med Biol 57:R161–R191

Kraft G (2000) Tumor therapy with heavy charged particles. Progr Particle Nucl Phys 45(Suppl 2): S473–S544

Kramer M (2001) Treatment planning for heavy-ion radiotherapy: biological optimization of multiple beam ports. J Radiat Res 42:39–46

Kusano Y, Kanai T, Yonai S, Komori M, Ikeda N, Tachikawa Y, Ito A, Uchida H (2007) Field-size dependence of doses of therapeutic carbon beams. Med Phys 34:4016–4022

Liu HH, Koch N, Starkschall G, Jacobson M, Forster K, Liao Z, Komaki R, Stevens CW (2004) Evaluation of internal lung motion for respiratory-gated radiotherapy using MRI: Part II-margin reduction of internal target volume. Int J Radiat Oncol Biol Phys 60:1473–1483

Mageras GS, Pevsner A, Yorke ED, Rosenzweig KE, Ford EC, Hertanto A, Larson SM, Lovelock DM, Erdi YE, Nehmeh SA, Humm JL, Ling CC (2004) Measurement of lung tumor motion using respiration-correlated CT. Int J Radiat Oncol Biol Phys 60:933–941

Malinen E, Sovik A (2015) Dose or 'LET'– painting – what is optimal in particle therapy of hypoxic tumors? Acta Oncol 54:1614–1622

Miyamoto T, Yamamoto N, Nishimura H, Koto M, tsujii H, Mizoe JE, Kamada T, Kato H, Yamada S, Morita S, Yoshikawa K, Kandatsu S, Fujisawa T (2003) Carbon ion radiotherapy for stage I non-small cell lung cancer. Radiother Oncol 66:127–140

Miyamoto T, Baba M, Sugane T, Nakajima M, Yashiro T, Kagei K, Hirasawa N, Sugawara T, Yamamoto N, Koto M, Ezawa H, Kadono K, Tsujii H, Mizoe JE, Yoshikawa K, Kandatsu S, Fujisawa T, Working Group for Lung C (2007) Carbon ion radiotherapy for stage I non-small cell lung cancer using a regimen of four fractions during 1 week. J Thorac Oncol 2:916–926

Mori S, Endo M, Komatsu S, Yashiro T, Kandatsu S, Baba M (2007) Four-dimensional measurement of lung tumor displacement using 256-multi-slice CT-scanner. Lung Cancer 56:59–67

Mori S, Asakura H, Kandatsu S, Kumagai M, Baba M, Endo M (2008) Magnitude of residual internal anatomy motion on heavy charged particle dose distribution in respiratory gated lung therapy. Int J Radiat Oncol Biol Phys 71:587–594

Mori S, Furukawa T, Inaniwa T, Zenklusen S, Nakao M, Shirai T, Noda K (2013) Systematic evaluation of four-dimensional hybrid depth scanning for carbon-ion lung therapy. Med Phys 40:031720

Mori S, Inaniwa T, Furukawa T, Takahashi W, Nakajima M, Shirai T, Noda K, Yasuda S, Yamamoto N (2014) Amplitude-based gated phase-controlled rescanning in carbon-ion scanning beam treatment planning under irregular breathing conditions using lung and liver 4DCTs. J Radiat Res 55:948–958

Mori S, Karube M, Shirai T, Tajiri M, Takekoshi T, Miki K, Shiraishi Y, Tanimoto K, Shibayama K, Yasuda S, Yamamoto N, Yamada S, Tsuji H, Noda K, Kamada T (2016) Carbon-ion pencil beam scanning treatment with gated markerless tumor tracking: an analysis of positional accuracy. Int J Radiat Oncol Biol Phys

Newhauser WD, Koch NC, Fontenot JD, Rosenthal SJ, Gombos DS, Fitzek MM, Mohan R (2007) Dosimetric impact of tantalum markers used in the treatment of uveal melanoma with proton beam therapy. Phys Med Biol 52:3979–3990

Ohara K, Okumura T, Akisada M, Inada T, Mori T, Yokota H, Calaguas MJ (1989) Irradiation synchronized with respiration gate. Int J Radiat Oncol Biol Phys 17:853–857

Paganetti H, Jiang H, Parodi K, Slopsema R, Engelsman M (2008) Clinical implementation of full Monte Carlo dose calculation in proton beam therapy. Phys Med Biol 53:4825–4853

Pan T, Lee TY, Rietzel E, Chen GT (2004) 4D-CT imaging of a volume influenced by respiratory motion on multi-slice CT. Med Phys 31:333–340

Pedroni E, Scheib S, Böhringer T, Coray A, Grossmann M, Lin S, Lomax A (2005) Experimental characterization and physical modelling of the dose distribution of scanned proton pencil beams. Phys Med Biol 50:541–561

Phillips MH, Pedroni E, Blattmann H, Boehringer T, Coray A, Scheib S (1992) Effects of respiratory motion on dose uniformity with a charged particle scanning method. Phys Med Biol 37:223–234

Rutherford RA, Pullan BR, Isherwood I (1976) Measurement of effective atomic number and electron density using an EMI scanner. Neuroradiology 11:15–21

Samavati N, Velec M, Brock K (2015) A hybrid biomechanical intensity based deformable image registration of lung 4DCT. Phys Med Biol 60:3359–3373

Schardt D, Elsasser T, Schulz-Ertner D (2010) Heavy-ion tumor therapy: physical and radiobiological benefits. Rev Mod Phys 82:383–425

Seco J, Robertson D, Trofimov A, Paganetti H (2009) Breathing interplay effects during proton beam scanning: simulation and statistical analysis. Phys Med Biol 54:N283–N294

Tsujii H, Kamada T (2012) A review of update clinical results of carbon ion radiotherapy. Jpn J Clin Oncol 42:670–685

Tsujii H, Kamada T, Shirai T, Noda K, Tsuji H, Karasawa K (2014) Carbon-ion radiotherapy. In: Tsujii H, Kamada T, Shirai T, Noda K, Tsuji H, Karasawa K (eds) Carbon-ion radiotherapy. Springer

Unkelbach J, oelfke U (2004) Inclusion of organ movements in IMRT treatment planning via inverse planning based on probability distributions. Phys Med Biol 49:4005–4029

Vanderstraeten B, Verstraete J, de Croock R, de Neve W, Lievens Y (2014) In search of the economic sustainability of Hadron therapy: the real cost of setting up and operating a Hadron facility. Int J Radiat Oncol Biol Phys 89:152–160

Yamamoto T, Langner U, Loo BW Jr, Shen J, Keall PJ (2008) Retrospective analysis of artifacts in four-dimensional CT images of 50 abdominal and thoracic radiotherapy patients. Int J Radiat Oncol Biol Phys 72:1250–1258

Zhang Y, Boye D, Tanner C, LOMAX AJ, Knopf A (2012) Respiratory liver motion estimation and its effect on scanned proton beam therapy. Phys Med Biol 57:1779–1795

Zietman AL (2007) The Titanic and the Iceberg: prostate proton therapy and health care economics. J Clin Oncol 25:3565–3566

Chapter 8
Computer-Assisted Treatment Planning Approaches for IMRT

Freddy Haryanto

Abstract This chapter gives an overview about the computer aided for IMRT. It will be begun with the historical of the evolution in radiotherapy techniques and then continuously with the comparison between 3DCRT and IMRT techniques. This chapter discusses the terminology in IMRT and also its techniques that are already implemented in clinical cases. This chapter will be closed with discussion about the optimization criteria that are used in IMRT.

Keywords IMRT • Terminology • Techniques • Optimization • Criteria

The purpose of radiation treatment planning system is to achieve maximum dose on the target and minimum dose on organs at risk. Based on this purpose, the development of delivery technique in radiotherapy becomes one of the important approaches. Table 8.1 shows the milestones of radiotherapy. Regarding the delivery technique in radiotherapy, there are three delivery techniques which are implemented based on the computer aid, namely, 2D, 3D conformal, and intensity-modulated radiation therapy (IMRT) techniques. Based on Table 8.1, the evolution of radiotherapy planning and delivery has changed very fast. Therefore, it brings the benefits for cancer patients, while new techniques or technologies have increased not only the probability of cure but also the efficiency of delivery. Here it can be seen that the development of computer technology always gives big impact on the evolution of radiation technique. Computer is needed not only to operate the linear accelerator but also to make better treatment plans.

Regarding the delivery techniques in radiotherapy, Fig. 8.1 shows illustrations on how the delivery techniques evolved. In the early stage, the external beams were implemented with a limited number of fields and arranged in simple ways that could be regularly repeated from case to case. The evolution on computer technologies brings also the influence into the delivery techniques in radiotherapy. In 1988, Andre Brahme had proposed a theory to modulate the fluence of beam radiation

F. Haryanto (✉)
Department of Physics, Faculty of Mathematics and Natural Sciences, Institut Teknologi Bandung, Bandung, Indonesia
e-mail: freddy@fi.itb.ac.id

H. Arimura (ed.), *Image-Based Computer-Assisted Radiation Therapy*,
DOI 10.1007/978-981-10-2945-5_8

Table 8.1 The milestones of radiotherapy

Stage	Modality	Delivery technique	Dose calculation
Early	Ortovolt – X ray	Conventional	Experiment based
Intermediate	Co – 60, low-energy Linac	2D and 3D conformal	Pencil beam
Advanced	High-energy Linac	IMRT	Pencil beam convolution
			Superposition
			Monte Carlo
			Analytical anisotropical algorithm (AAA)
			Boltzmann-based method

through the inverse method (Brahme 1988). This technique became a well-known technique which was called IMRT technique. However, the clinical implementation of this technique can be done around 12 years after Brahme's work (Webb 2005).

Nowadays, IMRT has many derivations. Regarding the radiation source, IMRT can be implemented not only for photons but also for other particles such as proton and electron. IMRT also evolves its technique with various methods. One of the new techniques has used image confirmation of the targets during treatment, namely, image-guided radiation therapy (IGRT) (Jaffray 2005). The other new technique based on the high-precision accelerated stereotactic modality is called stereotactic radiation therapy/surgery (SRT/S) (Blomgren et al. 1995; Hamilton et al. 1995). The newest delivery technique in IMRT was named intensity-modulated arc therapy (IMAT). These techniques implement rotational cone beams of varying shapes to achieve intensity modulations (Yu 1995). In this chapter, the discussion is focused only on the basic IMRT technique.

8.1 3D Conformal Radiation Therapy Versus IMRT

To understand the advantage of IMRT technique, it can be started by comparison between the 3D conformal radiation therapy (3DCRT) and IMRT (Webb 2000; Schlegel and Mahr 2001; Sternick 1997). Figure 8.2b shows that the IMRT is based on the inverse method to achieve the best dose distribution on the target. It differs from the 3DCRT which is based on forward method (Fig. 8.2a). IMRT has reformed the aims of treatment planning from the design of fields to the design of dose distributions.

IMRT also changes the paradigms in radiotherapy. Based on ICRU-50 recommendation, the dose distribution on the planning target volume (PTV) that is produced by 3DCRT should be uniformed (ICRU 50, 1993). But IMRT does not need to produce the uniform dose distribution on PTV. In the IMRT method, the ability to vary the fluence of radiation across the surface of the beam plays an important role. The IMRT technique should not produce the beams whose intensity

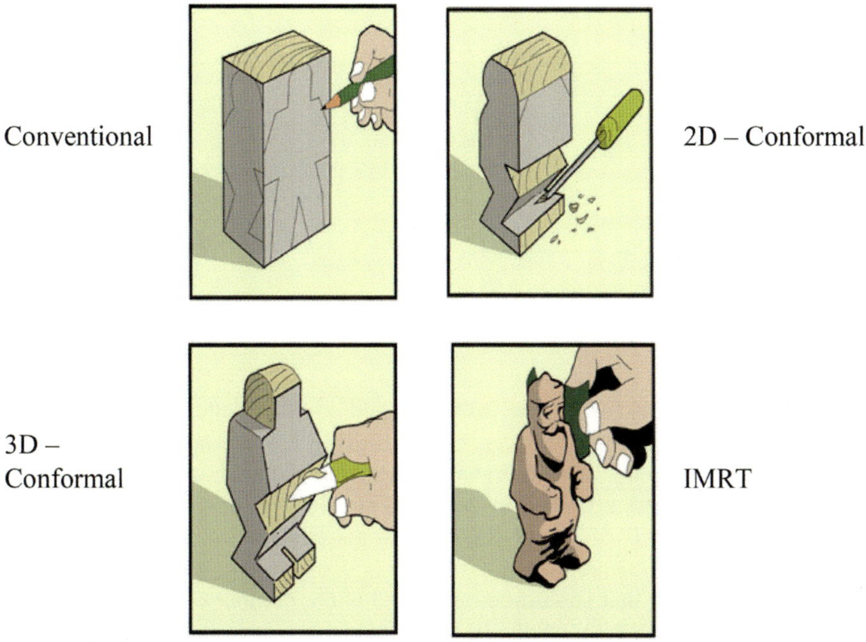

Fig. 8.1 The dose sculpting to illustrate the evolution of delivery techniques (Modified from John Schreiner 2006)

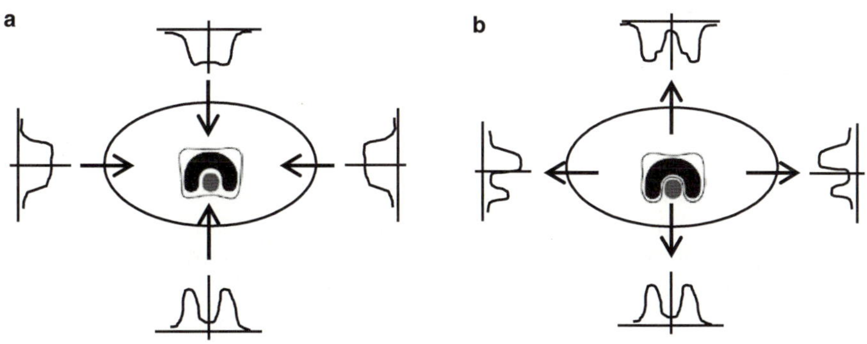

Fig. 8.2 Illustration for comparison of (**a**) 3DCRT and (**b**) IMRT (Modified from ICRU 83 2010)

is either uniform or changes uniformly, such as by the addition of a wedge filter. The other paradigm is also shifted in IMRT, namely, the dose at isocenter. In 3DCRT, the dose at isocenter should be reported but not in IMRT. The dose at isocenter in IMRT became an insignificant parameter. Table 8.2 shows the detailed comparison between the paradigms in 3DCRT and IMRT.

Table 8.2 The paradigms in 3DCRT and IMRT

	3DCRT	IMRT
Dose calculation	Forward method	Inverse method
Field composition	Simple	Complex
Region of interest (ROI)	No need to define	Target and organs at risk
Fluence distribution	Uniform	Nonuniform
Dose distribution	Uniform	High gradient
Monitor unit	Low	High

8.2 IMRT Terminology

As on the previous discussion, the IMRT method provides better dose distribution than 3DCRT method. Unfortunately, even with IMRT, it is impossible to deliver 100 % dose in target and 0 % in organs at risk. Bortfeld et al. confirmed that it is infeasible to make true inverse dose planning in IMRT. In this section, the IMRT terminology will be discussed. It is related to the physical variables that will be optimized and should be defined.

The first variable that should be optimized is the number of beams and their beam angles. Figure 8.3 shows the illustration of the number of beams and beam angles. The number of beams and beam angles depends on many factors such as anatomy, radiation tolerance, and the prescribed dose of target. Based on the image reconstruction in the CT scan, the early theoretical approaches to inverse planning assumed a very high number of coplanar beams (Brahme et al. 1982). It is related that the higher the number of beams is, the higher the dose conformation potential is. But Söderström and Brahme 1995 suggested using no more than three beams. Therefore, the question about the "optimum" number of beams in IMRT has been discussed frequently in the literature among the researchers (Brahme 1993, 1994; Mackie et al. 1994; Mohan and Ling 1995; Mohan and Wang 1996; Söderström and Brahme 1996). Regarding the optimization of orientation and the number of beams, it should be noted that the noncoplanar beams are unusually used in IMRT and the parallel-opposed beam should also be avoided (Stein et al. 1997).

In IMRT, the second variable that should be optimized is the intensity map for each beam. Usually, each beam is divided into a number of small areas which are called beam elements (bixels or beamlets). Each bixel or beamlet has a typical size of 0.5×0.5 to 1×1 cm^2, and the number of bixels or beamlets for all beams is normally in the order of 1000–10,000. Because it could be very difficult to deliver intensity-modulated beams directly with a linear accelerator (LINAC), the intensity maps are developed using a set configuration of multileaf collimator (MLC). One configuration of MLC is well known as segment. Figure 8.4 shows the illustration to understand bixels or beamlets and segments. Therefore, finding the best intensity maps is not only a high-dimensional problem in optimization but also a complex problem in "leaf sequencing." Many methods and techniques to optimize intensity

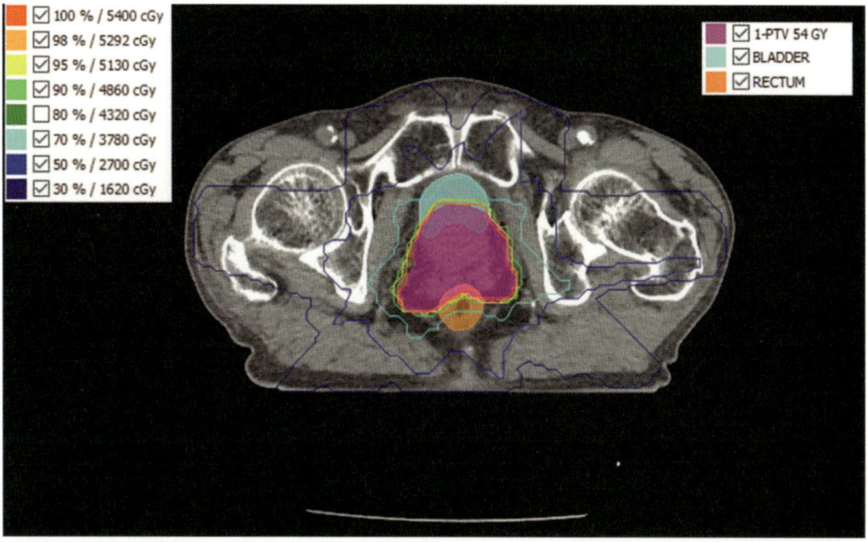

Fig. 8.3 An IMRT dose distribution for a prostate cancer from seven beam angles, namely, 25°, 85°, 129°, 180°, 223°, 275°, and 335°

maps have been developed and implemented (Cho and Marks 2000; Alber and Nüsslin 2001).

Instead of the intermediate step of using intensity maps altogether, there are two research groups that suggested to directly optimize MLC shapes (apertures) and their weights (DeNeve et al. 1996; Shepard et al. 2002). Based on the anatomy of the target or organs at risk, the MLC shapes can be generated. But the MLC shapes can be directly optimized together with the weights of the segments. The direct optimization of MLC shapes and weights becomes mathematically a difficult, non-convex problem.

The last optimization is related to the number of intensity levels. Many researchers agree that IMRT planning methods assume a continuous modulation of the intensity. But there are several researchers who have another idea to use a different approach. They suggested that promising results can be achieved "discreetly" like beam profile as well (Bortfeld et al. 1994a; Gustafsson et al. 1994; DeNeve et al. 1996). In fact, the results show no significant difference between using a moderate number of stairstep with 5–20 "intensity levels" in each beam profile and continuous modulation (Keller-Reichenbecher et al. Keller-Reichenbecher et al. 1999). Figure 8.5 shows the intensity levels that are produced by both methods. Therefore, it is unnecessary to use fully dynamic method in IMRT with MLC. To avoid the high-dose delivery to patients, IMRT can be realized in a step-and-shoot method. This method delivers the beams based on a number of static MLC-shaped segments from each direction of incidence. By this way, the total number of beam segments that is delivered is in the order of 100. Nowadays, the linac machine can implement this method automatically and quickly. More detailed

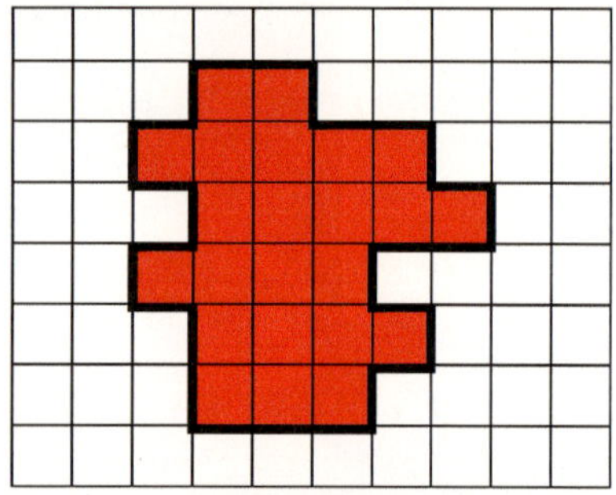

Fig. 8.4 One segment (*red* areas) consists of 23 bixels or beamlets

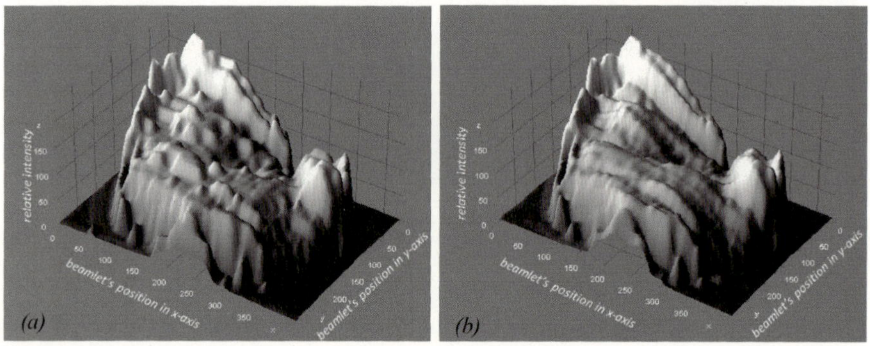

Fig. 8.5 The intensity levels based on the step-and-shoot method (**a**) and the sliding windows method (**b**)

information about the comparison of the features of dynamic versus step-and-shoot IMRT can be found in the publication from Chui et al. (2001).

8.3 Inverse Planning Techniques

After the discussion about the variables to be optimized, the inverse planning techniques became the next topic to discuss. The advantages of IMRT can only be taken into account through the implementation of these techniques. Using inverse planning, the aims of the treatments are not only the desired dose distribution but also the desired biological end points. The plan parameters which best reflect the treatment's aims are determined by optimization algorithms.

There are two well-known inverse planning techniques which are implemented in IMRT, namely, beamlet-based inverse planning and aperture-based inverse planning. The difference of both techniques is based on the treatment's variables that are optimized. Beamlet-based inverse planning begins with dividing the field into a grid of beamlets, and then the weights of these beamlets are optimized. The intensity map, which is a distribution of the beamlet's weights, is provided by the

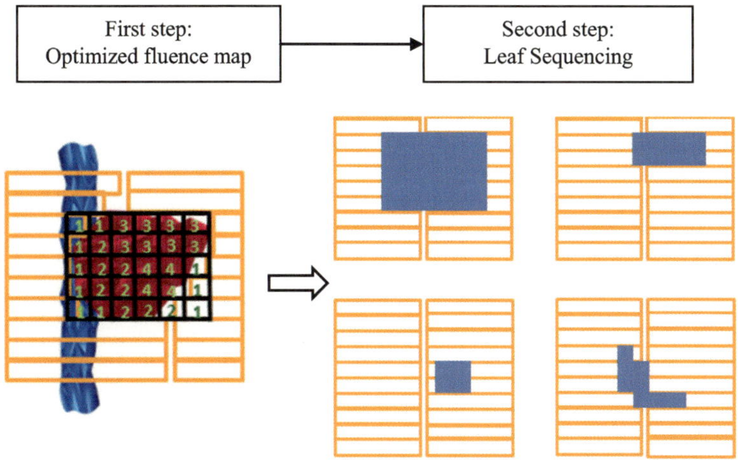

Fig. 8.6 An illustration of a two-step method on the beamlet-based inverse planning (Modified from Yu et al. 2006)

optimization. After the intensity maps are done, each intensity map is sequenced into a set of deliverable aperture shapes. Figure 8.6 shows the illustration of the two steps on the beamlet-based inverse planning. On the other hand, aperture-based inverse planning does not have the sequencing step, while a set of deliverable apertures is already included in the optimization.

Many researchers proposed beamlet-based inverse planning based on two major step approaches to produce an optimized treatment plan. In the first step, the pencil beam intensities of each beamlets are optimized (Bortfeld et al. 1994b; Chui et al. 1994; Galvin et al. 1993; Webb 1994, 1998a, b). During this process, the quality of the treatment plan is recorded based on an objective function. In the second step, this technique applied the leaf sequencing algorithm to implement each optimized intensity map into a set of deliverable beam apertures (Xia and Verhey 1998; Crooks et al. 2002; Langer et al. 2001; Saw et al. 2001; Convery and Webb 1998).

However, some problem appears from this two-step process (intensity optimization and leaf sequencing) employed in the beamlet-based inverse planning process for MLC-based IMRT. Cho et al. reported that a large number of complex field shapes lead to a loss in efficiency and an increase in collimator artifacts (Cho and Marks 2000). Some researcher tries to simplify the delivery and smoothing the intensity maps, but a loss in treatment plan quality occurred (Alber and Nüsslin 2000; Spirou et al. 2001). The other researcher used a large number of segments with a low number of monitor units (MUs) along with small off-axis fields (van Santvoort and Heijmen 1996; Webb et al. 1997). This approach not only brings new challenges for accurate dose calculation and unrealistic requirements for geometry accuracy of the MLC and dosimetric accuracy of the linear accelerator (Budgell et al. 2000; LoSasso et al. 1998) but also needs an intensively quality assurance to achieve the well-established safety and accuracy standards (LoSasso et al. 1998).

Aperture-based inverse planning is made as an inverse planning technique to solve the complexity of IMRT treatment plans. Each aperture that is considered by optimization process is determined to satisfy the delivery constraints. There is no leaf sequencing and no need to divide the final intensity maps into discrete intensity level. For this planning, there are two methods that already developed, namely, contour-based treatment planning and direct aperture optimization.

There are two approaches in contour-based treatment planning to define the aperture shapes. The first approach is based on the patient's anatomy (Xiao et al. 2000, 2003; Bednarz et al. 2002; Chen et al. 2002). Before the optimization, this approach constructed the aperture shapes based on a target and organ at risk for each beam angle from the beam's eye view (BEV). After the first aperture shape is confirmed for the target and its appropriate margin, the additional apertures are added to protect any OAR regarding the first aperture shape. Figure 8.7 demonstrates an illustration of these processes. After the dose calculation, the aperture weights are optimized. There are several algorithms, which have been performed for optimization, such as a simultaneous projection algorithm (Xiao et al. 2000), a mixed integer algorithm (Bednarz et al. 2002), and an iterative least-square algorithm (Chen et al. 2002). To produce the additional apertures, DeGersem developed an anatomy-based segmentation tool (ABST) (DeGersem et al. 2001a, b). In the second approach, isodose curves can be used to perform a contour-based treatment planning. At William Beaumont Hospital, this approach has been developed to increase the dose uniformity with tangential breast radiotherapy (Kestin et al. 2000; Remouchamps et al. 2003).

The second method, namely, direct aperture optimization (DAO), is an inverse planning technique where the aperture shapes and aperture weights are optimized simultaneously (Shepard et al. 2002). This technique is needed to specify not only the beam angles but also the number of apertures. In contrast with the contour-based planning methods described above, DAO takes account of the aperture shape as a parameter in the optimization. The optimization only considers aperture shapes that satisfy the constraints imposed by the MLC. But additional delivery considerations, such as the minimum aperture size and minimum number of monitor units (MUs), can also be included in the optimization. Before the process of optimization begins, DAO computed pencil beam dose distribution for each beam angle to increase the speed of its process. For this purpose, the rectangular MLC shape that covers the BEV of the target and its margin is used. In DAO algorithm, the beam angles, beam energies, and the number of apertures per beam angle became input parameter. The process of optimization begins to compute the objective function for the initial beam configuration. Then the leaf positions and aperture weights are to be optimized. At the end of the optimization, a final dose calculation is performed using the optimized aperture shapes and aperture weights. Then, the treatment plan is ready for delivery.

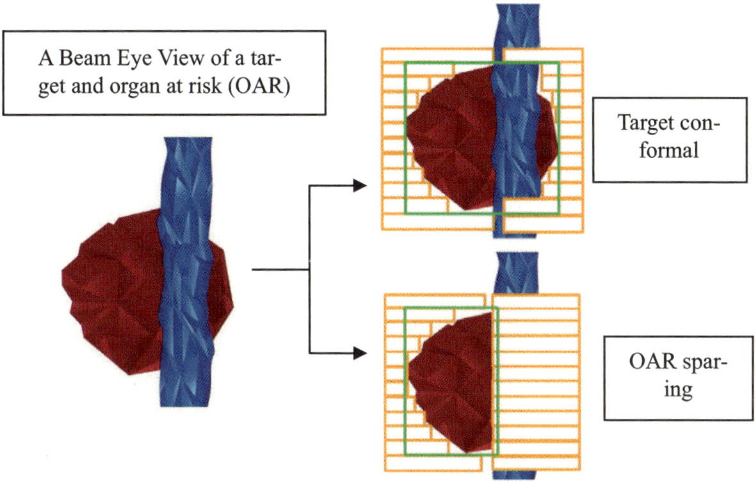

Fig. 8.7 An illustration of the processes to construct the aperture shapes based on a target and organ at risk from a beam's eye of view (BEV) (Modified from St-Hilaire et al. 2009)

8.4 Optimization Criteria

Although with IMRT it is impossible to guarantee that 100 % of the volume tumor or cancer will receive dose as it is prescribed by the doctor and 0 % of the volume of organ at risk, therefore, in this part, after the above discussion of optimization terminology and inverse planning techniques, optimization criteria will be discussed.

Regarding the optimization terminology, the optimization criteria belong to the component that is called the objective function. Beside this component, there are two other components in IMRT, namely, the driving variables and the driven variable. The driving variables are the variables that can be controlled. Beamlet or bixel of intensities of beam belongs to these variables. The other variables are the driven variable which would be changed and optimized. An example for this variable is dose distribution. Figure 8.8 shows a common flowchart of optimization algorithm.

In general, optimization criteria can be divided into physical and biological criteria (Niemierko 1992; Wang et al. 1995). All of these criteria can be taken account as constraints or objective function. As constraints, the criteria should have not over or below their limits. When the criteria act as objective, then the maximum or the minimum quantities of these criteria should be found. Physical criteria consist of the characteristic of radiotherapy dose distribution such as dose and volume of objects related to the characteristic of radiation source and geometrical object (Langer et al. 1996). Biological aspects are considered in the optimization process, if the effect of radiation on the living object is considered. There are three well-known biological criteria, namely, tumor control probability (TCP), normal

Fig. 8.8 A common flowchart of optimization algorithm

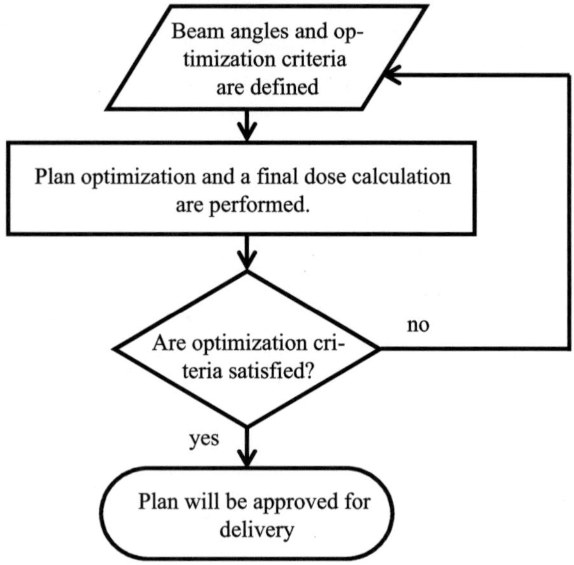

tissue complication probability (NTCP), uncomplicated TCP (UTCP), and equivalent uniform dose (EUD) (Niemierko 1999).

Generally, objective function is a function to describe the deviation from the prescribed dose. For tumor target, the objective functions can be expressed in terms of minimum dose, maximum dose, minimum dose to a given volume, maximum dose to a given volume, and uniform dose. A simple objective function for tumor target can be formulated as the following equation (Brahme 1993, 1994):

$$F_T = \sum_{k=1}^{N} \left(u_k [D_{P\min,k} - D_k]^2 + w_k [D_{P\max,k} - D_k]^2 \right) \tag{8.1}$$

where $D_{P\min,\,k}$ is the minimum prescribed dose at each voxel k and $D_{P\max,\,k}$ is the maximum prescribed dose at each voxel k. N is the number of voxels. u_k and $w_{k.}$ are the weighted factor of under- and overdose for each voxel k. Dk is the calculated dose at each voxel k, and it depends on the dose calculation that is implemented in the treatment planning system. In pencil beam convolution algorithm, as an example, the dose calculation can be expressed as the following equation (Storchi et al. 1999):

$$D(x,y,z) = \frac{(\mathrm{SSD} + z_{\mathrm{ref}})^2}{(\mathrm{SSD} + z)^2} \int_{-\infty}^{\infty} \int_{-\infty}^{\infty} I_F(u,v) I_P(u,v,z) K(x-u, y-v, z) \mathrm{d}u \mathrm{d}v \tag{8.2}$$

where SSD is the source to surface distance. $I_F(u,v)$ and $I_P(u,v,z)$ are the intensity of field and profile, respectively. K(x,y,z) is the pencil beam kernel, and z_{ref} is the reference depth that can be used for normalization.

Nowadays, there are many techniques to solve the optimization problem in IMRT. The common and easy technique is the gradient technique. In this technique, an iterative optimization is implemented, and then at every optimization step, the correction for each weighted factor is done. It is similar as a skier going down the hill into the valley (the valley represents the objective function). Therefore, this technique is also called "downhill technique." Many IMRT treatment planning systems used variations of gradient techniques for their optimization algorithm (Spirou and Chui 1998; Cotrutz et al. 2001). But many of the objective functions in radiotherapy plans contain many local minima. Therefore, alternative optimization algorithms such as simulated annealing are implemented (Langer et al. 1996; Webb 1992). These algorithms can reduce the probability that the solution is trapped in a nonoptimal local minima.

Constraints are the optimization criteria that the optimization algorithm attempts to meet. Constraints define the criteria for an acceptable solution, but they do not define an optimal solution. Generally, constraints are divided into two categories, namely, hard and soft constraints. Hard constraints must be attempted to meet by the optimization algorithm, but the soft constrains can be violated. The violation of the soft constraints will earn penalty for the constraints in the objective functions. By increasing or decreasing penalty of the constraints, the planner can control the level of "softness" of a constraint.

References

Alber M, Nüsslin F (2000) Intensity modulated photon beams subject to minimal surface smoothing constraint. Phys Med Biol 45(5):N49–N52

Alber M, Nüsslin F (2001) Optimization of intensity modulated radiotherapy under constraints for static and dynamic MLC delivery. Phys Med Biol 46(12):3229–3239

Bednarz G, Michalski D, Houser C, Huq MS, Xiao Y, Anne PR, Galvin J (2002) The use of mixed-integer programming for inverse treatment planning with pre-defined field segments. Phys Med Biol 47(13):2235–2245

Blomgren H, Lax I, Naslund I, Svanstrom R (1995) Stereotactic high dose fraction radiation therapy of extracranial tumors using an accelerator. Clinical experience of the first thirty-one patients. Acta Oncol 34:861–870

Bortfeld T, Boyer AL, Schlegel W, Kahler DL, Waldron TJ (1994a) Realization and verification of three-dimensional conformal radiotherapy with modulated fields. Int J Radiat Oncol Biol Phys 30(4):899–908

Bortfeld T, Haler DL, Waldron TJ, Boyer AL (1994b) X-ray compensation with multileaf collimators. Int J Radiat Oncol Biol Phys 28:723–739

Brahme A (1988) Optimisation of stationary and moving beam radiation therapy techniques. Radiother Oncol 12:129–140

Brahme A (1993) Optimization of radiation therapy and the development of multileaf collimation. Int J Radiat Oncol Biol Phys 25(2):373–375

Brahme A (1994) Optimization of radiation therapy. Int J Radiat Oncol Biol Phys 28(3):785–787

Brahme A, Roos JE, Lax I (1982) Solution of an integral equation encountered in rotation therapy. Phys Med Biol 27:1221–1229

Budgell GJ, Mott JHL, Williams PC, Brown KJ (2000) Requirements for leaf position accuracy for dynamic multileaf collimation. Phys Med Biol 45:1211–1227

Chen Y, Michalski D, Houser C, Galvin J (2002) A deterministic iterative least-squares algorithm for beam weight optimization in conformal radiotherapy. Phys Med Biol 47(10):1647–1658
Cho PS, Marks RJ II (2000) Hardware-sensitive optimization for intensity modulated radiotherapy. Phys Med Biol 45:429–440
Chui CS, LoSasso T, Spirou S (1994) Dose calculation for photon beams with intensity modulation generated by dynamic jaw or multileaf collimations. Med Phys 21:1237–1244
Chui CS, Chan MF, Yorke E, Spirou S, Ling CC (2001) Delivery of intensity modulated radiation therapy with a conventional multileaf collimator: comparison of dynamic and segmental methods. Med Phys 28:2441–2449
Convery DJ, Webb S (1998) Generation of discrete beam-intensity modulation by dynamic multileaf collimation under minimum leaf separation constraints. Phys Med Biol 43:2521–2538
Cotrutz C, Lahanas M, Kappas C, Baltas D (2001) A multiobjective gradient-based dose optimization algorithm for external beam conformal radiotherapy. Phys Med Biol 46(8):2161–2175
Crooks SM, McAven LF, Robinson DF, Xing L (2002) Minimizing delivery time and monitor units in static IMRT by leaf-sequencing. Phys Med Biol 47(17):3105–3116
DeGersem W, Claus F, DeWagter C, DeNeve W (2001a) An anatomy-based beam segmentation tool for intensity modulated radiation therapy and its application to head and neck cancer. Int J Radiat Oncol Biol Phys 51(3):849–859
DeGersem W, Claus F, DeWagter C, VanDuyse B, DeNeve W (2001b) Leaf position optimization for step-and-shoot IMRT. Int J Radiat Oncol Biol Phys 51(5):1371–1388
DeNeve W, DeWagter C, DeJaeger K, Thienpont M, Colle C, Derycke S, Schelfhout J (1996) Planning and delivering high doses to targets surrounding the spinal cord at the lower neck and upper mediastinal levels: static beam-segmentation technique executed with a multileaf collimator. Radiother Oncol 40(3):271–279
Galvin JM, Chen XG, Smith RM (1993) Combining multileaf fields to modulate fluence distributions. Int J Radiat Oncol Biol Phys 27:697–705
Gustafsson A, Lind BK, Brahme A (1994) A generalized pencil beam algorithm for optimization of radiation therapy. Med Phys 21(3):343–356
Hamilton A, Lulu B, Fosmire H, Stea B, Cassady J (1995) Preliminary clinical experience with linear accelerator-based spinal stereotactic radiosurgery. Technique and application. Neurosurgery 36:311–319
International Commission on Radiation Units and Measurements (ICRU) Report 50 (1993) Prescribing, recording, and reporting photon beam therapy. International Commission on Radiation Units and Measurements, Bethesda
International Commission on Radiation Units and Measurements (ICRU) Report 83 (2010) Prescribing, recording, and reporting photon beam intensity modulated radiation therapy. International Commission on Radiation Units and Measurements, Bethesda
Jaffray DA (2005) Emergent technologies for 3-dimensional image-guided radiation delivery. Semin Radiat Oncol 15:208–216
John Schreiner L (2006) Dosimetry in modern radiation therapy: Limitations and needs. J Phys Conf Ser 56:1–13
Keller-Reichenbecher MA, Bortfeld T, Levegrun S, Stein J, Prieser K, Schlegel W (1999) Intensity modulation with the 'step and shoot' technique using a commercial MLC: a planning study. Multileaf collimator. Int J Radiat Oncol Biol Phys 45:1315–1324
Kestin LL, Sharpe MB, Frazier RC, Vicini FA, Yan D, Matter RC, Martinez AA, Wong JW (2000) Intensity modulation to improve dose uniformity with tangential breast radiotherapy: initial clinical experience. Int J Radiat Oncol Biol Phys 48:1559–1568
Langer M, Morrill S, Brown R, Lee O, Lane R (1996) A comparison of mixed integer programming and fast simulated annealing for optimizing beam weights in radiation therapy. Med Phys 23:957–964
Langer M, Thai V, Papiez L (2001) Improved leaf sequencing reduces segments or monitor units needed to deliver IMRT using multileaf collimators. Med Phys 28(12):2450–2458

LoSasso T, Chui C-S, Ling CC (1998) Physical and dosimetric aspects of a multileaf collimation system used in the dynamic mode for implementing intensity modulated radiotherapy. Med Phys 25:1919–1927

Mackie R, Deasy J, Holmes T, Fowler J (1994) Optimization of radiation therapy and the development of multileaf collimation. Int J Radiat Oncol Biol Phys 28(3):784–785

Mohan R, Ling CC (1995) When becometh less more? Int J Radiat Oncol Biol Phys 33:235–237

Mohan R, Wang XH (1996) Physical vs. biological objectives for treatment plan optimization. Radiother Oncol 40:186–187

Niemierko A (1992) Random search algorithm (RONSC) for the optimization of radiation therapy with both physical and biological endpoints and constraints. Int J Radiat Oncol Biol Phys 23:89–98

Niemierko A (1999) A generalized concept of equivalent uniform dose (EUD). Med Phys 26 (6):1100

Remouchamps VM, Vicini FA, Sharpe MB, Kestin LL, Martinez AA, Wong JW (2003) Significant reductions in heart and lung doses using deep inspiration breath hold with active breathing control and intensity-modulated radiation therapy for patients treated with locoregional breast irradiation. Int J Radiat Oncol Biol Phys 55(2):392–406

Saw CB, Siochi RC, Ayyangar KM, Zhen W, Enke CA (2001) Leaf sequencing techniques for MLC-based IMRT. Med Dosim 26(2):199–204

Schlegel W, Mahr A (2001) 3D conformal radiation therapy: multimedia introduction to methods and techniques. Springer, Heidelberg (e-book)

Shepard DM, Earl MA, Li XA, Naqvi S, Yu C (2002) Direct aperture optimization: a turnkey solution for step-and-shoot IMRT. Med Phys 29(6):1007–1018

Söderström S, Brahme A (1995) What is the most suitable number of photon beam portals in coplanar radiation therapy. Int J Radiat Oncol Biol Phys 33:151–159

Söderström S, Brahme A (1996) Small is beautiful-and often enough. Int J Radiat Oncol Biol Phys 34(3):757–758

Spirou SV, Chui C-S (1998) A gradient inverse planning algorithm with dose-volume constraints. Med Phys 25:321–333

Spirou SV, Fournier-Bidoz N, Yang J, Chui CS, Ling CC (2001) Smoothing intensity-modulated beam profiles to improve the efficiency of delivery. Med Phys 28:2105–2112

Stein J, Mohan R, Wang XH, Bortfeld T, Wu Q, Preiser K, Ling CC, Schlegel W (1997) Number and orientation of beams in intensity-modulated radiation treatments. Med Phys 24(2):149–160

Sternick ES (ed) (1997) The theory and practice of intensity modulated radiation therapy. Advanced Medical Publishing, Madison

St-Hilaire J, Sévigny C, Beaulieu F, Gingras L, Tremblay D, Beaulieu L (2009) Optimization of photon beam energy in aperture-based inverse planning. J Appl Clin Med Phys 10(4):36–54

Storchi PRM, van Battum LJ, Woudsrta E (1999) Calculation of a pencil beam kernel from measured photon beam data. Phys Med Biol 44:2917–2928

van Santvoort JPC, Heijmen BJM (1996) Dynamic multileaf collimation without 'tongue and groove' underdosage effects. Phys Med Biol 41:2091–2105

Wang XH, Mohan R, Jackson A, Leibel SA, Fuks Z, Ling CC (1995) Optimization of intensity-modulated 3D conformal treatment plans based on biological indices. Radiother Oncol 37:140–152

Webb S (1992) Optimisation by simulated annealing of three-dimensional, conformal treatment planning for radiation fields defined by a multileaf collimator: 2. Inclusion of two-dimensional modulation of the x-ray intensity. Phys Med Biol 37:1689–1704

Webb S (1994) Optimizing the planning of intensity-modulated radiotherapy. Phys Med Biol 39 (12):2229–2246

Webb S (1998a) Configuration options for intensity-modulated radiation therapy using multiple static fields shaped by a multileaf collimator. II: constraints and limitations on 2D modulation. Phys Med Biol 43(6):1481–1495

Webb S (1998b) Configuration options for intensity-modulated radiation therapy using multiple static fields shaped by a multileaf collimator. Phys Med Biol 43(2):241–260

Webb S (2000) Advances in three-dimensional conformal radiation therapy physics with intensity modulation. Lancet Oncol 1:30–36

Webb S (2005) Contemporary IMRT: developing physics and clinical implementation. Institute of Physics Publishing, Bristol/Philadelphia

Webb S, Bortfeld T, Stein J, Convery D (1997) The effect of stair-step leaf transmission on the 'tongue-and-groove problem' in dynamic radiotherapy with multileaf collimator. Phys Med Biol 42:595–602

Xia P, Verhey LJ (1998) Multileaf collimator leaf sequencing algorithm for intensity modulated beams with multiple static segments. Med Phys 25:1424–1434

Xiao Y, Galvin J, Hossain M, Valenti R (2000) An optimized forward-planning technique for intensity modulated radiation therapy. Med Phys 9:2093–2099

Xiao Y, Censor Y, Michalski D, Galvin J (2003) The least-intensity feasible solution for aperture-based inverse planning in radiation therapy. Ann Oper Res 119:183–203

Yu CX (1995) Intensity-modulated arc therapy with dynamic multileaf collimation – an alternative to tomotherapy. Phys Med Biol 40(9):1435–1449

Yu CX, Shepard D, Earl M, Cao D, Luan S, Wang C, Chen DZ (2006) New developments in intensity modulated radiation therapy. Technol Cancer Res Treat 5(5):451–464

Part III
Image-Guided Patient Positioning

Chapter 9
X-Ray Image-Based Patient Positioning

Akihiro Haga

Abstract Recent progressed image-guided radiation therapy (IGRT) has improved both accuracy and precision in patient positioning. Because a setup margin considered to deliver a prescribed dose to a target becomes small, the dose for normal tissues surrounding a target can be substantially reduced or the dose for a target can be escalated as an expected complication probability of normal tissues is kept. Consequently, the X-ray imaging have played a central role in modern IGRT technologies. In this chapter, several techniques with the X-ray-based patient positioning will be introduced, including physics and mathematics regarding digitally reconstructed radiograph, cone-beam computed tomography reconstruction, and patient registration. In addition, the treatment verification will be given from the viewpoint of dose reconstruction and in-treatment X-ray imaging. In the last of this chapter, the development of a quality assurance/quality control program in IGRT system will also be described.

Keywords Image-guided radiation therapy (IGRT) • X-ray imaging • Computed tomography (CT) • Patient registration • Treatment verification

9.1 Introduction to Image-Guided Radiation Therapy (IGRT) and the Use of X-Ray Images

The progress of radiation therapy over the years has achieved an ideal dose distribution with high-dose gradients to spare the normal tissue close to the target. However, there is a concern that the steep dose gradients offered by these high-precision radiotherapies can provide a lower dose to the target and a higher dose than expected to organs at risk (OARs) in the actual delivery, if the patients and their anatomies differ from the treatment planning situation. The uncertainties arising from patient positioning, including anatomical changes, are considered as the "margin" for the target and the OARs. The dose intended for the target,

A. Haga (✉)
Department of Radiology, The University of Tokyo Hospital, 7-3-1 Hongo, Bunkyo-ku, Tokyo 113-8655, Japan
e-mail: haga-haga@umin.ac.jp

H. Arimura (ed.), *Image-Based Computer-Assisted Radiation Therapy*,
DOI 10.1007/978-981-10-2945-5_9

including the margin, is often inadvertently delivered to surrounding tissues; therefore, the achievable dose for the tumor is often compromised to spare these tissues. Intensity-modulated radiation therapy (IMRT) and its rotational version (volumetric modulated arc therapy; VMAT), combined with image-guided radiation therapy (IGRT), allow for tighter margins than conventional radiotherapy.

Three-dimensional (3D) volumetric imaging using computed tomography (CT), which is equipped in the treatment room, represents the latest development in the IGRT armamentaria (Jaffray et al. 1999; Jaffray and Siewerdsen 2000; Jaffray et al. 2002). Cone-beam CT (CBCT) imaging mounted on a linear accelerator (LINAC) is accompanied with multiple kilovoltage (kV) two-dimensional (2D) radiographs acquired by a large flat-panel detector (FPD). The CBCT was also extended to four-dimensional (4D) imaging by sorting kV radiographs from the respiratory signals of the patient before reconstruction (Sonke et al. 2005; Li et al. 2006; Dietrich et al. 2006). Using the 2D–4D information obtained immediately prior to treatment, the patient location can be corrected remotely by controlling the treatment couch, and the treatment can be quickly started. Numerous articles report the clinical utility and benefits of IGRT (Bujold et al. 2012; Van Herk 2008; Wikström et al. 2014; Barney et al. 2011; Deegan et al. 2014; Kestin et al. 2014; Zelefsky et al. 2012).

This chapter focuses on X-ray image-based IGRT. The typical IGRT process is shown in Fig. 9.1. First, treatment planning CT is performed around a week before the radiation therapy course is started. Then, the structures for the target and its surrounding OAR are delineated on the resulting image sets, and a treatment plan is created with a fiducial point that indicates the positon difference from the corresponding point of the registration image acquired immediately prior to treatment. The plan isocenter can be defined as the fiducial point to be registered in the normal LINAC, whereas, similarly to TomoTherapy®, it can be arbitrary defined within a region allowed by the system. For the patient positioning, assuming that the patient is rigid and that no structures change from the planning CT, a pair of projection images with each different angle is necessary. In this case, a reprojection 2D image of the planning CT from the corresponding angle direction is created in advance. This is called the digitally reconstructed radiograph (DRR). The DRR can be created by kV cone beams as well as treatment beams. Unlike a CBCT image, a DRR image cannot visualize the 3D volumetric image and clear anatomical structures, especially the soft tissues inside a patient body. Nevertheless, this method plays a central role in the X-ray image-based patient-positioning scheme. In the next section, the concept of the DRR is discussed, along with 3D/4D CBCT reconstruction. In Sect. 9.3, the image registration algorithm often used in the commercial IGRT system is introduced. The nonrigid registration is inapplicable to online patient positioning; therefore, it is not included here. The verification of the patient positioning is crucial for clinical practice. This gives, for example, the site-specific margin of the planning target volume (PTV) unified according to the treatment data. With such analyses, it is reported that a state-of-the-art IGRT can reduce the positioning uncertainty to the extent that a 1- to 2-mm PTV margin is often sufficient to account for this uncertainty, especially if adequate immobilization and motion management are available (Bujold et al. 2012). With adaptive

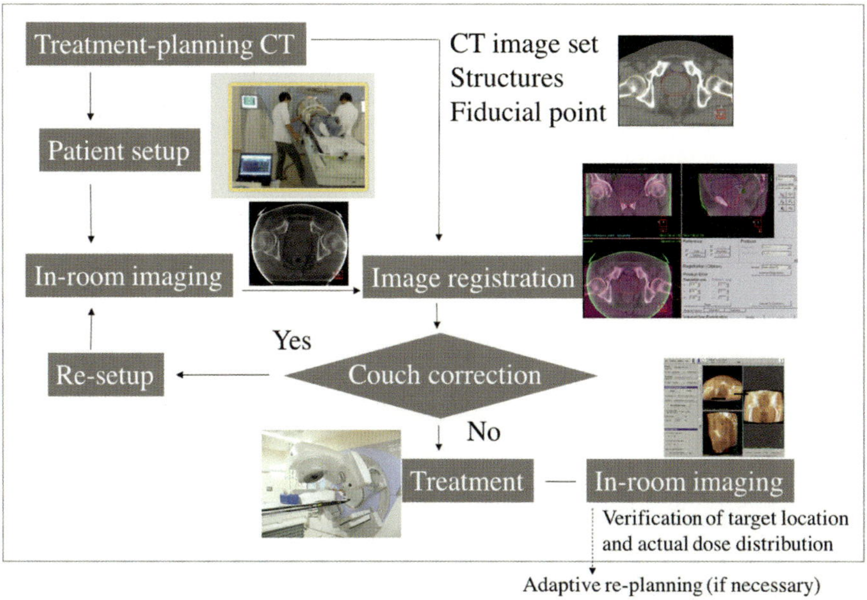

Fig. 9.1 IGRT workflow. Treatment planning CT; the structures and fiducial point of the treatment planning are included in a reference set of the image registration for in-room imaging. After the remote couch correction, the treatment is immediately started. During or immediately after the treatment, in-room imaging is performed for verification, including margin analysis. This post analysis triggers adaptive replanning. The imaging loop after the remote couch correction can be omitted with the validation of the accuracy of the remote couch correction

radiotherapy, the analysis of the actual treatment provides an opportunity to modify the margin assumed at the beginning of treatment session (Yan et al. 2000). The robust adaptive strategies must be based on multiple data sets acquired during treatment (Timmerman and Xing 2009). To fully exploit the information provided by the IGRT system used, it should be ensured that the system maintains a high performance. General issues of quality assurance (QA) and quality control (QC) for the CT-based IGRT systems are discussed toward the end of this chapter.

9.2 Image Preparation

In precise radiation therapy, the patient setup is crucial; the patient position during treatment planning CT acquisition must be reproduced during each treatment session as well as possible. The IGRT is helpful for this, providing images acquired immediately prior to treatment. The dimensionalities for the image registration in X-ray image-based IGRT are divided into the following categories (Hajnal et al. 2001).

- 2D-to-2D

If projection images with several angle directions of the X-ray cone-beam source are obtained independently in the treatment planning CT, they can be used as reference images to be registered in the treatment session. It may be necessary to use the same geometry for the acquisition of projection images as is used for the reference image or to correct for the geometrical differences. In the past, this type of registration was frequently used with X-ray simulators. However, in modern radiation therapy, the use of this registration is rare.

- 3D-to-3D

Currently, it is typical to use one or several volumetric CT images for treatment planning. The CT images can be obtained by the standard equipment of the radiation therapy system immediately prior to treatment (kV/MV CBCT, fan-beam MVCT, CT-on-rail, etc.). In clinical applications, CT images offer a distinct advantage over projection images in that they allow the direct imaging of soft tissue structures. Even for prostate cancer, which is not directly targeted with projection imaging without implanted fiducial markers, the patient positioning can be performed flexibly with 3D-to-3D registration around the target area while viewing the rectal gases and/or bladder size and shape for both the treatment planning CT and the registration one.

- 3D/4D-to-4D

Especially for stereotactic body radiotherapy (SBRT) of the lung and liver, 4D CT imaging is indispensable for target delineation in treatment planning. With the requirement of the imaging of the target motion in the registration, 4D CBCT has been utilized in IGRT systems. In the currently available IGRT tool, 4D CBCT is registered into one 3D CT out of the treatment planning 4D CT set or the averaged 3D CT. The operator verifies that the target trajectory is covered by the PTV, which includes the consideration of the motion in the treatment plan, and then the treatment is started. In principle, 4D-to-4D registration is possible; however, it is not practically implemented, because of reasons including its ineffectiveness.

- 3D/4D-to-2D

This case may be required for establishing a correspondence between 3D/4D volumes used for treatment planning and projection images acquired for IGRT. In this case, the DRRs are created from 3D/4D CT in advance and used in the patient registration as reference images to register acquired projection images with the same angle views. This type of registration has a drawback: it can reproduce only skeletal features without implanted fiducial markers. However, some radiation machines provide a real-time monitoring function for motion tracking using the projection images acquired during treatment beam delivery.

All modern IGRT technologies using X-ray images are based on projection images (and corresponding DRRs) and/or CT reconstructed from projection data.

In the following subsections, the physics and principles of the DRR and CT reconstruction are described.

9.2.1 DRR

In modern radiation therapy, the DRR technique is predominantly used in image-guidance systems to monitor the patient setup during clinical routines. The geometrical accuracy of the patient setup is guaranteed by superimposing a portal image of a megavoltage (MV) treatment beam or kV projection image acquired immediately prior to treatment onto the corresponding DRR created in the treatment planning. Thus, the common anatomical features on both images must be matched after the image registration. In this registration, various metrics, such as the least mean squares of the intensity difference, the normal cross correlation, and mutual information, can be employed. Each metric has advantages and disadvantages. Even if a metric is employed, the contrast mismatch between the portal image and the DRR affects the registration accuracy. Therefore, the generation of the DRR should be as realistic as possible, according to the fundamental physical process of the X-ray quanta (Staub and Murphy 2013).

The basic component of a DRR generation model is ray tracing with information on the linear attenuation coefficient from CT images. The observed projection in a detector element at a certain projection angle, y_i, is related to the corresponding photon count n_i as follows:

$$n_i = n_0 e^{-y_i}, \qquad i = 1, 2, \ldots, M. \tag{9.1}$$

Here, M is the number of total projection elements given by the pixel number of the detector, and n_0 is the constant photon number generated in the X-ray source. Assuming a monoenergetic spectrum in the X-ray beam, the relationship between the linear attenuation coefficient and the projection is linear, and the projection y_i can be evaluated by performing a line integral of the linear attenuation coefficient distribution $\mu(\boldsymbol{x})$ in 3D space vector $\boldsymbol{x}$, along with a line between the X-ray source and the detector element i, as follows:

$$y_i = \ln(n_0/n_i) = \int da\, \mu(\boldsymbol{x}) \sim \sum_j \Delta a_{ij}\mu_j, \quad i = 1, \cdots, M. \tag{9.2}$$

where the variable da is taken along with this line. The integration is approximately expressed by the summation of $\Delta a_{ij}\mu_j$ over j, which means the sampling point in the line, with the fact that Δa_{ij} is sufficiently small. The step size Δa_{ij} could be constant, but, with the use of CT voxels, it would be more efficient to calculate it analytically from the coordinates of X-ray source and detector element i. A schematic illustration is shown in Fig. 9.2, where μ_j and Δa_{ij} are the line attenuation coefficient and

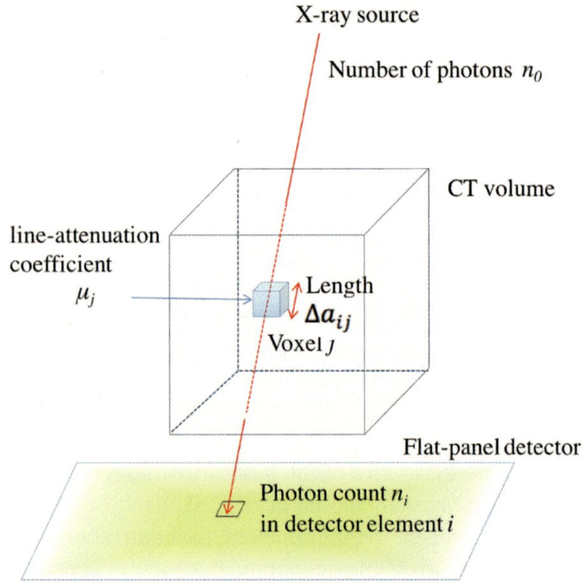

Fig. 9.2 Schematic of ray tracing with information about the attenuation coefficient from CT images

the length of the photon (which dives into the detector element i) trace in the voxel j, respectively. Although μ_j is converted from Hounsfield units (HUs) in CT, the X-ray energy in the IGRT system can differ from that in the treatment planning CT, and this conversion is possibly necessary. Here, the geometrical uncertainty of the X-ray source and detectors must be avoided. Uncertainty may arise with the use of an onboard FPD; therefore, the geometrical shift values should be measured in a QA/QC program and recorded for the correction for clinical imaging. This is one of the simplest ways to create a realistic DRR image.

The projection y_i can be influenced by additional physical effects. One such effect is the scattering, which is considerably large for FPDs in cone-beam projections. There are various methods for estimating the scattering, including experimental (e.g., beam stop arrays (Ning et al. 2004; Siewerdsen et al. 2004; Schörner et al. 2011; Zhu et al. 2009)), theoretical (e.g., scatter kernel methods (Yao and Leszczynski 2009a, b; Zhao et al. 2015), and Monte Carlo simulation (Zbijewski et al. 2006; Jarry et al. 2006) methods, as well as combinations of these. Another important effect influencing projections is beam hardening (Hsieh et al. 2000; Grimmer et al. 2009). In Eq. (9.2), a monoenergetic spectrum was assumed for an X-ray beam, but, the actual X-ray spectra are polyenergetic. As the X-ray passes deeply through the body of the patient, the spectrum becomes "hard" owing to the large cross sections for low X-ray energy. The scatter and beam-hardening corrections are discussed in the next subsection, where a simple correction method for CBCT reconstruction is introduced.

The other effects are relatively unimportant, but a rigorous reproduction requires them. One representative challenge for a realistic DRR is the consideration of the X-ray absorption due to the treatment couch, if a different couch is used in the treatment planning CT system. This attenuation is considered by inserting the virtual treatment couch. Other effects, such as veiling glare and signal leakage, can be considered in the DRR creation (Staub and Murphy 2013).

9.2.2 *CBCT*

Since it was introduced by Jaffray et al., the CBCT system has taken on a very important role in IGRT (Jaffray et al. 2002; Dawson and Jaffray 2007; Létourneau et al. 2005; Boda-Heggemann et al. 2011). Figure 9.3 shows a typical cone-beam X-ray imaging system, which consists of a kV X-ray tube and an FPD unit perpendicular to the treatment MV beam, mounted on a LINAC gantry. Volumetric images can be reconstructed from 2D projection images on the FPD with a half rotation + fan angle range. Before the introduction of the CBCT imaging system, orthogonal pairs of portal images of the posterior–anterior and lateral directions using portal films or electric portal imaging devices (EPIDs) played the main role in the patient setup workflow (Mongioj et al. 2011; Birkner et al. 2007; Hawkins et al. 2011). In contrast, CBCT visualizes the anatomical information (shapes and locations) inside the body with a high contrast. After the in-room CBCT system was established, the accuracy of patient setup, i.e., the accuracy of dose delivery, drastically improved (Bujold et al. 2012).

In this subsection, the basic formalism of the CBCT reconstruction using an FPD is briefly introduced, but it can be easily extended to fan-beam CT and other geometrical cases. Further details are provided in the literature (Kak and Slaney 2001; Buzug 2008). First, we consider a parallel X-ray beam. As shown in Fig. 9.4, a projection $P(\theta, p)$ measured in the detectors aligned perpendicularly to the X-ray direction, p, in the projection angle θ, is expressed as

$$P(\theta, p) = \int dxdy \;\; f(x, y)\delta(x\cos\theta + y\sin\theta - p), \tag{9.3}$$

where $\delta(x)$ is the Dirac delta function, i.e., the line integral of the photon path, and $f(x, y)$ is the 2D image of an object. The range of the integral for (x, y) is obvious—from the X-ray source to each detector element—and is therefore omitted throughout this chapter.

Equation (9.3) can be transformed as

$$f(x, y) = \int d\theta dp \;\; P(\theta, p)h(x\cos\theta + y\sin\theta - p), \tag{9.4}$$

where the integral range regarding projection angle θ is $[0, \pi]$ and the kernel function $h(x\cos\theta + y\sin\theta - p)$ is defined as

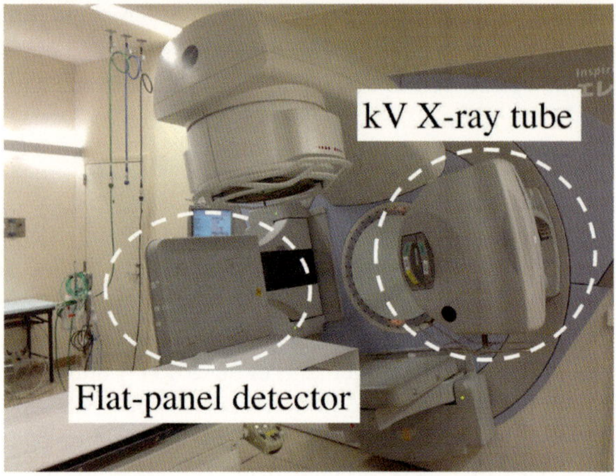

Fig. 9.3 CBCT system mounted on the LINAC (Elekta Synergy system)

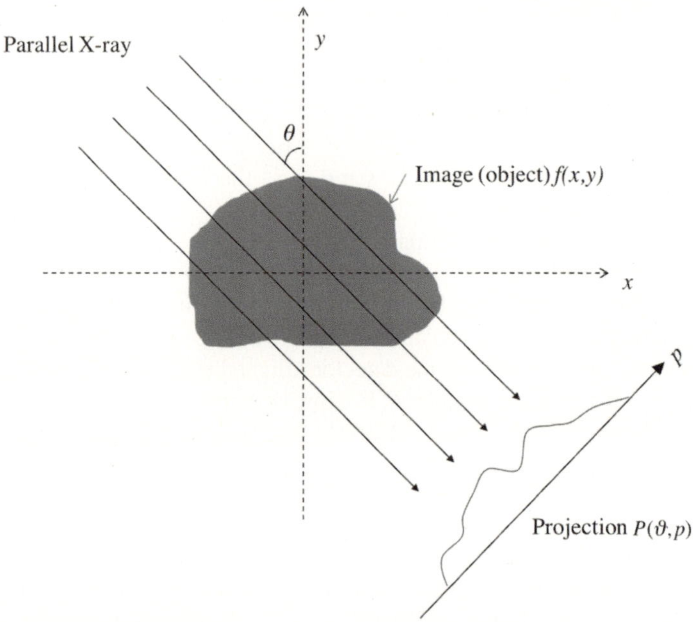

Fig. 9.4 Geometry of a CT reconstruction using a parallel X-ray beam

$$h(x\cos\theta + y\sin\theta - p) = \int_{-\infty}^{+\infty} d\omega|\omega|e^{i\omega(x\cos\theta+y\sin\theta-p)}. \tag{9.5}$$

Equation (9.4) can be ascertained by multiplying both sides of Eq. (9.3) by $h(x' \cos\theta + y' \sin\theta - p)$ and integrating them with respect to p, obtaining

$$\int dp\ \ P(\theta,p)h(x^{'}\cos\theta+y^{'}\sin\theta-p)=\int dxdy\ \ f(x,y) \\ \times\ \ h(x^{'}\cos\theta+y^{'}\sin\theta-(x\cos\theta+y\sin\theta)). \tag{9.6}$$

Then, integrating the projection angle θ over the range of $[0, \pi]$ yields Eq. (9.4), where the relation

$$\begin{aligned}&\int_0^{\pi} d\theta\ \ h(x^{'}\cos\theta+y^{'}\sin\theta-(x\cos\theta+y\sin\theta))\\ &=\int_0^{2\pi} d\theta \int_0^{+\infty} d\omega|\omega|e^{i\omega\cos\theta(x^{'}-x)+i\omega\sin\theta(y^{'}-y)}=\int_{-\infty}^{+\infty} dudv\ \ e^{iu(x^{'}-x)+iv(y^{'}-y)}\\ &=\delta(x^{'}-x)\delta(y^{'}-y)\end{aligned} \tag{9.7}$$

is used (here, $u = |\omega| \cos\theta$ and $v = |\omega| \sin\theta$).

The image $f(x, y)$ is reconstructed by the convolution integral of the kernel h with the projection. Assuming a monoenergetic X-ray, the relation of the attenuation coefficient $\mu(x, y)$ in the object to observed photons is given as,

$$n(\theta,p)=n_0\exp\left[-\int dxdy\ \mu(x,y)\delta(x\cos\theta+y\sin\theta-p)\right] \tag{9.8}$$

or

$$y(\theta,p)=\ln\left(n_0/n(\theta,p)\right)=\int dxdy\ \ \mu(x,y)\delta(x\cos\theta+y\sin\theta-p). \tag{9.9}$$

Here, n_0 and $n(\theta, p)$ are the numbers of photon generated in the X-ray source and detected by the detector with (θ, p), respectively. A comparison with Eq. (9.3) reveals that the reconstructed image $f(x, y)$ corresponds to $\mu(x, y)$ when $y(\theta, p) = \ln(n_0/n(\theta, p))$ is used as $P(\theta, p)$.

The reconstruction formula for a parallel beam can be easily extended to a fan beam with a line-detector geometry. As exhibited by the geometry shown in Fig. 9.5, the projection of the off-axis beam SP is regarded as $P(\theta, p')$ in the parallel-beam geometry. Therefore, the reconstruction formula can be represented as

$$f(x,y)=\int d\theta dp' P\left(\theta,p^{'}\right)h(x\cos\theta+y\sin\theta-p'), \tag{9.10}$$

where

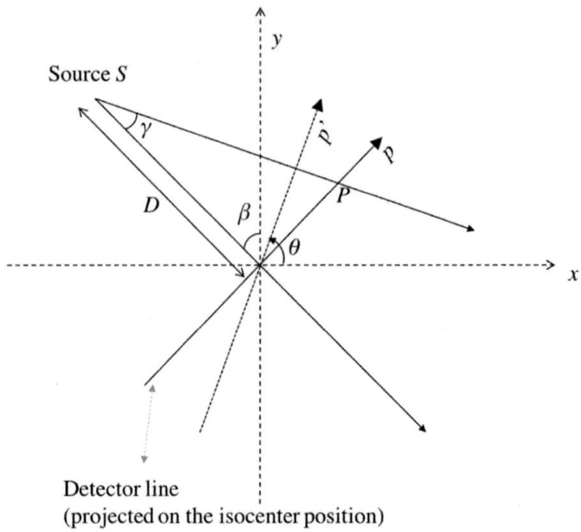

Fig. 9.5 Geometry for a fan-beam CT reconstruction, where γ is the fan angle, and β is regarded as the source angle instead of θ

$$\theta = \beta + \gamma, \qquad p^{'} = p\cos\gamma = p\frac{D}{\sqrt{D^2 + p^2}} \quad . \tag{9.11}$$

By replacing the integrating variables θ and p' with β and p, respectively, we obtain

$$f(x,y) = \int d\beta \frac{D^2}{(D-s)^2} \int dp \mathcal{R}(\beta,p) \frac{D}{\sqrt{D^2+p^2}} h\left(\frac{Dt}{D-s} - p\right), \tag{9.12}$$

where $s = -x\sin\beta + y\cos\beta$, $t = x\cos\beta + y\sin\beta$, and the projection in the fan-beam geometry is expressed as $\mathcal{R}(\beta,p)$.

Now, the formula for CBCT reconstruction with an FPD can be obtained by extending the aforementioned fan-beam CT reconstruction formula. The modifications are the distance from the source to the reconstruction points on the plane perpendicular to the s-axis ($D^2+p^2 \rightarrow D^2+p^2+\zeta^2$), and the projection $\mathcal{R}(\beta,p,\zeta)$ depends on the z-axis through ζ (see Fig. 9.6):

$$f(x,y,z) = \int d\beta \frac{D^2}{(D-s)^2} \times \int dp \mathcal{R}(\beta,p,\zeta) \frac{D}{\sqrt{D^2+p^2+\zeta^2}} h\left(\frac{Dt}{D-s} - p\right). \tag{9.13}$$

This is the final expression for the CBCT reconstruction. If ζ is fixed, the sinogram required in the reconstruction on the cone-beam projection $\mathcal{R}(\beta,p,\zeta)$ is a line with v in the FPD corresponding to ζ. For instance, this formula reproduces the fan-beam

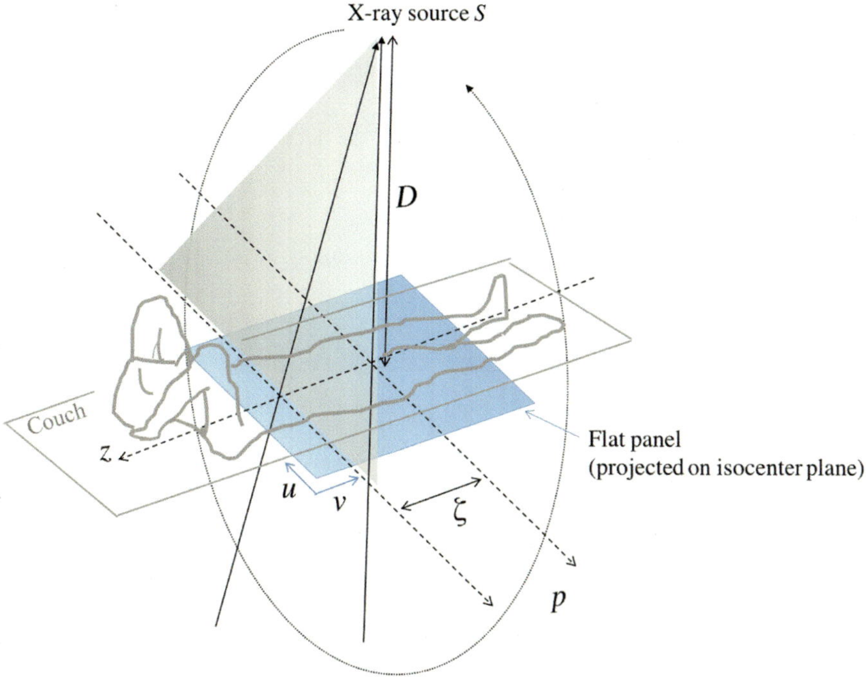

Fig. 9.6 Geometry for a CBCT reconstruction, where (u, v) constructs an FPD plane with its intrinsic coordinates. This corresponds to the representation using (p, ζ)

reconstruction formula (Eq. (9.12) at $\zeta = 0$, where the sinogram is constructed from the projection lines in the middle of the v-axis.

In an actual computation, the aforementioned integration is replaced by a summation. In the case of slow gantry rotation, the summation of the angle β can be performed during the rotation. Therefore, the reconstruction is processed during the acquisition of the projection data, allowing the rapid reconstruction of volumetric images.

Well-known artifacts are observed in the LINAC-mounted CBCT reconstruction image. One of them is a "cupping artifact," which is caused by several factors, the most dominant being the scattering of the X-ray for CBCT reconstruction using an FPD. Because of the photons scattered by the human body, *the X-ray intensity measured in each pixel of the FPD becomes higher than that expected without scattering*. This is more serious for the pixel in which the photon passes through the long range of highly dense materials. The CBCT formula described here does not consider any scattered photons. Therefore, when Eq. (9.13) is used in the reconstruction, the strategy of the correction is to remove the scattered photons in the measured projections. Although there are various methods for estimating the CBCT scattering, including beam stop aperture/moving blockers, scatter kernel models, and Monte Carlo simulation, one of the simplest methods is to multiply the detector count $n(\theta, p)$ by a factor κ $(0 < \kappa \leq 1)$. Then, the corrected projection is obtained as

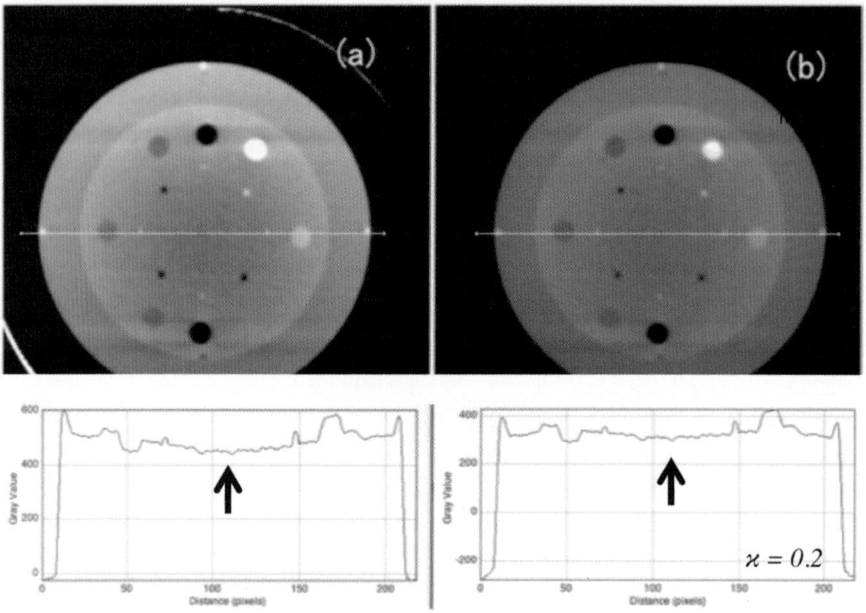

Fig. 9.7 Reduction of the cupping artifact: (**a**) no correction and (**b**) correction with $\kappa = 0.2$ in Eq. (9.14). The *bottom frames* show the profiles corresponding to the *yellow lines* in the top images

$$y_{\mathrm{corr}}(\theta, p) = \ln(n_0/\kappa n(\theta, p)). \tag{9.14}$$

This means that the number of scattered photons in the detector decreases depending on the photon number. Thus, this factor can be used to correct the measured X-ray intensity, which is higher than that predicted with no photon scattering.

Figure 9.7 shows the effectiveness of this simple correction. Here, the cupping artifact shown in Fig. 9.7 (a) is visually corrected as shown in Fig. 9.7 (b). The center gray value profiles support this.

The beam-hardening effect may also yield a cupping artifact. The attenuation of an X-ray passing through the same tissue depends on the length of the path, owing to the change of the X-ray spectrum. Because a low-energy (soft) X-ray is attenuated more than a high-energy (hard) one, the magnitude of attenuation coefficient decreases as the path length increases. Thus, *without beam-hardening correction, the measured X-ray intensity is always higher than the expected one*. This also occurs in the case of scattering. The scattering and hardening of X-rays have similar influences on the projection image. Therefore, Eq. (9.14) can also be used for the correction of beam hardening. Of course, the physics differ between the two effects, and more quantitative corrections should be performed for both. There is a considerable amount of literature concerning beam hardening (Herman 1979; Nalcioglu and Lou 1979; Search et al. 1985; Hsieh et al. 2000; Ct et al. 2015).

Radar artifacts resulting from image lag are the other type of artifact commonly observed in CBCT. Image lag is defined as a residual signal present in image frames subsequent to the frame in which the residual signal is generated. The effect called "ghosting" (Mail et al. 2007) is similar to image lag and refers to the change in the detector pixel sensitivity as a long-term effect. Correction methods for image lag have been proposed in the literature. One of the practical methods is to subtract from the current projection frame previous frames weighted by a temporal response function (Mail et al. 2008). The reduction of the X-ray exposure on the detector using a "bow-tie filter" can be effective because the image lag depends on the X-ray intensity.

The geometrical uncertainty of the FPD, as well as the X-ray source during gantry rotation, causes the blurring of the reconstructed image. The distance between the center of the FPD and the projected point of the object pin located on the beam isocenter must be recorded for all projection angles, and it should be applied to correct the coordinates of the detector position or projection image. This is known as "flexmap correction" (Jaffray et al. 2002), and an example is shown in Fig. 9.8. Flexmap correction not only removes the blurring but also aligns the resulting image with the beam isocenter.

9.2.3 4D CBCT

For periodic motions such as breathing or a heartbeat, motion-correlated CBCT images can be reconstructed by dividing projection images into several phase bins according to the motion signal (see Fig. 9.9). This technique is called "4D CBCT" and consists of four dimensions, including space (3D) as well as time. The 4D CBCT technique is widely utilized in IGRT, especially for SBRT requiring a more careful patient setup than the conventional treatment.

There are several conditions to implement a 4D CBCT reconstruction. The most important condition is the stability, i.e., the reproducibility, of periodic breathing. Generally, in 4D CBCT acquisition using an IGRT system, it takes several minutes to acquire a sufficient number of projections, which are classified into respective phases, owing to the slow gantry rotation. This means that the projection images in a certain phase are acquired at different moments. Therefore, breathing stability is required to correctly reconstruct images, including the location and shape of tumor and the surrounding normal tissues, for each phase. This type of 4D CBCT is regarded as "averaged" 4D CBCT because the projections in each phase are collected over several minutes. Notably, this does not reflect temporary motions such as a cough or sneeze. On the other hand, *real-time* 4D CBCT reconstruction techniques, including an approach for nonperiodic time-ordered motions, are under investigation. Hereafter, we focus on the periodic motion.

The acquisition time for the projection images in 4D CBCT is relatively long with a slow gantry rotation (typically 3–4 min) compared with normal 3D CBCT acquisition (1–2 min). This is because if the normal gantry rotation speed is used,

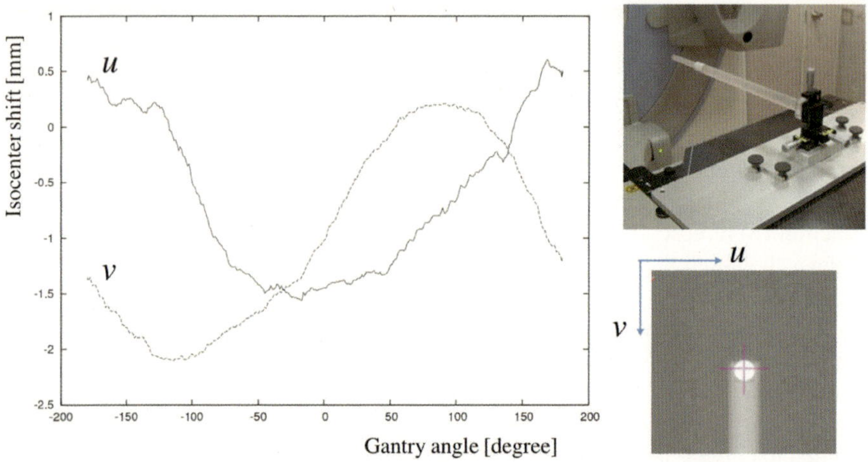

Fig. 9.8 Flexmap (*left*), which is a plot of the distance between the center of the FPD and the projected point of the object center located on the beam isocenter (*top and bottom right*)

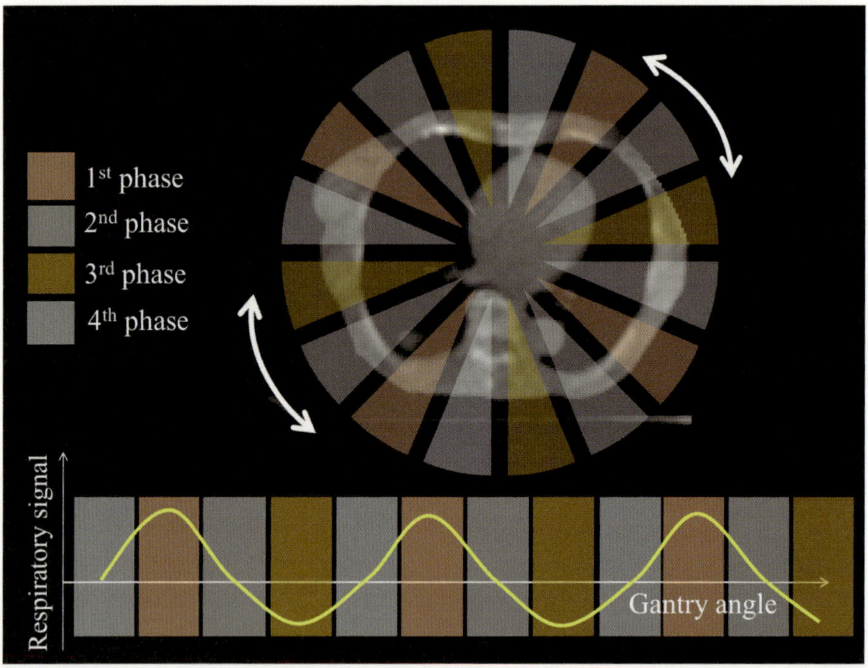

Fig. 9.9 Phase-sorting concept for motion-correlated 4D CBCT reconstruction. A certain phase of CT is reconstructed by only using the projections with the same phase bin (*upper*), which are classified by respiratory-signal analysis (*bottom*)

the gantry-angle gap between the projection images becomes large in each phase bin, depending on the respiratory-cycle period, where the relationship between the gantry-angle gap (phase) $\Delta\theta$ [degrees] and the gantry rotation speed (angular velocity) v_{gan} [degree/s] is

$$\Delta\theta = R_{\mathrm{cycle}} v_{\mathrm{gan}}. \tag{9.15}$$

Here, R_{cycle} [s] is the respiratory-cycle period. For example, in the condition of $R_{\mathrm{cycle}} = 3$ s and 60 s for 360° rotation ($v_{\mathrm{gan}} = 6$ [degree/s]), the gantry-angle gap $\Delta\theta$ is 18°. On the other hand, the typical gantry-angle gap for normal 3D CBCT is 0.5°–1.0°, assuming that the signal-acquisition interval of the FPD is 0.2 s. Such a large gantry-angle gap in acquiring projections for 4D CBCT yields a severe streak artifact in the reconstructed image. Thus, for the improvement of the image quality, the adaptation of slow gantry rotation is simple and effective.

Controlling the patient breathing can also reduce the artifacts. There are forced and unforced methods for this. Among the former, external breathing control is a representative example (Wong et al. 1999). This is performed with two pairs of flow monitors and scissor valves, by using one of each to control the inspiration and expiration paths to the patient through a mouthpiece. Among the latter methods, rhythmical sounds (e.g., metronome) or visual indications (e.g., Abches device) can be useful (Matsuo et al. 2013). Breath control is advantageous for 4D CBCT imaging, to reduce not only streak artifacts but also the blurring by stabilizing the breathing depth and cycle.

The 4D CBCT reconstruction method is based on the phase classification of acquired projections. Here, the knowledge of the respiratory phase during kV imaging plays a key role. There are several methods for measuring a respiratory signal synchronized with image acquisition, for example, external respiratory monitoring and real-time position management (Dietrich et al. 2006; Lu et al. 2007). Additionally, the utility of extracting respiratory signals using kV radiographs by monitoring the trajectory of a radio-opaque fiducial marker was reported (Li et al. 2006). Image-processing algorithms for projections obtained without external devices have been proposed by some groups. One such method is the "Amsterdam Shroud" (Fig. 9.10), which projects edge-enhanced projection images perpendicular to the axis of gantry rotation, leaving one-dimensional (1D) information in the cranio-caudal direction (Zijp et al. 2004). The advantage of the image-based recognition technique is that the respiratory signal can be detected with a high efficiency without an external system that synchronizes with projection images. The Amsterdam Shroud method was employed with the Elekta XVI system. Other methods are available, and respiratory-signal acquisition using the normal cross correlation with a limited area of projections was adapted to *in-treatment* 4D CBCT reconstruction performed during rotational treatment (Kida et al. 2012).

There are few methods for 4D CBCT reconstruction for nonperiodic motion. Nevertheless, a recent development of reconstruction methodology with compressive sensing (Donoho 2006) enables us to reconstruct images with a limited

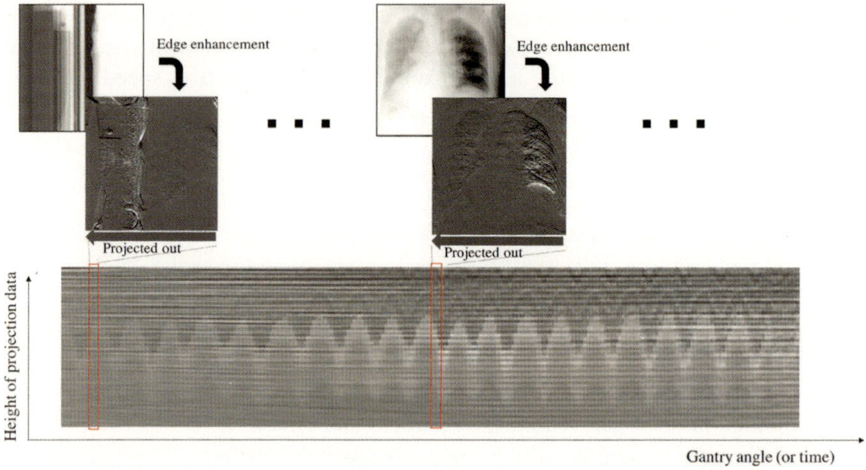

Fig. 9.10 Amsterdam Shroud method for deriving a respiratory signal. This method first projects edge-enhanced projection (such as a logarithm operation with a Sobel filter) images perpendicular to the axis of gantry rotation, leaving 1D information in the cranio-caudal direction, and then sorts them with respect to the gantry angle (or time)

projection range. The prior image constrained compressive sensing (PICCS) method (Chen et al. 2008) and, more recently, a reconstruction method based on the chain-graph model (Nakano 2016) were proposed for slow-gantry-scan CBCT systems. An iterative reconstruction framework is needed for these methods, which requires a large computational cost. Therefore, the utility of this type of 4D CBCT is limited. It is suitable not for online patient registration but for post analysis, including margin analysis and dose verification.

9.3 Image Registration

Image registration is an essential part of IGRT. The patient positioning is performed by acquiring an image set (2D projection, 3D or 4D CBCT image, etc.), while the patient is in the posture in which he/she undergoes the treatment and by shifting a moveable treatment couch according to a value indicated by the image registration between planning CT (or its DRR) and the acquired image.

An image registration system for IGRT requires a comprehensive database to ensure that the patient positioning matches that of the treatment plan. Treatment planning CT, structure set, and isocenter (or some reference point) information are commonly necessary in modern IGRT systems. With treatment planning CT and its isocenter location, the absolute value of the couch correction is calculated on the basis of the image registration. Displaying the structures enables the visual verification of this match.

A state-of-the-art treatment couch can move with six degrees of freedom (DOFs)—three translational and three rotational—but this is usually optional. Couches with three DOFs—for translation only—are widely installed for various reasons, including cost reduction. Nevertheless, we consider a six-DOF couch because it includes the functions of a three-DOF couch with no rotation. A 3D space vector $\boldsymbol{x}$ is then transformed into $\boldsymbol{x}_T$ as

$$\boldsymbol{x}_T = R\boldsymbol{x} + \boldsymbol{t}, \tag{9.16}$$

where R and $\boldsymbol{t}$ are the rotation matrix and the translation vector, respectively. The rotation matrix can be expressed using the Euler angle (α, β, γ) as

$$\begin{aligned} R &= R_{z''} R_{y'} R_z \\ &= \begin{pmatrix} \cos\gamma & \sin\gamma & 0 \\ -\sin\gamma & \cos\gamma & 0 \\ 0 & 0 & 1 \end{pmatrix} \begin{pmatrix} \cos\beta & 0 & -\sin\beta \\ 0 & 1 & 0 \\ \sin\beta & 0 & \cos\beta \end{pmatrix} \begin{pmatrix} \cos\alpha & \sin\alpha & 0 \\ -\sin\alpha & \cos\alpha & 0 \\ 0 & 0 & 1 \end{pmatrix}, \end{aligned} \tag{9.17}$$

where α, β, and γ represent rotations about the original z-axis, the new y-axis (y'), and the final z-axis (z''), respectively (Fig. 9.11). This is one representation of the Euler rotation; a different representation can be employed without any change in the physics. On the other hand, the translation vector is given as

$$\boldsymbol{t} = \begin{pmatrix} t_x \\ t_y \\ t_z \end{pmatrix}. \tag{9.18}$$

This type of transformation, which cannot include any scale change or deformation of the space, is called a "rigid transformation." A rigid registration is only meaningful for online patient positioning, owing to the limitations of transformation by couch movement.

A rigid transformation has six variables $\{\alpha, \beta, \gamma, t_x, t_y, t_z\}$. Once these variables (i.e., R and $\boldsymbol{t}$) are known, the patient positioning can be performed. The variables R and $\boldsymbol{t}$ are given by the image registration via optimization. The term "optimization" implies the minimization (or maximization) of a cost function (or objective function) by tuning the six variables. In general, a "similarity measure" is employed as the cost function. Thus, this process is conducted by decreasing the similarity measure by taking the derivative of the variables in the iteration step. As an example of a similarity measure, we consider a least-squares measure. Suppose that an image $\boldsymbol{I}_T = \psi(\boldsymbol{I})$ is a transformed CBCT set to be registered with a reference image $\boldsymbol{I}_R$, which is a treatment planning CT set. Then, the least-squares measure F_{LS} is given as

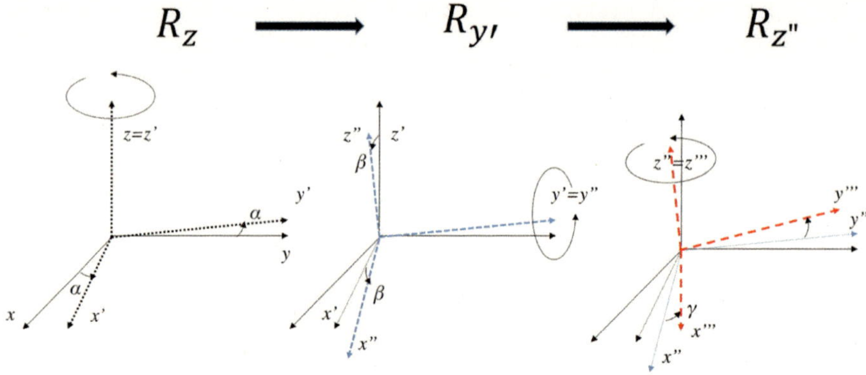

Fig. 9.11 Euler angles α , β, and γ and the three Euler rotations R_z (*left*), $R_{y'}$ (*middle*), and $R_{z''}$ (*right*) that carry the initial (x, y, z) coordinates into the final (x''', y''', z''') coordinate system

$$F_{LS} = \sum_{\omega \in \Omega} (I_T(\omega) - I_R(\omega))^2. \tag{9.19}$$

This summation is performed within the volume of interest (VOI) Ω on $\boldsymbol{I}_R$. If the image $\boldsymbol{I}$ has a similar intensity/feature to the image $\boldsymbol{I}_R$, it is safe to assume that the minimum value of F_{LS} searched by the possible transformation ψ of the image $\boldsymbol{I}$ yields the best registration results.

Once the similarity measure is determined, the image registration is implemented using an optimization scheme. There are several numerical methods for solving optimization problems. For instance, in the case of matching images of the brain, the horizontal translation and the rotation around the vertical axis are more constrained by the shape of the head than the pitching rotation around the left-to-right horizontal axis. Therefore, aligning the images in the horizontal plane by optimizing the in-plane parameters may facilitate the optimization of the out-of-plane parameters. However, as the optimization proceeds, the Powell algorithm may introduce other optimization directions and change the order in which these are considered (Maes et al. 1997).

In clinical applications, it is important for the image registration to be conducted rapidly. Automatic image registration should take less than a few seconds, and the subsequent visual verification and approval should be completed within a few minutes. The image registration algorithm must be valid for patient positioning, with robustness and little computational effort.

A limited overview of the image registration algorithm used in IGRT is presented in the following subsections, including three examples frequently used in clinical practice.

9.3.1 Landmarks

The most intuitively obvious registration method employs corresponding landmarks in the two images (Peters et al. 2000; West et al. 1997). Histologically or morphologically clear points (top of nasal bone, external protuberance of occipital bone, etc.) and fiducial markers can be useful as landmarks. With rigid image registration, three landmarks that are not aligned are sufficient to determine the transformation between two 3D images. Including additional landmarks may yield more reliable results.

The algorithm for calculating the transformation is very simple:

- First, the centroid positions of all or a part of the landmarks in the two images are calculated. The 3D difference between the centroids represents the translation vector $\boldsymbol{t}$. This translation is applied to one image and the corresponding landmark set.
- Second, this translated landmark set is rotated until the sum of the squared distances between each pair of corresponding landmarks is minimized.

With more than four landmarks, the root-mean-square error is meaningful for the reliability of the registration. Although the landmark registration is intuitive, fast, and easy, a limited number of landmarks can yield a mismatch, depending on the landmark positions. Moreover, with a limited image quality of the IGRT system, the registration for soft tissues is quite difficult without the placement of invasive markers.

9.3.2 Chamfer Matching

Chamfer matching (Borgefors 1988) is a bone-registration algorithm that employs CT images, whereby regions with densities that are the same as bone densities are detected and transferred (and rotated) . The chamfer matching algorithm is not very sensitive to image noise. In addition, the calculation is quick. A schematic workflow of chamfer matching is shown in Fig. 9.12. Here, the edge detection both to the reference and input images is first performed. The distant transformation allows the edge-input image to be converted into a distance image, which has a pixel value that is a measure of the distance to the nearest edge pixel. This distance is called the chamfer distance. Finally, the matching between the chamfer-distance image and the edge-reference image produces the registration result.

Several edge detection algorithms are available. For the present purpose—bone edge detection—one of the simple methods is threshold adaptation, which sets a certain range for the bone edge detection. After the edge detection, the images are binarized. For the input image (i.e., CBCT image), this binarized image is converted into a distance image:

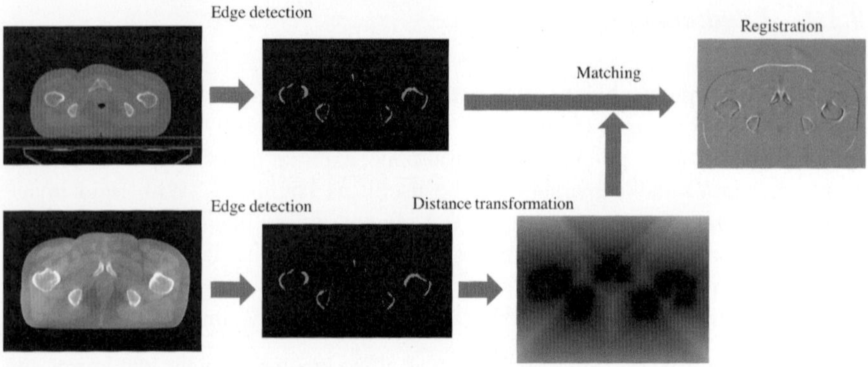

Fig. 9.12 Schematic workflow of chamfer matching. First, binary images are created by an edge detection algorithm such as the Sobel filter, the threshold setting, and so on, for both the registration and reference images. Second, distance transformation is performed, typically for the registration binary image. Finally, matching yields the optimization of the transformation parameters

$$D(\omega) = \psi_{DT}(B(\omega)), \tag{9.20}$$

where $D(\omega)$ and $B(\omega)$ are the distance and the input binary image, respectively. While it is not difficult to create a Euclidean distance image, the 3–4 distance transformation ψ_{DT} (Fig. 9.13) can be easier and quicker than the Euclidean distance transformation. The cost function in image registration using chamfer matching is then

$$F_{CM} = \sum_{\omega \in \Omega} I_R(\omega) D_T(\omega), \tag{9.21}$$

where D_T means the distance image transformed by Eq. (9.16). The couch correction is determined by minimizing F_{CM} with the transformation parameters (the gradient decent method is typically applied). This algorithm can be used together with markers made of metals such as titan, by setting the proper edge detection threshold.

The chamfer matching algorithm was improved by embedding a hierarchical resolution pyramid: the matching is performed not only in the original image resolution but in a series of images, where each image is a low-resolution representation of the original scene.

9.3.3 *Gray Value Matching*

Gray value matching (Roche et al. 1998; Hristov and Fallone 1996) is registration that employs the pixel intensity values of the volumetric images to calculate the

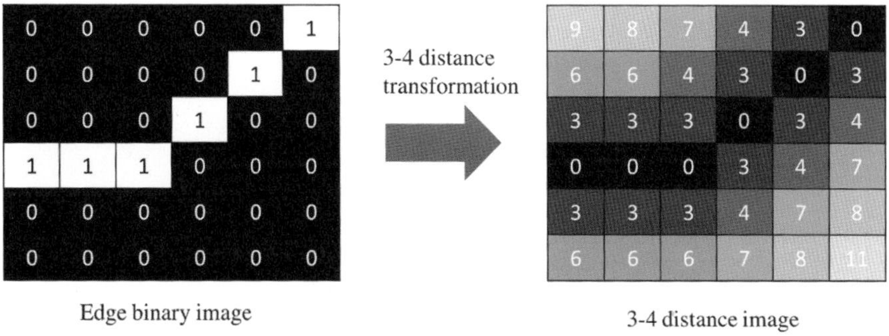

Fig. 9.13 A 3–4 distance transformation. The pixel value is converted depending on the distance from "1" indicated in a binary image (*left*). The two local distances in a 3-by-3 neighborhood are the distance between horizontal/vertical neighbors ("3") and that between diagonal neighbors ("4"). This is an approximation of the Euclidean distance transformation

translations and rotations. Gray value matching has a similar workflow to the aforementioned two algorithms. That is, the registration involves optimization with respect to a similarity measure.

Many similarity measures have been proposed for gray value matching, including a least-squares criterion, correlation ratio criterion, cross correlation criterion, and mutual information criterion. The cost function in the least-squares criterion is explicitly given in Eq. (9.19). For the other criteria, the cost functions are described as follows:

- Correlation ratio

$$F_{CR} = \frac{1}{N\sigma^2}\sum_j N_j {\sigma_j}^2, \tag{9.22}$$

where

$$\sigma^2 = \frac{1}{N}\sum_{\omega\in\Omega} I_R(\omega)^2 - \widetilde{I_R}^2, \quad \widetilde{I_R} = \frac{1}{N}\sum_{\omega\in\Omega} I_R(\omega), \tag{9.23}$$

$${\sigma_j}^2 = \frac{1}{N_j}\sum_{\omega\in\Omega_j} I_R(\omega)^2 - \widetilde{I_R}_j^{\,2}, \quad \widetilde{I_R}_j = \frac{1}{N_j}\sum_{\omega\in\Omega_j} I_R(\omega). \tag{9.24}$$

Here, N is the number of voxels in the VOI (Ω) for image registration; Ω_j is the subset regarding the transformed image $\boldsymbol{I}_T = \psi(\boldsymbol{I})$, defined as $\Omega_j = \{\omega \in \Omega, I_T(\omega) = j\}$; and the N_j values are the cardinals $N_j = \mathrm{Card}(\Omega_j)$.

- Cross correlation

$$F_{CC} = \frac{\mathrm{Cov}(I_T, I_R)}{\sigma(I_T)\sigma(I_R)}, \tag{9.25}$$

where

$$\mathrm{Cov}(I_T, I_R) = \frac{1}{N}\sum_{\omega \in \Omega}\left(I_R(\omega) - \widetilde{I_R}\right)\left(I_T(\omega) - \widetilde{I_T}\right), \tag{9.26}$$

$$\sigma(I_R) = \sqrt{\frac{1}{N}\sum_{\omega \in \Omega}\left(I_R(\omega) - \widetilde{I_R}\right)^2}, \tag{9.27}$$

$$\sigma(I_T) = \sqrt{\frac{1}{N}\sum_{\omega \in \Omega}\left(I_T(\omega) - \widetilde{I_T}\right)^2}, \tag{9.28}$$

- Mutual information

$$F_{MI} = H_{I_R} + H_{I_T} - H_{I_R I_T}, \tag{9.29}$$

where

$$H_{I_R} = -\sum_i p(i)\log p(i), \tag{9.30}$$

$$H_{I_T} = -\sum_j p(j)\log p(j), \tag{9.31}$$

$$H_{I_R I_T} = -\sum_{i,j} p(i,j)\log p(i,j), \tag{9.32}$$

and $p(i) = N_i/N$ is the probability of the image $\boldsymbol{I}_R$ having intensity i, whereas $p(i,j)$ is the joint probability of the images $\boldsymbol{I}_R$ and $\boldsymbol{I}_T$ having intensities i and j, respectively.

The correlation ratio works with the images obtained in the different modalities as well as the mutual information. The mutual information requires a 2D histogram, whereas the correlation ratio does not. This causes an important difference in the computational efficiency. Classical algorithms for computing the mutual information have an $O(n_A n_B)$ complexity, where n_A and n_B are the numbers of intensity levels in the A and B images, respectively, whereas correlation ratio computation has only an $O(n_A)$ complexity and is independent from n_B (Roche et al. 1998).

9.4 In-Treatment Verification and Post Analysis

Intra- and inter-fractional motion analysis can be performed by various methods, including CBCT or ultrasound imaging before and after treatment, embedded fiducial markers with a portal imager, and electromagnetic coil systems. The reported displacement of a target during treatment exceeded a few millimeters with an increasing probability for a longer delivery time (Ueda et al. 2012), indicating that the PTV margin is underestimated if it is based on pretreatment positioning errors.

An in-room CT system can play a central role in margin analysis, as volumetric images allow the identification of the target or OAR location and the shape during the treatment. However, a recent study revealed that postdelivery CBCT imaging overestimated the localization errors due to the delay between the end of the treatment delivery and posttreatment CBCT (Adamson et al. 2011). Ideally, CBCT acquisition must be performed during treatment delivery, or combined cone-beam X-ray projections with online motion measurements must be employed. Currently, these methods are available for clinical treatment cases (Nakagawa et al. 2009). In the following subsections, *in-treatment* CBCT imaging and real-time projection image analysis acquired concurrently with the treatment delivery are introduced. For the latter, online motion measurement typically requires fiducial markers and may not be always desirable. Thus, we focus on a recently developed markerless technique in that subsection. Although these two topics are based on the use of X-rays in the kV energy range, it is possible to analyze portal images of the treatment X-ray beam. Volumetric image visualization by portal imaging is discussed toward the end of this section.

9.4.1 In-Treatment CBCT

Although the CBCT system mounted on the LINAC is intended to provide image registration with accurate patient setup immediately prior to treatment, it is also applicable for image volume acquisition in the state of delivered beams. This method, called "in-treatment CBCT," can be performed with rotational treatments, such as VMAT, wherein the gantry of a LINAC rotates continuously during the radiation therapy. With in-treatment CBCT, the displacement of the target from the treatment planning can be evaluated. Previously, CBCT reconstruction during VMAT was not available in any commercial software. Currently, however, in-treatment CBCT images, including their 4D versions, can be reconstructed using the equipped IGRT system immediately after treatment.

The principle of in-treatment CBCT reconstruction is the same as that of normal CBCT reconstruction, which is described in Sect. 9.2.2. However, unlike the case of normal CBCT acquisition, the gantry rotation speed can vary depending on the beam-intensity modulation at each angle, so that the sampling interval of sequential projections is generally not constant. This is not a serious problem, provided that the numerical integration over the angle β in Eq. (9.13) is properly performed with unequal sampling.

The largest concern regarding in-treatment CBCT is the scattering photons from the MV treatment beam (Ling et al. 2011). The magnitude of the impact of scattering photons on the image quality depends on the treatment plan. However, according to several clinical reports, the scattering does not to cause any difficulties in post analysis (Kida et al. 2012; Shiraishi et al. 2014; Takahashi et al. 2013). Nevertheless, correction methods have been proposed. One of them involves the assumption that the scattering effect is homogeneous on the FPD, that is, the whole projection image (Kida et al. 2012). Then, the projection image is normalized during the treatment by subtracting the difference between the minimum pixel value taken immediately prior to the treatment and that during the treatment at the isocenter line (crossline of the FPD, the line used in the reconstruction of one axial plane). Prior to the treatment, the projection image is chosen at the angle closest to the projection image during the treatment. This is applied for all the projections. In the 4D CBCT case, the respiratory phase during treatment may differ from that prior to treatment at the same angle. However, such an inconsistency is negligible because the normalization is performed with the minimum pixel value, which means that the ray passes through the air.

An alternative approach is to evaluate the scattering photon number at the FPD with a realistic geometry of the LINAC and patient, according to basic theory. A Monte Carlo calculation provides an almost complete result but requires an impractical computation effort in clinical applications. Therefore, in practice, a lowest-order approximation, i.e., the Compton scattering formula, or a convolution model may be employed.

Margin analysis using in-treatment CBCT is directly performed by comparing the daily data with the corresponding treatment planning CT data. Here, the volume center of in-treatment CBCT is considered to agree with the isocenter of the treatment plan. The maximum lengths required to cover the target volume during treatment in each direction of the 3D space are regarded as a part of the component for the PTV margin (which should also include the treatment dose uncertainty, geometrical uncertainty in the IGRT system, dose simulation uncertainty, etc.). For instance, the region protruding outside the target volume can be evaluated by manually delineating the regions of interest (ROIs) in the treatment planning CT and the in-treatment CBCT and comparing them. The results of a margin evaluation using in-treatment CBCT are presented in the literature (Shiraishi et al. 2014; Takahashi et al. 2013), for prostate cancer and lung cancer, respectively. The results of a margin analysis for a state-of-the-art 4D CBCT registration system were also reported (Haga et al. 2015). The current radiation treatment seems to require a maximum PTV margin of ~5 mm. Of course, this depends on the IGRT equipment, delivery technique, and patient-immobilization tools; therefore, it should not be generalized.

At end of this subsection, we emphasize the usefulness of in-treatment CBCT with regard to dose verification in actual treatment. That is, the actual dose distribution in patients can be reconstructed via in-treatment CBCT by using delivery data such as LINAC logs or portal images. A difficulty arises from the fact that the HU in CBCT is substantially unreliable. To avoid this uncertainty, a patient-specific ROI mapping method can be applied (van Zijtveld et al. 2007; Hu et al. 2010). In this method, the relative densities in the anatomical regions defined by ROI contouring are measured for an individual patient by using the treatment planning CT data. Then, these densities are substituted into the corresponding anatomies delineated in in-treatment CBCT, and the beams are delivered.

For a moving target, the dose reconstruction is not as simple as it is in the static case. This is mainly because the beam delivery data must link with the motion phase to reconstruct the 4D dose distribution. This process is summarized as follows (Saotome 2013):

- The cone-beam projection images and the beam delivery data are acquired during treatment.
- The motion signal is derived from the cone-beam projection images.
- According to the motion signal, the projection images and beam delivery data are classified into motion phase bins.
- The 4D CBCT sets are reconstructed with these phase bins.
- The beam data form of the treatment planning system is created from the beam delivery data for each phase. Thus, beam data sets corresponding to the 4D CBCT sets are produced for each treatment fraction.
- The image region of the 4D CBCT is extended as much as possible, so as to include the patient surface in the calculation region.
- The ROIs (e.g., GTV, lung, cord, airway, and soft tissue) are delineated in each phase.
- Dose calculation is performed for each in-treatment 4D CBCT set, where the patient-specific ROI mapping method is applied.
- The dose distribution is accumulated into a certain phase of CBCT (e.g., maximum exhale CBCT) by a nonrigid transformation.

Because the actual beam information corresponding to the acquisition time of the projection images is used for the dose calculation in each phase of in-treatment 4D CBCT, the absolute dose distribution can be reconstructed by using only the observed data.

9.4.2 Markerless Tracking for Moving Tumor Using Cone-Beam Projections

In the previous section, the utility of in-treatment CBCT is described. One of the disadvantages of in-treatment CBCT is that it cannot be used for real-time treatment analysis. With in-treatment CBCT, the image is reconstructed completely after all the projections are acquired. Another possible limitation is that anomalous motions (e.g., cough) that occur during the CBCT scan are hidden because of the slow gantry rotation, yielding "averaged" images. Therefore, to verify and control the target location in real time, the direct use of cone-beam projections must be considered.

Although many studies have reported the detection of the patient or tumor location by real-time X-ray imaging, it is challenging to track a location in three dimensions without markers. In particular, continuous markerless tracking during rotational delivery (e.g., VMAT) is quite difficult without markers, as the image contrast of the ROI, such as lung tumor in X-ray projections, depends on the gantry angle.

One strategy for markerless tracking for all gantry-angle directions involves utilizing prior information or a model for the motion. The general method for this employs treatment planning 4D CT, wherein DRRs are generated with all angle views (e.g., 360° with 1° intervals) for reference or template images for cone-beam projections in advance. Figure 9.14 shows a schematic workflow to classify the projections into the motion phase bins defined by the treatment planning 4D CT phases. The projection image is immediately compared with all the phase DRRs at the same angle, and the DRR phase with the maximum matching score is regarded as the actual phase of that projection. This can be performed in real time because no image registration is required.

The aforementioned method works only if the tumor or VOI is contained within the region traced in the treatment planning 4D CT. For tracking nonstationary and nonperiodic motion, this assumption is invalid. In such cases, image registration is required. Hugo et al. investigated several template tracking-based methods and reported that the introduction of templates reduces the search area for the registration (Hugo et al. 2010). Other groups investigated the possibility of a real-time tracking solution based on the acquisition of CBCT projection images during lung VMAT (Zhuang et al. 2013; Lewis et al. 2010; Koste et al. 2015). Although a single 2D–2D registration does not cause a shift about the depth from the isocenter, the position error induced by this cause is negligible because the projected direction is always perpendicular to the cranio-caudal axis of the patient, which is the normal dominant direction of the tumor motion for lung and liver cancers. Alternatively, 2D matching is followed by the triangulation of the target position from multiple 2D registrations, e.g., of similar breathing cycle phases, for the 3D localization of the target. The simultaneous use of portal imaging of the treatment beam is an alternative solution for 3D target tracking (Liu et al. 2008; Yan et al. 2012).

9.4.3 Visualization of Treatment Area Using Treatment Beam

Volumetric visualization using MV beams is not new. Tomotherapy and other MVCT systems have been employed to reconstruct patient images for setup and

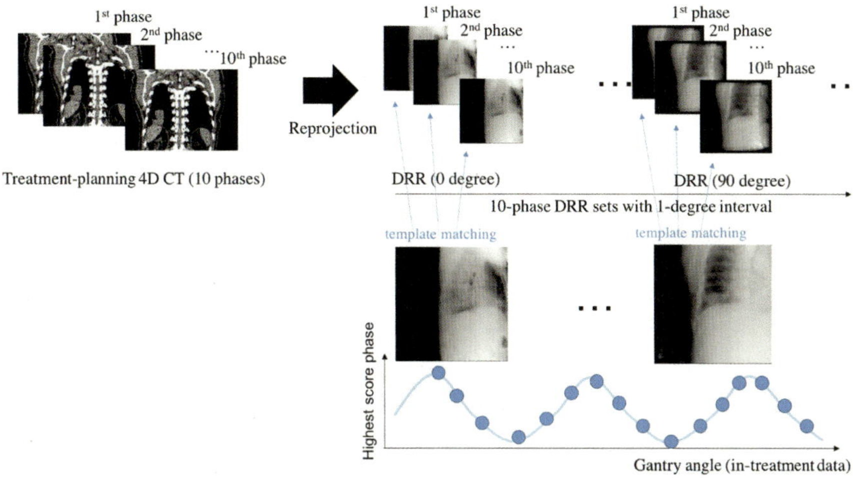

Fig. 9.14 Example of real-time markerless phase recognition. Template DRR images are generated by 10-phase 4D CT with all the angle views used in the treatment plan. During the treatment, cone-beam projections are acquired and matched with the DRR images in real time. The template DRR creation is limited to the target area

dose reconstruction (Ruchala et al. 2000). However, the studies aiming to visualize the treatment area using portal images of the treatment beam are limited.

It is mathematically impossible to perform a *correct* reconstruction with the field of view (FOV) partially blocked by a multileaf collimator when a filtered back projection (FBP) algorithm is employed. The blocked area has a lower X-ray intensity than the area inside the FOV; thus, the conventional reconstruction scheme does not successfully visualize the imaging object. Instead, it yields an unrealistically high-attenuation area outside the irradiated site in the object (Poludniowski et al. 2010).

For successful reconstruction, the PICCS algorithm is promising because modern radiation therapy always accompanies treatment planning CT and MVCT/CBCT used in the patient registration, which are the best types of prior information for this type of algorithm. The PICCS method is not described in this chapter; details are found in the literature (Chen et al. 2008). Rather, we discuss the possibility and limitations of applying the FBP algorithm.

For visualization of treatment area using the FBP algorithm, two corrections are necessary. One is a masking correction, which masks the area outside the FOV so as not to include this area in the back projection process. For a conventional LINAC, the corrected portal image $\tilde{y}(\beta, p, \zeta)$ is

$$\tilde{y}(\beta, p, \zeta) = \begin{cases} 0, & \textit{if } n(\beta, p, \zeta)/n_0 < p' \\ \ln(n_0/n(\beta, p, \zeta)), & \text{otherwise} \end{cases} \tag{9.33}$$

where β is the gantry angle, p and ζ are the same as in Fig. 9.6, and $n(\beta, p, \zeta)$ indicates the photon number detected in the EPID with the coordinates (p, ζ) at the gantry angle of β. In Eq. (9.33), p'defines the threshold for the masking region. With this threshold, the outside field is regarded as vacuum ($\tilde{y}\,(\beta, p, \zeta) = 0$), and the boundary of the masking region is discontinuous. Of course, this is not true, but it enhances the information from the irradiated area in the FBP reconstruction scheme.

The other correction is a ray-passing adjustment, which normalizes each voxel of the reconstructed image to the number of X-rays passing through the corresponding voxel. This is expressed by

$$R_{\beta'}(x, y, z) = \frac{\theta\left(\int d\beta\, M(\beta, p, \zeta) - \beta'\right)}{\frac{1}{2\pi}\int d\beta\, M(\beta, p, \zeta),} \tag{9.34}$$

with $p = Dt/(D-s)$ (where $s = -x\sin\beta + y\cos\beta$, $t = x\cos\beta + y\sin\beta$) and $\zeta = z\sqrt{D^2 + p^2}/\sqrt{(D-s)^2 + t^2}$. The coordinates (β, p, ζ) correspond to the projected point of (x, y, z) on the detector plane (p, ζ) at the gantry angle β. The masking function is

$$M(\beta, p, \zeta) = \begin{cases} 0, & \textit{if } n(\beta, p, \zeta)/n_0 < p' \\ 1, & \text{otherwise} \end{cases}. \tag{9.35}$$

The back projection generates stronger signals when the angles pass more X-ray quanta. The ray-passing correction corrects this effect. The reconstruction area can be controlled according to β'.

The reconstruction formula using MV portal images can be expressed by making the replacement

$$\mathcal{R}(\beta, p, \zeta) \rightarrow R_{\beta'}(x, y, z)\tilde{y}\,(\beta, p, \zeta) \tag{9.36}$$

in Eq. (9.13). Figure 9.15 shows the reconstructed image with portal images acquired during VMAT delivery. Here, the delivery area is visualized. In principle, 4D visualization for periodic motion (e.g., lung tumor) can be developed without difficulty. The requirement is the link between the portal images and the phase bins in the motion signal. After the periodic-motion signal is somehow acquired, the 4D images are reconstructed by sorting the portal images in each phase (Kida et al. 2011).

The actual treatment area is visualized by portal imaging of the treatment beam X-rays. However, the image quality is insufficient for diagnosis and quantitative margin analysis with an image correlation, as can be done with in-treatment CBCT. In this context, the aforementioned approach using the FBP algorithm has some limitations. To increase the reliability of the volume reconstruction obtained by portal imaging, the use of an a posteriori estimation algorithm, as typified by

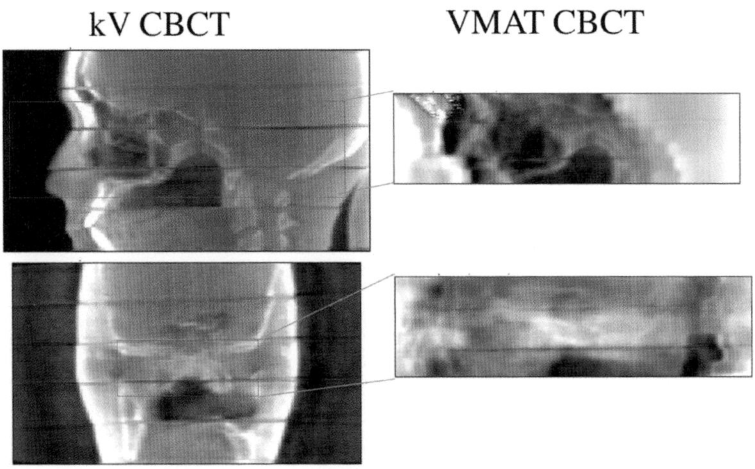

Fig. 9.15 kV CBCT (*left*) and corresponding VMAT CBCT (*right*) for a head phantom. The irradiated area is only visualized in the VMAT CBCT

PICCS, is desired. In particular, the image series acquired for the patient positioning can be used in this algorithm as prior information.

9.5 QA for IGRT

The accuracy requirements for patient positioning in radiation therapy have recently increased in order to ensure a high accuracy for treatments designed to achieve adequate tumor control and the reduction of normal-tissue complications. In this context, IGRT is essential for every type of modern radiation therapy. All commercially available IGRT systems provide precise patient setup; however, this assumes the continuation of the appropriate QA/QC of the system. The QA issues for IGRT are summarized as follows:

- Geometric accuracy
- Image quality
- Image registration (including remote couch control)
- Imaging dose

The AAPM TG-179 (Bissonnette et al. 2012) reviews the clinical implementations and QA aspects for commercially available CT-based IGRT, each having unique capabilities and underlying physics. The following subsections cite this review, which readers can refer to for a detailed discussion.

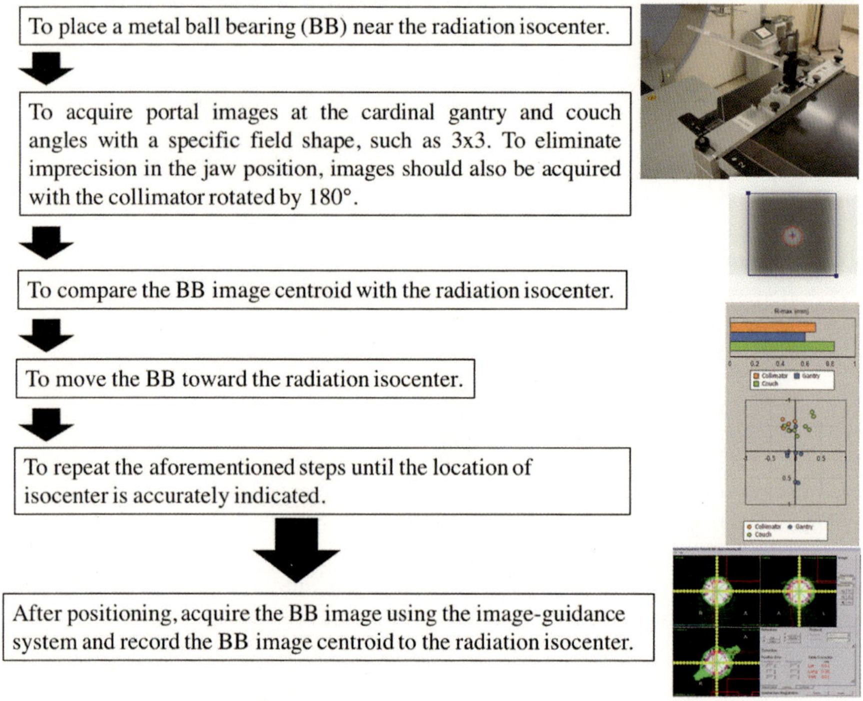

Fig. 9.16 Example of the Winston–Lutz test procedure

9.5.1 Geometric Accuracy

LINAC-mounted kV CBCT systems may have a different isocenter location from that of the treatment beam, owing to the different sources. This discrepancy should be small, i.e., less than ± 1 mm. A convenient method for performing kV CBCT system geometric calibration is derived from the Winston–Lutz procedure. This procedure is briefly described in Fig. 9.16.

For fan-beam MVCT units, the imaging beam is generated by the same source that generates the treatment beam, and the two beams share a common geometry. Spatial accuracy and geometry tests for fan-beam MVCT are described in AAPM TG-148 (Langen et al. 2010).

The geometric accuracy affects directly the accuracy of the patient setup; therefore, it is recommended that the simplified geometric calibration be tested daily to identify sudden performance changes or gross errors.

9.5.2 *Image Quality*

The QA program of a CT-based IGRT system is based on the utilization of the system. For image-quality issues, the QA program should focus on localizing the targets and OARs and executing correction strategies to minimize geometric uncertainties. The soft tissue detectability is an important aspect, whereas the CT number linearity and accuracy are only important if the CT scans are also used for dose calculation.

The QA program recommended by AAPM TG-179 includes the verification of the following:

- Scale and distance accuracy
- Low contrast resolution
- Spatial resolution
- Uniformity and noise
- Accuracy of CT numbers

These image QC tests can be performed using commercially available phantoms that contain multiple inserts tailored to test various aspects of the image quality (Fig. 9.17).

AAPM TG-179 recommends that image-quality tests be performed on a monthly basis initially, and ultimately on a semiannual basis, after the parameter stability is demonstrated by the users.

9.5.3 *Image Registration and Accuracy of Remote Couch Control*

Automatic image registration is convenient in clinical practice of CT-based IGRT. Because of the nonrigid nature of the anatomy of the patients and the limited correction methods, the ideal alignment may depend on the clinical case and frequently involves manual registration. Therefore, the QA program of image registration is ineffective, and an offline review of the clinical data is recommended. It is also highly recommended by AAPM TG-179 that the user establishes site-specific clinical protocols to explicitly describe the VOI, alignment goals, and evaluation criteria.

The accuracy of remote couch control is a key component in any image-guidance system. The couch position accuracy can be measured using high-precision calipers, optical navigation systems, and film. Of course, this is confirmed by the IGRT system by analyzing two scanned images in which the target location has a known different length and rotation angle.

The accuracy and precision of correction movements should be assessed during commissioning, and the long-term accuracy should be verified through post analysis of the IGRT procedure (see Sect. 9.4).

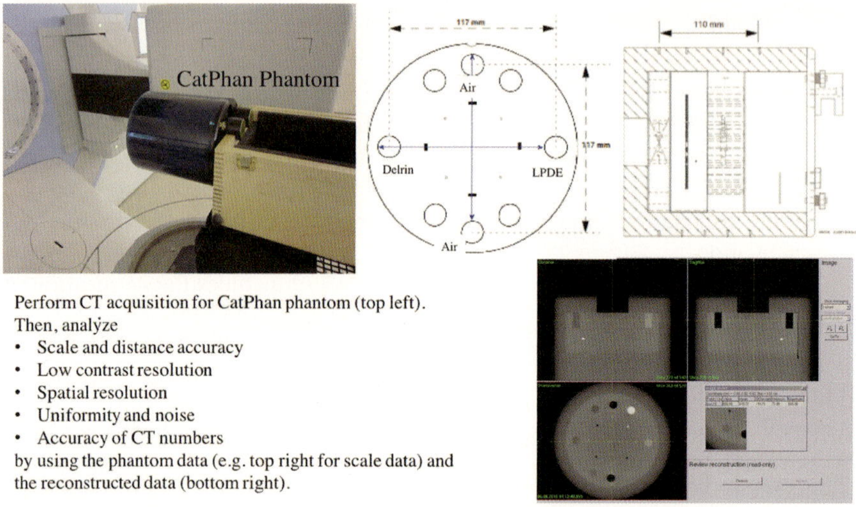

Fig. 9.17 Example of multifunctional imaging phantom (CatPhan500 phantom (The Phantom Laboratory, Salem)) designed to provide a comprehensive evaluation for different CT scanning technologies

A couch with six DOFs (three translational and three rotational) is commercially available. Using this equipment, the accuracy of the volumetric image registration algorithm should be tested with regard to both rotational and translational shifts.

9.5.4 Imaging Dose

One concern regarding daily CT imaging is the additional exposure to the entire imaged volume, which may cause a secondary malignancy. There is an interplay between the increased use of CT imaging and the improvement of the patient setup. In this context, imaging dose as well as the therapeutic dose must be evaluated.

The measurement of the imaging dose consists of several steps (Ma et al. 2001; Murphy et al. 2007). For dosimetric CT-based imaging studies, the reported doses were from 0.1 to 2 cGy/scan for kV CBCT and 0.7 to 10.8 cGy/scan for MV CBCT. For fan-beam MVCT images, the doses range from 0.7 to 4 cGy, depending on the selected CT pitch and the imaged anatomy thickness (Bissonnette et al. 2012). These values are generally small compared with the therapeutic doses. Nevertheless, the medical staff must reduce them as much as possible within the IGRT framework. The image quality is intimately linked to the X-ray energy, tube current, and gantry rotation speed and range. Therefore, it is desired to establish several protocols depending on the treatment site and the patient body size.

9.6 Summary

This chapter introduced the basic concept of X-ray-based patient positioning in radiation therapy. All modern IGRT systems attempt to reproduce the patient position during treatment planning CT acquisition. For patient registration, treatment planning CT is used directly or indirectly, depending on the IGRT system used. If the IGRT system allows the reconstruction of a CT image, the image is registered to the treatment planning CT as is, whereas if the X-ray projection image is only available in the IGRT system, it is registered to the DRR image created from treatment planning CT. The former requires CT reconstruction immediately after or during the projection-image acquisition. On the other hand, the latter requires a reprojection process for DRR creation during the treatment planning. These processes are discussed in Sect. 9.2.

The accuracy of patient positioning in radiation therapy is drastically improved by the automatic registration system with IGRT, and the remote couch function is established. The sequential flow of the patient setup and image acquisition, registration, correction, verification, and approval is now sophisticated and provides fast and comfortable treatment for patients and medical staff. In addition, a huge data set of X-ray images may enable the further development of IGRT technology. The analysis of medical-image big data and its feedback for following treatments or other patients can provide a considerable benefit. The detection of outlier or anomalies by machine learning for sudden motions or unexpected situations is also important for the next-generation system. This chapter introduced a few examples of post analysis using X-ray images acquired in an IGRT system; however, we did not discuss the utility of IGRT beyond margin analysis. Knowledge from the analysis of past treatments is utilized for the improvement of the sequential treatment and for the other patients. For this purpose, the development of quantitative imaging in IGRT must continue.

Finally, the IGRT system must be validated thorough QA/QC. This is important for the successful operation of everything discussed herein. The development of a QA/QC program is not separate from the other topics discussed. It would be exciting to develop an efficient and effective QA/QC process for quantitative image analysis based on mathematical and computational physics.

References

Adamson J, Wu Q, Yan D (2011) Dosimetric effect of intrafraction motion and residual setup error for hypofractionated prostate intensity-modulated radiotherapy with online cone beam computed tomography image guidance. Int J Radiat Oncol Biol Phys 80(2):453–461

Barney BM et al (2011) Image-Guided Radiotherapy (IGRT) for prostate cancer comparing kV imaging of fiducial markers with Cone Beam Computed Tomography (CBCT). Int J Radiat Oncol Biol Phys 80(1):301–305

Birkner M et al (2007) Analysis of the rigid and deformable component of setup inaccuracies on portal images in head and neck radiotherapy. Phys Med Biol 52(18):5721–5733

Bissonnette J-P et al (2012) Quality assurance for image-guided radiation therapy utilizing CT-based technologies: A report of the AAPM TG-179. Med Phys 39(4):1946

Boda-Heggemann J et al (2011) kV cone-beam CT-based IGRT: a clinical review. Strahlentherapie und Onkologie : Organ der Deutschen Röntgengesellschaft [et al] 187 (5):284–291

Borgefors G (1988) Hierarchical Chamfer matching: a parametric edge matching algorithm. IEEE Trans Pattern Anal Mach Intell 10:849–865

Bujold A et al (2012) Image-guided radiotherapy: has it influenced patient outcomes? Semin Radiat Oncol 22(1):50–61

Buzug TM (2008) Computed tomography: from photon statistics to modern cone-beam CT. Springer, Berlin

Chen G-H, Tang J, Leng S (2008) Prior image constrained compressed sensing (PICCS): A method to accurately reconstruct dynamic CT images from highly undersampled projection data sets. Med Phys 35(2):660

Ct X et al (2015) A model-based image reconstruction algorithm with simultaneous beam hardening correction for X-ray CT. IEEE Trans Computational Imaging 1(3):1–16

Dawson LA, Jaffray DA (2007) Advances in image-guided radiation therapy. J Clin Oncol 25 (8):938–946

De Koste JRVS et al (2015) Markerless tracking of small lung tumors for stereotactic radiotherapy Markerless tracking of small lung tumors for stereotactic radiotherapy. Med Phys 42 (4):1640–1652

Deegan T et al (2014) Assessment of cone beam CT registration for prostate radiation therapy: fiducial marker and soft tissue methods. J Med Imaging Radiat Oncol 59:91–98

Dietrich L et al (2006) Linac-integrated 4D cone beam CT: first experimental results. Phys Med Biol 51(11):2939–2952

Donoho DLL (2006) Compressed sensing. IEEE Trans Inf Theory 52(4):1289–1306

Grimmer R, Maaß C, Kachelrieß M (2009) A new method for cupping and scatter precorrection for flat detector CT. IEEE Nucl Sci Symp Conf Rec:3517–3522

Haga A, Kida S, Saotome N (2015) Four-dimensional cone-beam CT during SBRT. In: Nagata Y (ed) Stereotactic body radiation therapy. Springer, Tokyo, pp 225–239

Hajnal J, Hill D, Hawkes D (2001) Medical image registration. CRC Press, New York

Hawkins MA et al (2011) Set-up errors in radiotherapy for oesophageal cancers--is electronic portal imaging or conebeam more accurate? Radiother Oncol: J Eur Soc Ther Radiol Oncol 98 (2):249–254

Herman GT (1979) Correction for beam hardening in computed tomography. Phys Med Biol 24 (1):81–106

Hristov DH, Fallone BG (1996) A grey-level image alignment algorithm for registration of portal images and digitally reconstructed radiographs. Med Phys 23(1):75–84

Hsieh J et al (2000) An iterative approach to the beam hardening correction in cone beam CT. Med Phys 27(1):23–29

Hu W et al (2010) Use of kilovoltage X-ray volume imaging in patient dose calculation for head-and-neck and partial brain radiation therapy. Radiat Oncol 5(29):1–10

Hugo GD, Liang J, Yan D (2010) Marker-free lung tumor trajectory estimation from a cone beam CT sinogram. Phys Med Biol 55(9):2637–2650

Jaffray DA, Siewerdsen JH (2000) Cone-beam computed tomography with a flat-panel imager: initial performance characterization. Med Phys 27(6):1311–1323

Jaffray DA et al (1999) A radiographic and tomographic imaging system integrated into a medical linear accelerator for localization of bone and soft-tissue targets. Int J Radiat Oncol Biol Phys 45(3):773–789

Jaffray DA et al (2002) Flat-panel cone-beam computed tomography for image-guided radiation therapy. Int J Radiat Oncol Biol Phys 53(5):1337–1349

Jarry G et al (2006) Characterization of scattered radiation in kV CBCT images using Monte Carlo simulations. Med Phys 33(11):4320
Kak AC, Slaney M (2001) Principles of computerized tomographic imaging (Classics in applied mathematics). Society of Industial and Applied Mathematics, Philadelphia
Kestin L et al (2014) Dose-response relationship with clinical outcome for lung stereotactic body radiotherapy (SBRT) delivered via online image guidance. Radiother Oncol 110(3):499–504
Kida S et al (2011) 4D-CBCT reconstruction using MV portal imaging during volumetric modulated arc therapy. Radiother Oncol 100:380–385
Kida S, Masutani Y, Yamashita H (2012) In-treatment 4D cone-beam CT with image-based respiratory phase recognition. Radiol Phys Technol 5:138–147
Langen KM et al (2010) QA for helical tomotherapy: report of the AAPM Task Group 148. Med Phys 37(9):4817–4853
Létourneau D et al (2005) Cone-beam-CT guided radiation therapy: technical implementation. Radiother Oncol 75(3):279–286
Lewis JH et al (2010) Markerless lung tumor tracking and trajectory reconstruction using rotational cone-beam projections: a feasibility study. Phys Med Biol 55:2505–2522
Li T et al (2006) Four-dimensional cone-beam computed tomography using an on-board imager. Med Phys 33(10):3825–3833
Ling C et al (2011) Acquisition of MV-scatter-free kilovoltage CBCT images during RapidArc™ or VMAT. Radiother Oncol 100(1):145–149
Liu W et al (2008) Real-time 3D internal marker tracking during arc radiotherapy by the use of combined MV-kV imaging. Phys Med Biol 53(24):7197–7213
Lu J et al (2007) Four-dimensional cone beam CT with adaptive gantry rotation and adaptive data sampling. Med Phys 34(9):3520
Ma CM et al (2001) AAPM protocol for 40-300 kV x-ray beam dosimetry in radiotherapy and radiobiology. Med Phys 28(6):868–893
Maes F et al (1997) Multimodality image registration by maximization of mutual information. IEEE Trans Med Imaging 16(2):187–198
Mail N, O'Brien P, Pang G (2007) Lag correction model and ghosting analysis for an indirect conversion flat panel imager. J Appl Clin Med Phys 8(3):137–146
Mail N et al (2008) An empirical method for lag correction in cone-beam CT. Med Phys 35 (11):5187–5196
Matsuo Y et al (2013) Guidelines for respiratory motion management in radiation therapy. J Radiat Res 54(3):561–568
Mongioj V et al (2011) Set-up errors analyses in IMRT treatments for nasopharyngeal carcinoma to evaluate time trends, PTV and PRV margins. Acta Oncol 50(1):61–71
Murphy MJ et al (2007) The management of imaging dose during image-guided radiotherapy: report of the AAPM Task Group 75. Med Phys 34(10):4041–4063
Nakagawa K et al (2009) First clinical cone-beam CT imaging during volumetric modulated arc therapy. Radiother Oncol 90(3):422–423
Nakano M (2016) Time-ordered cone-beam CT image reconstruction. The University of Tokyo, Tokyo
Nalcioglu O, Lou RY (1979) Post-reconstruction method for beam hardening in computerised tomography. Phys Med Biol 24(2):330–340
Ning R, Tang X, Conover D (2004) X-ray scatter correction algorithm for cone beam CT imaging. Med Phys 31(5):1195
Peters AR et al (2000) The accuracy of image registration for the brain and the nasopharynx using external anatomical landmarks. Phys Med Biol 45(8):2403–2416
Poludniowski G et al (2010) CT reconstruction from portal images acquired during volumetric-modulated arc therapy. Phys Med Biol 55(19):5635–5651
Roche A et al (1998) The correlation ratio as a new similarity measure for multimodal image registration. Proc Int Conf Medical Image Computing and Computer-Assisted Interventation (MICCAI) 1496:1115

Ruchala KJ et al (2000) Megavoltage CT image reconstruction during tomotherapy. Phys Med Biol 45:3545–3562

Saotome N (2013) Four-dimensional dose calculation using in-treatment cone beam computed tomography and linear accelerator log data. The University of Tokyo, Tokyo

Schörner K, Goldammer M, Stephan J (2011) Comparison between beam-stop and beam-hole array scatter correction techniques for industrial X-ray cone-beam CT. Nucl Instrum Methods Phys Res, Sect B 269(3):292–299

Search H et al (1985) A beam-hardening correction using dual-energy computed tomography. Phys Med Biol 30:1251–1261

Shiraishi K et al (2014) Validation of planning target volume margins by analyzing intrafractional localization errors for 14 prostate cancer patients based on Three-Dimensional cross-correlation between the prostate images of planning CT and intrafraction cone-beam CT during volumetric modulated arc therapy. Biomed Res Int 2014:1 960928

Siewerdsen JH et al (2004) The influence of antiscatter grids on soft-tissue detectability in cone-beam computed tomography with flat-panel detectors. Med Phys 31(12):3506–3520

Sonke J-J et al (2005) Respiratory correlated cone beam CT. Med Phys 32(4):1176

Staub D, Murphy MJ (2013) A digitally reconstructed radiograph algorithm calculated from first principles. Med Phys 40(1):011902

Takahashi W et al (2013) Verification of planning target volume settings in volumetric modulated arc therapy for stereotactic body radiation therapy by using in-treatment 4-Dimensional cone beam computed tomography. Int J Radiat Oncol Biol Phys 86(3):426–431

Timmerman RD, Xing L (2009) Image-guided and adaptive radiation therapy. Lippincott Williams & Wilkins, Philadelphia

Ueda Y et al (2012) Craniocaudal safety margin calculation based on interfractional changes in tumor motion in lung SBRT assessed with an EPID in cine mode. Int J Radiat Oncol Biol Phys 83(3):1064–1069

Van Herk M (2008) Will IGRT live up to its promise? Acta Oncol (Stockh) 47(7):1186–1187

van Zijtveld M, Dirkx M, Heijmen B (2007) Correction of conebeam CT values using a planning CT for derivation of the "dose of the day.". Radiother Oncol 85(2):195–200

West J et al (1997) Comparison and evaluation of retrospective intermodality brain image registration techniques. J Comput Assist Tomogr 21(4):554–568

Wikström K et al (2014) A comparison of patient position displacements from body surface laser scanning and cone beam CT bone registrations for radiotherapy of pelvic targets. Acta Oncol 53(2):268–277

Wong JW et al (1999) The use of active breathing control (ABC) to reduce margin for breathing motion. Int J Radiat Oncol Biol Phys 44(4):911–919

Yan D et al (2000) An off-line strategy for constructing a patient-specific planning target volume in adaptive treatment process for prostate cancer. Int J Radiat Oncol Biol Phys 48(1):289–302

Yan H et al (2012) Hybrid MV-kV 3D respiratory motion tracking during radiation therapy with low imaging dose. Phys Med Biol 57(24):8455–8469

Yao W, Leszczynski KW (2009a) An analytical approach to estimating the first order scatter in heterogeneous medium. II. A practical application. Med Phys 36(7):3157–3167

Yao W, Leszczynski KW (2009b) An analytical approach to estimating the first order x-ray scatter in heterogeneous medium. Med Phys 36(7):3145–3156

Zbijewski W, Beekman FJ, Member S (2006) Efficient Monte Carlo based scatter artifact reduction in Cone-Beam Micro-CT. IEEE Trans Med Imaging 25(7):817–827

Zelefsky MJ et al (2012) Improved clinical outcomes with high-dose image guided radiotherapy compared with non-IGRT for the treatment of clinically localized prostate cancer. Int J Radiat Oncol Biol Phys 84(1):125–129

Zhao W et al (2015) Patient-specific scatter correction for flat-panel detector-based cone-beam CT imaging. Phys Med Biol 60(3):1339–1365

Zhu L et al (2009) Scatter correction for cone-beam CT in radiation therapy. Med Phys 36(6):2258

Zhuang L et al (2013) An optimization algorithm for 3D real-time lung tumor tracking during arc therapy using kV projection images. Med Phys 40(10):101710

Zijp L, Sonke J, van Herk M (2004) Extraction of the respiratory signal from sequential thorax Cone-Beam X-ray images. International Conference on the Use of Computers in Radiation Therapy, pp 507–509.

Chapter 10
Surface-Imaging-Based Patient Positioning in Radiation Therapy

Mazen Soufi and Hidetaka Arimura

Abstract The accelerating advancement in surface-imaging technology has led to promising possibilities with respect to monitoring patient positioning during radiation therapy without the use of radiographic imaging. The aim of this chapter is to introduce theoretical aspects and key computational techniques utilized in estimating positioning errors and analysing the patient's surface during radiation treatment. In particular, we provide an overview of current surface-imaging technologies. Next, we introduce quantitative approaches for mathematical reconstruction of a patient's surface using non-uniform rational B-spline (NURBS) modelling and subsequently characterizing of the local shapes of the patient's surface based on differential geometry. In addition, an iterative closest point (ICP) registration algorithm, which is a basic technique for estimating positioning errors, is explained. We hope that the topics covered in this chapter will be assistive in understanding the current applications in the field and will create launching points for the development of novel solutions.

Keywords Radiation therapy • Patient positioning errors • Surface imaging • Anatomical feature points • Differential geometry features

10.1 Introduction

Surface-imaging systems have become essential in-room imaging modalities in the era of high-precision radiation therapy (Timmerman and Xing 2009). Modern external radiation treatments, such as intensity-modulated radiation therapy (IMRT) and stereotactic body radiation therapy (SBRT), have enabled the dose directed at the tumours to be escalated while sparing the neighbouring normal tissues. Nevertheless, the challenging problem of the patient positioning errors (i.e. the discrepancies in the patient position between the treatment planning time and the radiation treatment time) has simultaneously attracted an increasing amount

---

M. Soufi (✉) • H. Arimura
Computer-aided Diagnosis and Radiotherapy Laboratory, Graduate School of Medical Sciences, Kyushu University, 3-1-1, Maidashi, Higashi-ku, Fukuoka 812-8582, Japan
e-mail: mazen_soofi@yahoo.com

H. Arimura (ed.), *Image-Based Computer-Assisted Radiation Therapy*,
DOI 10.1007/978-981-10-2945-5_10

of attention. The reason is that small position errors (a few millimetres) might deviate the steep dose distribution towards the neighbouring normal tissues, thereby raising the probability of complications in the normal tissues and reducing the dose directed at the target tumour. Therefore, technologies of high-precision radiation therapy have required the development of accompanying solutions for wisely controlling the radiation process and compensating for the discrepancies in the patient position during the patient setup and treatment (Willoughby et al. 2012).

In this context, surface-imaging systems have been suggested for two main applications: (1) positioning the patient on the treatment couch (for reducing *inter-fractional* patient setup error) and (2) monitoring of the patient's motion during treatment (for decreasing *intra-fractional* patient setup error) (Bert et al. 2005). In both applications, errors in the patient's position are detected by estimating the displacements in the surface point coordinates between a reference image acquired in treatment planning and images acquired just before and during the radiation treatment. Figure 10.1 illustrates the two applications of surface-imaging systems in radiation therapy for reducing inter- and intra-fractional setup errors.

The main advantages of surface-imaging systems are (1) non-ionization and (2) real-time acquisition. Intuitively, the non-ionizing approaches can be considered to be the most important motivation in the employment of surface-imaging systems in radiation therapy. The conventional radiographic imaging-based methods provide information about internal body structures and thus enable an accurate target-based positioning. However, the additional radiation dose that the patient receives during the CT scan is inevitable.

The current techniques for patient positioning using surface imaging can be divided in terms of the imaging principle into techniques based on projected light patterns, techniques based on laser scanning and techniques based on infrared ray time-of-flight (TOF) imaging. One might think of ultrasound (US) imaging as a feasible technique for patient positioning because it can produce three-dimensional (3D) images of body structures without the use of ionizing radiation. However, despite its advantages, US imaging is limited by its low image quality, as well as the fact that it deforms the surface and internal structures as a result of the pressure of the probe. Therefore, US imaging is not discussed in this chapter.

Surface-imaging systems are generally 'marker-less' because they do not require reflective markers (which are used in conventional approaches) to be attached to the patient's surface (Wang et al. 2001, Meeks et al. 2005, Wagner et al. 2007, Yoshitake et al. 2008). Instead of using the reflective markers, the patient's surface is illuminated with light rays (e.g. low-energy infrared laser rays) from a light source installed on an imaging unit, and the rays reflected from the patient's surface are detected by cameras installed on the same unit. Measurements of the detected rays are used to generate a 3D surface image – i.e. a 3D point distribution of the patient's surface. The main advantage of the surface image is that it represents the topography of the patient's surface, which enables us to estimate the positioning errors using image registration algorithms.

In this chapter, we introduce the theoretical aspects of surface image registration and analysis techniques, which are useful for patient positioning in radiation

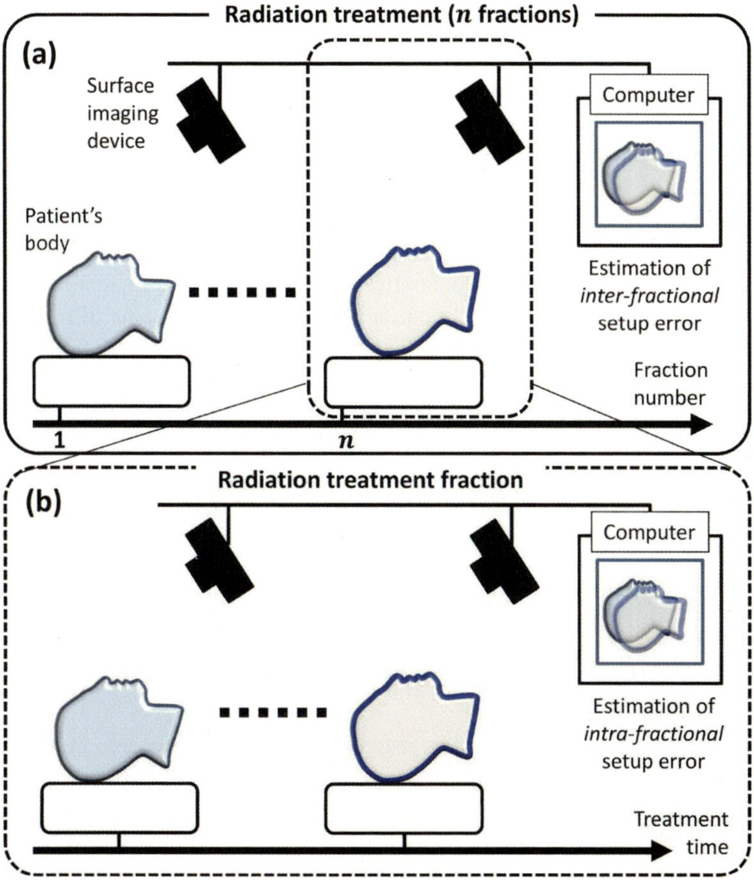

Fig. 10.1 Illustration of the applications of surface-imaging systems in radiation therapy in the estimation of (**a**) inter-fractional and (**b**) intra-fractional setup errors

therapy. We explain fundamental approaches for mathematical reconstruction of the patient's surface by using non-uniform rational B-spline (NURBS) modelling. Besides, we introduce an approach for analysing the topography of the patient's surface based on differential geometry in order to localize anatomical feature points on the patient's surface. Finally, we explain the concept of an iterative closest point (ICP) algorithm, which is a widely adopted algorithm in the estimation of patient positioning errors.

10.2 Surface-Imaging-Based Patient Positioning

A surface-image-based patient positioning and motion detection system consists of two main components: a surface-imaging device and a surface-image processing unit (e.g. a personal computer). During the radiation treatment time, the imaging device captures images of the patient's surface, which are fed to the personal computer. Next, these treatment images are preprocessed in order to reduce spatial and temporal noise, such as that caused by the imaging circuitry. In addition, optical distortions, which are caused by the optical components of the imaging device, are corrected using pre-calculated calibration parameters. At the same time, reference images are retrieved from a database or a storage device. In the context of this chapter, the reference image is a surface image that can be acquired either at the beginning of the treatment session or at the planning phase. Another option is to obtain the reference image from the planning CT image. The moving image, on the other hand, is the surface image acquired during treatment. Since the surface image is the essential element in this computational pipeline, we start with its mathematical definition.

10.2.1 Definition of Surface Image

A surface image can be expressed by using a position vector located in a Cartesian coordinate system. Let a position vector be $\boldsymbol{p} = (x, y, z(x, y)) \in \mathbb{R}^3$. Thus, a surface image $\boldsymbol{I}$ consisting of N position vectors on the patient's surface can be expressed as follows (Colombo et al. 2006):

$$\boldsymbol{I} = \begin{bmatrix} x_1 & y_1 & z_1(x_1, y_1) \\ \vdots & \vdots & \vdots \\ x_N & y_N & z_N(x_N, y_N) \end{bmatrix}. \tag{10.1}$$

This vector-based representation of the surface image enables the implementation of shape-modelling techniques and image registration algorithms that can be used to calculate patient positioning errors using both rigid and nonrigid transformations. A rigid transformation entails a translation vector and a rotation matrix, whereas a nonrigid transformation includes scaling and nonlinear deformations represented as pointwise displacement vectors. For simplicity, we will hereafter refer to a position vector representing a point on a surface as a *point*. Next, we introduce basic technologies for the acquisition of surface images.

10.2.2 Surface Imaging Based on Projected Light Pattern

Surface-imaging systems based on projected light pattern (e.g. AlignRT, Vision RT, Ltd., UK) have been widely used to monitor of patient's positioning. Such systems consist of two imaging units (pods) suspended at the ceiling of the treatment room.

In surface-imaging systems based on projected light pattern, the patient's surface image is acquired based on the stereovision imaging principle (Bert et al. 2005). In stereovision imaging, an epipolar geometrical model is used for computing the 3D coordinates of a point on the object's surface. This model is based on the cameras' internal parameters and the relative position of the point in two images captured from different viewpoints. Therefore, this principle requires a correspondence between the pixels of the object's surface points in the acquired images. As the patient's skin might not include sufficient information for establishing this correspondence, a speckle pattern is projected on the surface during the acquisition of the stereo images, and the pattern is detected in the images in order to estimate the required correspondence.

10.2.3 Surface Imaging Based on Laser Scanning

Surface-imaging systems based on laser scanning have also been developed in order to monitor patient positioning. Typically, a laser scanner consists of a laser source, a mirror attached to a motor, and a camera. A laser fan beam is swept over the patient's surface by changing the mirror angle using the motor. With each sweep of the laser beam, the camera captures an image of the reflected laser light over the patient's surface. The surface image is then reconstructed by estimating the distance between the camera and the object based on a triangulation principle (Brahme et al. 2008).

10.2.4 Infrared Ray-Based Time-of-Flight Camera

Recently, low-cost range (distance) imaging systems (e.g. TOF cameras) have been suggested for use in monitoring patient positioning in radiation therapy (Placht et al. 2012, Bauer et al. 2013). The TOF camera consists of infrared light-emitting diodes (IR-LEDs), which irradiate the surface of the patient's body with infrared rays, and an imaging sensor that receives the reflected rays.

The TOF camera produces surface images based on measurements of the distance between the object and the camera. The distance is measured by calculating the phase shift between the irradiated and reflected infrared light rays over the patient's surface according to the following equation:

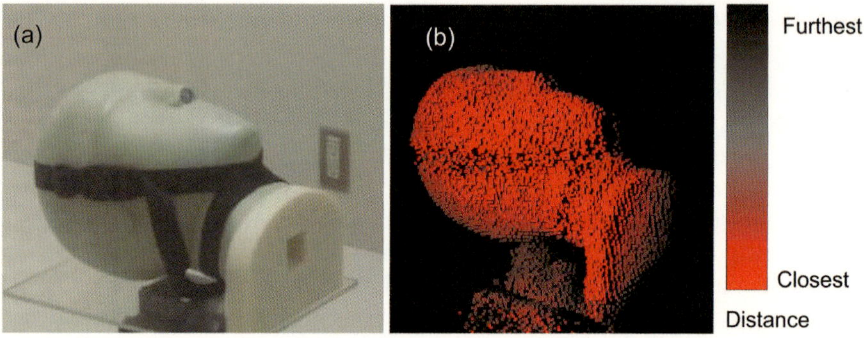

Fig. 10.2 Example of a surface image acquired by using a time-of-flight (TOF) camera: (**a**) anthropomorphic head phantom. (**b**) Surface image of the head phantom acquired by a TOF camera. *Red points* belong to closer regions, whereas *black points* belong to further regions

$$d = \frac{c}{4\pi f_{\mathrm{mod}}}\varphi, \tag{10.2}$$

where d is the estimated distance, φ is the phase shift, $c \approx 3 \times 10^8$ m/s is the speed of light and f_{mod} is the modulation frequency of irradiated rays (Büttgen and Seitz 2008).

Figure 10.2 shows an example of a surface image acquired by using a TOF camera. Figure 10.2a shows a picture of an anthropomorphic head phantom, and Fig. 10.2b shows a surface image of the phantom acquired by a TOF camera (CamCube 3.0, PMD Technologies, Siegen, Germany). The colours represent the distance between the camera and phantom's surface.

10.3 Mathematical Reconstruction of Patient's Surface Using NURBS

The mathematical reconstruction of the patient's surface is a useful technique for compensating for the sparsity and discontinuity in surface images. More specifically, the sparsity in the surface image originates from the low spatial resolution of the imaging sensor (number of pixels in the image) and distance between the camera and the object. In addition, owing to the noise produced by imaging circuitry and reflectivity characteristics of the surface, the smoothness of the acquired surface image may become deteriorated. Such limitations affect the quality of the acquired image by creating outliers and/or changing the topographic attributes of the surface image. Consequently, image analysis approaches based on differential vectors and image registration techniques (explained later) are frustrated by the appearance of outliers and/or changes in the topographic attributes. By using an appropriate reconstruction technique, it is possible to obtain dense and smooth surfaces (i.e. continuously differentiable surfaces) that improve the outcome of the aforementioned processes. However, first, we must define the principle of surface parameterization, as it is essential for the following topics.

10.3.1 Parameterized Surface

Let S be a surface consisting of points $\boldsymbol{p}\in\mathbb{R}^3$, as shown in Fig. 10.3. A parameterization of the surface is a map $\boldsymbol{S}:\mathbb{R}^2\rightarrow\mathbb{R}^3$. In other words, it can be obtained by assigning two values of parametric variables $(u,v)\in\mathbb{R}^2$ to each point $\boldsymbol{p}\in\mathbb{R}^3$ in the surface. Thus, the parameterization of the surface S can be expressed as follows:

$$\boldsymbol{p}(u,v)=\boldsymbol{p}(x(u,v),y(u,v),z(x(u,v),y(u,v))). \tag{10.3}$$

10.3.2 NURBS Surface Reconstruction

The basic idea of NURBS modelling is to calculate a smooth approximation for the position of a query point $\widehat{\boldsymbol{S}}(u,v)$ on the object's surface by using a set of neighbouring points derived from the original image, which are called control points, and n-degree piecewise B-spline functions that determine the influence of each control point on the query point's position. Given control points $\boldsymbol{p}_{i,j}$, the query point $\widehat{\boldsymbol{S}}(u,v)$ can be calculated using the following equation:

$$\widehat{\boldsymbol{S}}(u,v)=\frac{\sum\limits_{i=0}^{n}\sum\limits_{j=0}^{m}N_{i,c}(u)N_{j,d}(v)w_{i,j}\boldsymbol{p}_{i,j}}{\sum\limits_{i=0}^{n}\sum\limits_{j=0}^{m}N_{i,c}(u)N_{j,d}(v)w_{i,j}}, \tag{10.4}$$

where $u,v\in\mathbb{R}$ are the parametric variables; $m+1$ and $n+1$ are the number of the control points in the u and v directions, respectively; w is a weighting factor; and $N_{i,c}(u)$ and $N_{j,d}(v)$ are the basis functions of degrees c and d in the u and v directions, respectively (Piegl and Tiller 1997). The numerator of Eq. (10.4) can be seen as a locally weighted summation of the control points, whereas the denominator can be seen as a normalization term.

The degree of the basis function is an important factor in determining the shape of the obtained surface. Cubic functions – for example – produce smoother surfaces than linear or quadratic functions. The basis functions of the parametric variable u can be calculated by using the following Cox-de boor recursive formulas (Cox 1972, de Boor 1972):

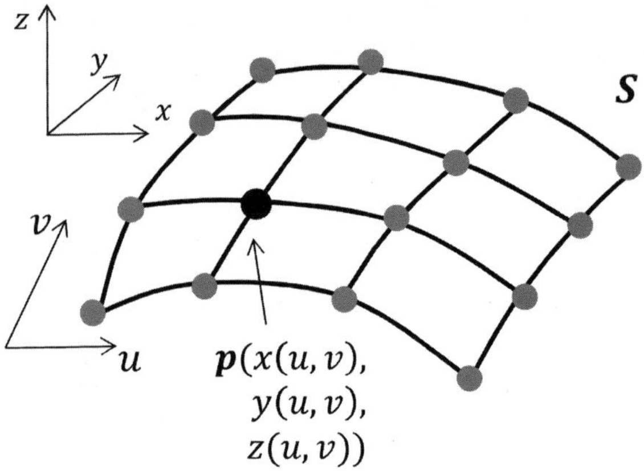

Fig. 10.3 A surface in a Cartesian coordinate system parameterized using two parametric variables u and v

$$N_{i,0}(u) = \begin{cases} 1 & \text{if } u_i \leq u < u_{i+1} \\ 0 & \text{otherwise} \end{cases}, \tag{10.5}$$

$$N_{i,c}(u) = \frac{u - u_i}{u_{i+c} - u_i} N_{i,c-1}(u) + \frac{u_{i+c+1} - u}{u_{i+c+1} - u_{i+1}} N_{i+1,c-1}(u). \tag{10.6}$$

Similarly, the basis functions of the parametric variable v can be computed as

$$N_{j,0}(v) = \begin{cases} 1 & \text{if } v_j \leq v < v_{j+1} \\ 0 & \text{otherwise} \end{cases}, \tag{10.7}$$

$$N_{j,d}(v) = \frac{v - v_j}{v_{j+d} - v_j} N_{j,d-1}(v) + \frac{v_{j+d+1} - v}{v_{j+d+1} - v_{j+1}} N_{j+1,d-1}(v). \tag{10.8}$$

For simplicity, we show examples for one-dimensional B-spline functions and NURBS curves. Figure 10.4 illustrates B-spline functions of the 1st (linear), 2nd (quadratic) and 3rd (cubic) degrees, which were calculated for five control points with respect to the parametric variable u.

Figure 10.5 illustrates the effect that the degree of the basis functions has upon the shape of a reconstructed NURBS curve $\boldsymbol{c}(u)$. In Fig. 10.5, linear basis functions were used for reconstructing the curve $\boldsymbol{c}_1$, whereas quadratic and cubic functions were used for reconstructing the curves $\boldsymbol{c}_2$ and $\boldsymbol{c}_3$, respectively. The smoothest curve was $\boldsymbol{c}_3$, which shows the advantage of using cubic basis functions.

The elements ui and v_j in Eqs. (10.5, 10.6, 10.7, 10.8) are called 'knots' because they define the connection between the basis functions in the parametric space. The knots, concatenated and ordered in ascending order, are called 'knot vectors'. For the parametric variables u and v, the knot vectors normalized in the range between 0 and 1 can be expressed as

$$\dot{\boldsymbol{u}} = [0, \ldots, 0, \ldots, u_k, u_{k+1}, \ldots, 1, \ldots, 1]; k = 1, \ldots, c + m + 2, \tag{10.9}$$

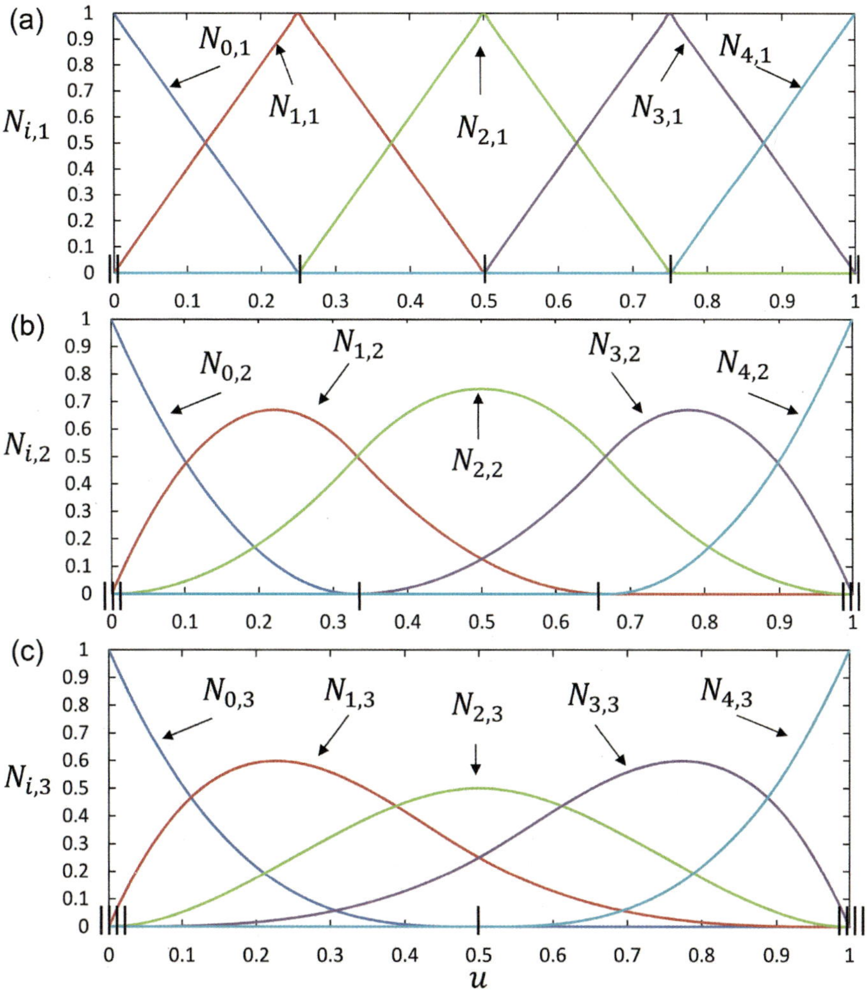

Fig. 10.4 Basis functions calculated for five control points with respect to the parametric variable *u*: (**a**) 1st (*linear*), (**b**) 2nd (*quadratic*) and (**c**) 3rd (*cubic*) degree functions

$$\dot{\boldsymbol{v}} = [0, \ldots, 0, \ldots, v_l, v_{l+1}, \ldots, 1, \ldots, 1]; l = 1, \ldots, d + n + 2. \tag{10.10}$$

The design of the knot vectors (i.e. location and spacing of the knots) has an effect on the shape of the computed surface. The number of repetitions of knots in both ends of vectors $\dot{\boldsymbol{u}}$ and $\dot{\boldsymbol{v}}$ is referred to as the multiplicity of the knot. By increasing the multiplicity of a knot, the control points on its side will have larger influence on the shape, because more basis functions will be connected at that knot. A multiplicity equal to the degree of the basis functions plus one is needed for the first and last elements in order to allow the surface to pass through the boundary control points. In Fig. 10.4, knot vectors of $\dot{\boldsymbol{u}} = [0, 0, 0.25, 0.5, 0.75, 1, 1]$,

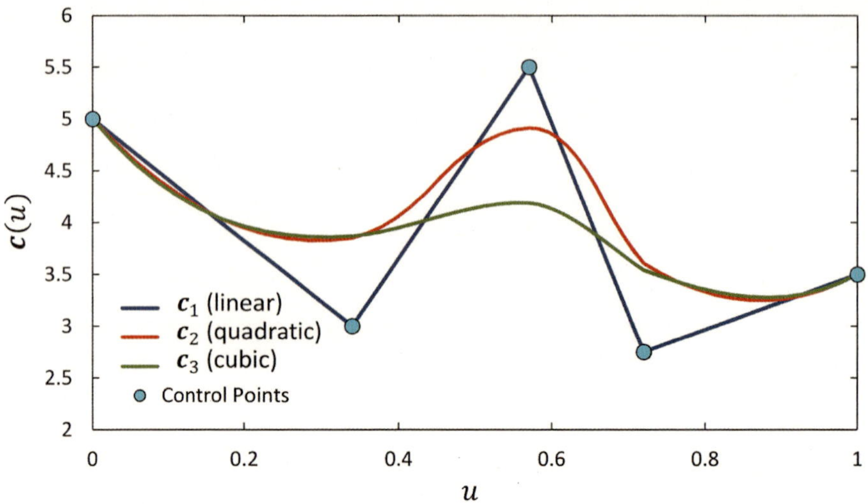

Fig. 10.5 Effect of degree of the basis functions on the smoothness of the reconstructed NURBS curves

$\dot{\boldsymbol{u}} = [0, 0, 0, 0.33, 0.67, 1, 1, 1]$ and $\dot{\boldsymbol{u}} = [0, 0, 0, 0, 0.5, 1, 1, 1, 1]$ were used for computing the linear, quadratic and cubic basis functions, respectively (the knots were represented as black bars in the u axis).

The algorithm of computing a point $\widehat{\boldsymbol{S}}(u, v)$ on the reconstructed NURBS surface can be summarized as follows:

Step 1: Select the control points from the original surface image parametrized with two parametric variables u and v.
Step 2: Set the degrees of the surface in u and v directions – i.e. c and d.
Step 3: Set the knot vectors in the u and v directions.

For the parametric value u, perform the following steps:

Step 4: Find the knot span – i.e. the interval $[u_k, u_{k+1})$ in which u lies.
Step 5: Compute the basis functions $N_{k-c,c}(u) \ldots N_{k,c}(u)$.

For the parametric value v, perform the following steps:

Step 6: Find the knot span – i.e. the interval $[v_l, v_{l+1})$ in which v lies.
Step 7: Compute the basis functions $N_{l-d,d}(v) \ldots N_{l,d}(v)$.
Step 8: Compute the query point $\widehat{\boldsymbol{S}}(u, v)$ using Eq. (10.4).

Figure 10.6 shows a reconstructed surface of the nose region of a head phantom surface obtained using NURBS modelling. The control points were derived from an image of the phantom's surface, as shown in Fig. 10.6b. A smooth surface of the nose region was obtained by using cubic basis functions, as shown in Fig. 10.6c.

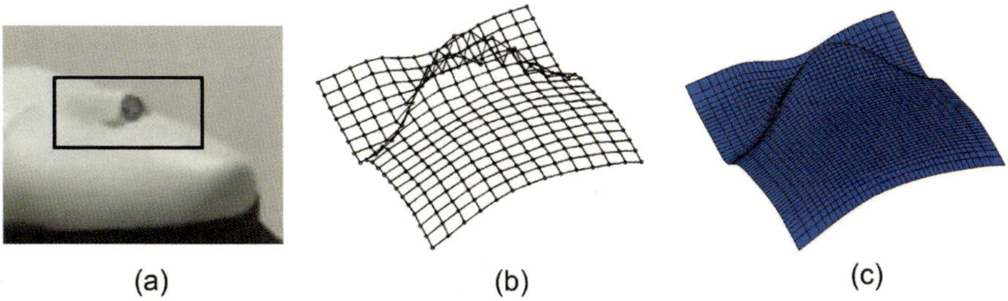

Fig. 10.6 An example for reconstruction of a patient's surface using NURBS modelling from a surface image. (**a**) Nose region defined on a head phantom. (**b**) Control points obtained from the surface image. (**c**) The reconstructed NURBS surface of the nose region

10.4 Analysis of a Patient's Surface Using Differential Geometry

The localization of anatomical landmarks on patient surfaces is beneficial for monitoring patient positioning during radiation therapy, particularly in the image registration step. Feature points on the localized landmarks can be used to accelerate the image registration process by dividing it into two steps: coarse registration and fine registration. During the coarse registration, the feature points are used to identify initial transformation parameters in a short time, as they constitute a subset of the original point distribution. Then, the fine registration boosts the estimation of the transformation parameters by further minimizing the error function (Placht et al. 2012).

One of the intuitive approaches for the localization of anatomical landmarks in a surface image is to compute differential geometry (curvature) features. The mathematical field of differential geometry includes theories for analysing the geometrical characteristics of a surface in a 3D space (Pressley 2010). Differential geometry uses differential vectors of surface points to identify and analyse the surface characteristics. However, this method of analysis is limited by its sensitivity to noise in the surface (Agam and Tang 2005). As a result, this sensitivity affects the accuracy of the estimated features and, consequently, the stability of the localized points. Aside from the use of appropriate spatial and filtering techniques, NURBS surface reconstruction is expected to improve the outcome of such analysis (Soufi et al. 2016).

In order to localize of anatomical landmarks, we focus on the property of the surface curvature. The assumption here is that anatomical landmarks on the surface of patient's body – especially the surface of the head – have distinctly curved shapes. For example, Fig. 10.7 shows anatomical landmarks at the nose region of a head phantom. Apparently, the apex and alae of the nose have convex shapes, whereas the nasolabial and nasofacial sulci have concave shapes.

We introduce the principles of analysing the patient's surface based on its curvature by first defining the curvature of a curve. Next, we explain the concept

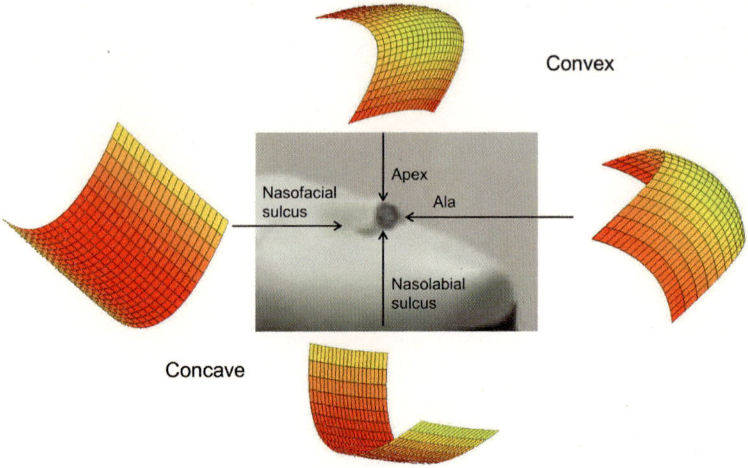

Fig. 10.7 Anatomical landmarks of the nose region with corresponding curvature types

of the curvature of a surface, which will help us to measure the local shape of surface regions analytically and localize the feature points.

10.4.1 Curvature of a Curve

The curvature of curve can be obtained by studying the changes in a position vector representing a point's position on the parameterized curve. Suppose that $\boldsymbol{c}(s)$ is a parameterized regular curve (i.e. the curve is differentiable, and $\|\dot{\boldsymbol{c}}(s)\| \neq 0$ at all the points, where $\dot{\boldsymbol{c}}(s)$ indicates the first derivative (velocity) of $\boldsymbol{c}(s)$). The parameter $s \in \mathbb{R}$ is called *arc length* and indicates the length of the curve's segment measured between two points of it. Then, the curvature of $\boldsymbol{c}(s)$ can be calculated as

$$\kappa = \frac{\|\ddot{\boldsymbol{c}}(s) \times \dot{\boldsymbol{c}}(s)\|}{\|\dot{\boldsymbol{c}}(s)\|^3}, \tag{10.11}$$

where '×' denotes the outer product operator and $\ddot{\boldsymbol{c}}(s)$ indicates the second derivative (acceleration) of $\boldsymbol{c}(s)$.

Now, assume that a short segment of $\boldsymbol{c}(s)$ can be approximated to an arc of a circle, as shown in Fig. 10.8, and we want to calculate its curvature. In this case, $\boldsymbol{c}(s)$ can have the following parameterization at that segment:

$$\boldsymbol{c}(s) = (x_0 + r\cos(\theta), y_0 + r\sin(\theta)). \tag{10.12}$$

where $\boldsymbol{m}(x_0, y_0)$ is the centre of the circle, r is its radius and θ is the central angle of the arc in Radians. By using the arc-length relationship ($s = \theta r$), Equation (10.12) can be rewritten as

$$\boldsymbol{c}(s) = \left(x_0 + r\cos\left(\frac{s}{r}\right), y_0 + r\sin\left(\frac{s}{r}\right)\right). \tag{10.13}$$

Thus, the first and second derivatives can be derived as shown in Eqs. (10.14) and (10.15), respectively:

$$\dot{\boldsymbol{c}}\,(s) = \left(-\sin\left(\frac{s}{r}\right),\ \cos\left(\frac{s}{r}\right)\right), \tag{10.14}$$

$$\ddot{\boldsymbol{c}}(s) = \left(-\frac{1}{r}\cos\left(\frac{s}{r}\right), -\frac{1}{r}\sin\left(\frac{s}{r}\right)\right). \tag{10.15}$$

By using the cross product formula:

$$\boldsymbol{a} \times \boldsymbol{b} = \|\boldsymbol{a}\|\|\boldsymbol{b}\|\sin(\alpha)\boldsymbol{n}, \tag{10.16}$$

where α is the angle between $\boldsymbol{a}$ and $\boldsymbol{b}$ (α is a right angle because $\dot{\boldsymbol{c}}\,(s)$ and $\ddot{\boldsymbol{c}}(s)$ are perpendicular) and $\boldsymbol{n}$ is a unit normal vector to the plane spanned by $\dot{\boldsymbol{c}}\,(s)$ and $\ddot{\boldsymbol{c}}(s)$; the curvature of $\boldsymbol{c}(s)$ can be calculated as

$$\kappa = \frac{\sqrt{\left(-\frac{1}{r}\cos\left(\frac{s}{r}\right)\right)^2 + \left(-\frac{1}{r}\sin\left(\frac{s}{r}\right)\right)^2}\sqrt{\left(\cos\left(\frac{s}{r}\right)\right)^2 + \left(\sin\left(\frac{s}{r}\right)\right)^2}}{\left(\sqrt{\left(\cos\left(\frac{s}{r}\right)\right)^2 + \left(\sin\left(\frac{s}{r}\right)\right)^2}\right)^3},$$
$$\kappa = \frac{1}{r}. \tag{10.17}$$

Equation (10.17) indicates an inverse relationship between the curvature of the curve and the radius of the approximated circle. In order to clarify this relationship, let us compare two curves $\boldsymbol{c}_1$ and $\boldsymbol{c}_2$, where $\boldsymbol{c}_2$ has a larger curvature at point $\boldsymbol{p}_2$ than the curvature of $\boldsymbol{c}_1$ at a point $\boldsymbol{p}_1$, as shown in Fig. 10.9. This implies that the approximated circle at $\boldsymbol{p}_1$ must have a larger radius r_1 than r_2 in order to fit within the curve. On the other side, if $\boldsymbol{c}_1$ were almost flat, then r_1 would have to be very large in order to allow the circle to approximate a flat surface, in which case the curvature would approach zero.

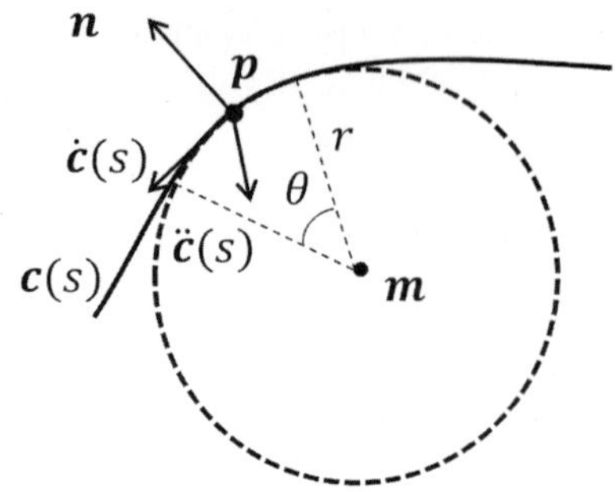

Fig. 10.8 Definition of the curvature of a parameterized curve

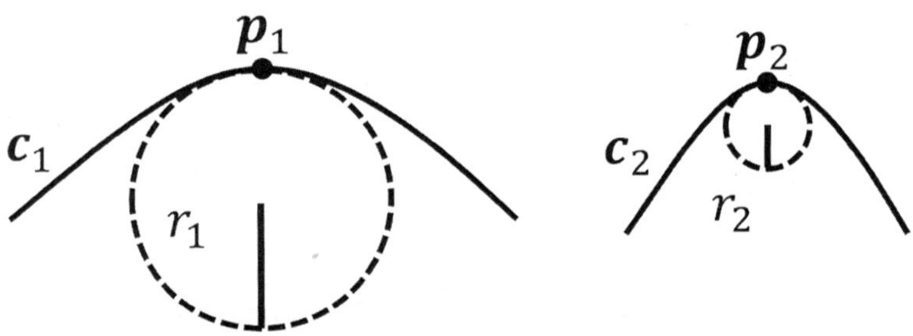

Fig. 10.9 Relationship between the radius of the circle used to approximate the curve at a point and the curvature of the curve at that point

10.4.2 Curvature of a Surface

Now, we advance to the concept of surface curvature. At an arbitrary point $\boldsymbol{p}_s$ of the surface $\boldsymbol{S}$, there can be an infinite number of curves passing through $\boldsymbol{p}_s$ and lying on the surface. As a result, there can be an infinite number of tangential vectors $\boldsymbol{g}$ to the surface at that point. However, there is a single normal vector $\boldsymbol{n}$ to the surface, which is oriented at a certain direction from the surface (upwards or downwards). This normal vector, combined with an arbitrary tangential vector, spans a normal plane P, which intersects with the surface to form a curve C, as shown in Fig. 10.10. The curvature of C is called the normal curvature.

Among the normal planes, there exist two planes whose normal curves have special characteristics. Those are the planes whose normal curves have either the maximum curvature, κ_1, or the minimum curvature, κ_2, of the surface at $\boldsymbol{p}_s$, as shown in Fig. 10.11. The curvatures κ_1 and κ_2 are called the principal curvatures, and together with their associated tangential vectors (also called principal directions), they can be used to define a local quadratic approximation to the surface. In other words, they define a new coordinate system with axes $\widehat{x}$ and $\widehat{y}$ in the principal directions, and $\widehat{z}$ in the normal direction. The new coordinate system can be used to characterize the shape of the surface at the local neighbourhood of the point $\boldsymbol{p}_s$.

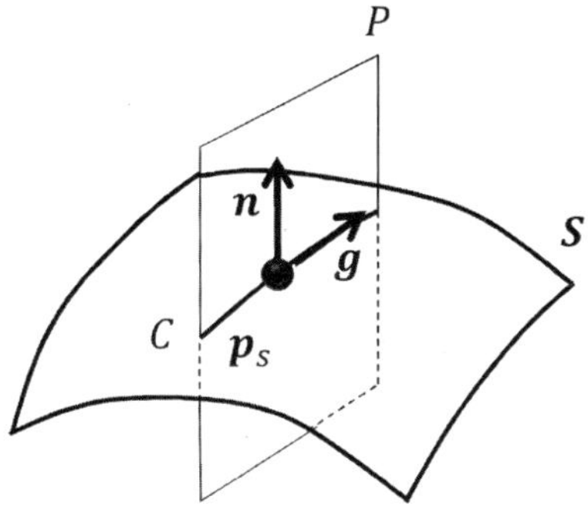

Fig. 10.10 Definition of the normal curvature of a surface S at point p_s as the curvature of the curve C that results from the intersection of plane P with the surface. Plane P (the normal plane) is spanned by a tangential vector g and the normal vector n

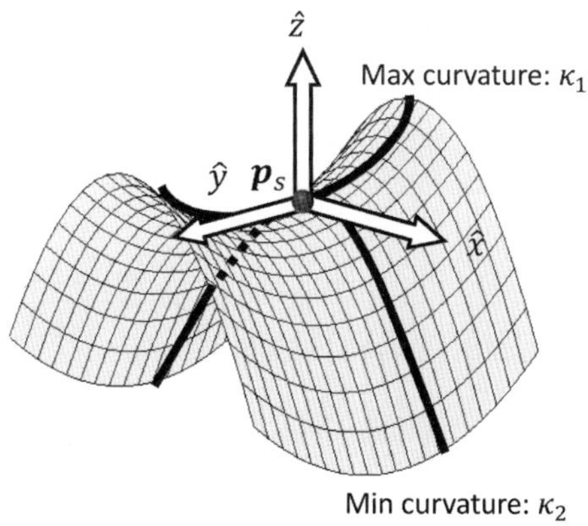

Fig. 10.11 Definition of the principal curvatures – i.e. maximum and minimum curvatures and principal directions at a point p_s of an object's surface

Using the new coordinate system, the local shape of a surface, which is represented by its principal curvatures, can be approximated as a paraboloid described by the following equation:

$$\widehat{z} = -\left(\kappa_1\widehat{x}^2 + \kappa_2\widehat{y}^2\right). \tag{10.18}$$

The paraboloid can have one of two shapes at the neighbourhood of p_s based on the signs of the principal curvatures. If both signs are identical, the shape will be elliptic – i.e. convex if both signs are negative and concave if the signs are positive – as shown in Fig. 10.12a, b, respectively. If the signs are opposite, the shape will be hyperbolic (i.e. saddle-shaped), as shown in Fig. 10.12c.

The principal curvatures at a point of a parametric surface can be calculated as the eigenvalues of a fundamental matrix, which is computed by using first and second fundamental forms. The first fundamental form is calculated by using first-order differential vectors of the surface at the point, whereas the second fundamental form is computed by using the second-order differential vectors and the normal vector at that point (Pressley 2010).

The calculation procedure of the principal curvatures by using the fundamental matrix can be summarized as follows:

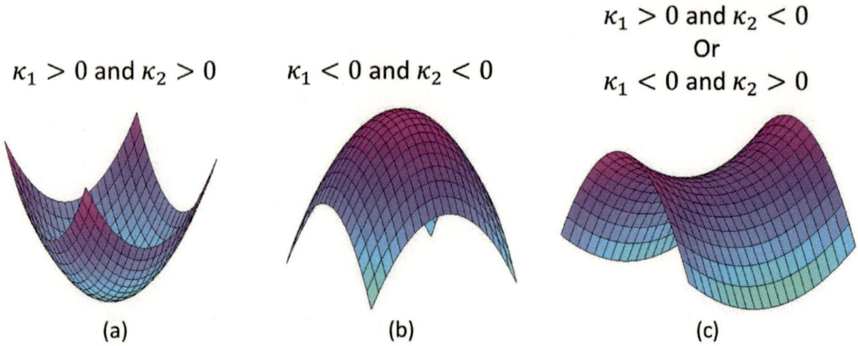

Fig. 10.12 Classification of the local shape type based on the sign of the principal curvatures. (**a**) Elliptic concave shape. (**b**) Elliptic convex shape. (**c**) Hyperbolic (saddle) shape

Step 1: Calculate the first-order differential vectors of the surface with respect to the parametric variables u and v:

$$\boldsymbol{p}_u = \left(\frac{\partial x}{\partial u}, \frac{\partial y}{\partial u}, \frac{\partial z}{\partial u}\right), \boldsymbol{p}_v = \left(\frac{\partial x}{\partial v}, \frac{\partial y}{\partial v}, \frac{\partial z}{\partial v}\right). \tag{10.19}$$

Step 2: Calculate the second-order differential vectors of the surface with respect to the u and v directions:

$$\boldsymbol{p}_{uu} = \left(\frac{\partial^2 x}{\partial u^2}, \frac{\partial^2 y}{\partial u^2}, \frac{\partial^2 z}{\partial u^2}\right), \boldsymbol{p}_{uv} = \left(\frac{\partial^2 x}{\partial u \partial v}, \frac{\partial^2 y}{\partial u \partial v}, \frac{\partial^2 z}{\partial u \partial v}\right), \boldsymbol{p}_{vv} = \left(\frac{\partial^2 x}{\partial v^2}, \frac{\partial^2 y}{\partial v^2}, \frac{\partial^2 z}{\partial v^2}\right). \tag{10.20}$$

Step 3: Calculate the coefficients of the first fundamental form:

$$E = \| \boldsymbol{p}_u \|^2, \;\; F = \langle \boldsymbol{p}_u, \boldsymbol{p}_v \rangle \;\; G = \| \boldsymbol{p}_v \|^2, \tag{10.21}$$

where $\langle \cdot, \cdot \rangle$ denotes the inner product operator.

Step 4: Calculate the normal vector perpendicular to the surface at the point $\boldsymbol{p}_s$:

$$\boldsymbol{n} = \frac{\boldsymbol{p}_u \times \boldsymbol{p}_v}{\|\boldsymbol{p}_u \times \boldsymbol{p}_v\|}, \tag{10.22}$$

where '×' denotes the outer product operator.

Step 5: Calculate the coefficients of the second fundamental form:

$$L = \langle \boldsymbol{p}_{uu}, \boldsymbol{n} \rangle, M = \langle \boldsymbol{p}_{uv}, \boldsymbol{n} \rangle, N = \langle \boldsymbol{p}_{vv}, \boldsymbol{n} \rangle. \tag{10.23}$$

Step 6: Calculate the fundamental matrix $\boldsymbol{A}$:

$$\boldsymbol{A} = \begin{bmatrix} E & F \\ F & G \end{bmatrix}^{-1} \begin{bmatrix} L & M \\ M & N \end{bmatrix}, \tag{10.24}$$

with $\begin{vmatrix} E & F \\ F & G \end{vmatrix} \neq 0.$

Step 7: Calculate the eigenvalues of $\boldsymbol{A}$ that represent the principal curvatures κ_1 and κ_2 of the surface at $\boldsymbol{p}_s$.

The coefficients of the first fundamental form quantify deformations in the surface patches that result from non-uniform distribution of the points on the object's surface in the surface image. Figure 10.13 shows the effect of the surface patch on the coefficients of the first fundamental form. The coefficients E and G represent the length of the first-order differential vectors, whereas the coefficient F is related to the angle between the two vectors. In Fig. 10.13a, the patch is deformed into a parallelogram, which leads to positive coefficients. However, the rectangular patch has F value of zero because the differential vectors are orthogonal, as shown in Fig. 10.13b.

In order to further understand the coefficients of the first fundamental form, let us examine the computed vectors on the object's surface. Figure 10.14 shows an example of the first-order differential vectors and normal vectors in an image of the nose region of a head phantom's surface. On the left-hand side, the patches, which were deformed as a result of the irregular distribution of the points at the nasal wall, are depicted. On the right-hand side, the rectangular patches on the apex of nose region are depicted. The effect of the deformation can be observed through the colour-coded maps of the coefficients of the first fundamental form, as shown in Figs. 10.15a–c. We can note that large values were obtained at the deformed patches at the nasal wall. In Figs. 10.15a, c, large values were obtained due to the large magnitudes of the derivatives in the u and v directions, respectively, at the deformed patches. In Fig. 10.15b, the colour-coded map is asymmetric owing to the different signs of the first-order differential vectors between the ascending and descending regions – i.e. the sign of the differentials of the z-coordinate.

The coefficients of the second fundamental form, which were estimated in Eq. (10.23), represent the variations in the angle between the second-order differential vectors and normal vectors. Figures 10.15d–f show colour-coded maps of the coefficients of the second fundamental form. At the sulci and edges of the object's surface, the variations in the angle between the second-order differential vectors and normal vectors have a larger magnitude than those at the flat regions.

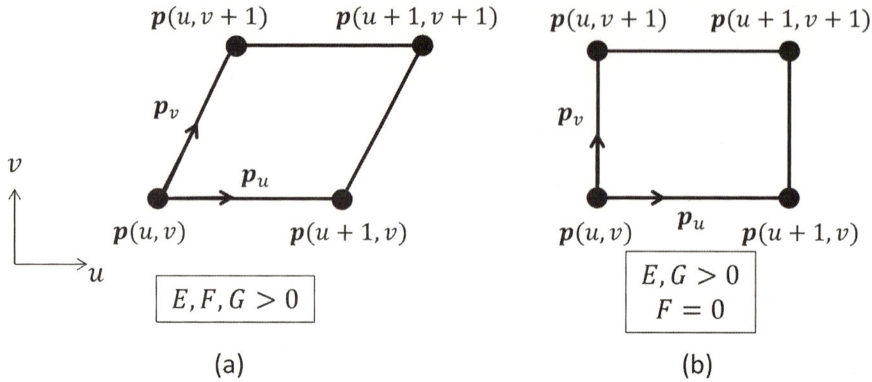

Fig. 10.13 Illustration of the meaning of the coefficients of the first fundamental form, whose values represent the deformation in the patches of a parameterized object's surface. (**a**) Deformed patch. (**b**) Rectangular (underformed) patch

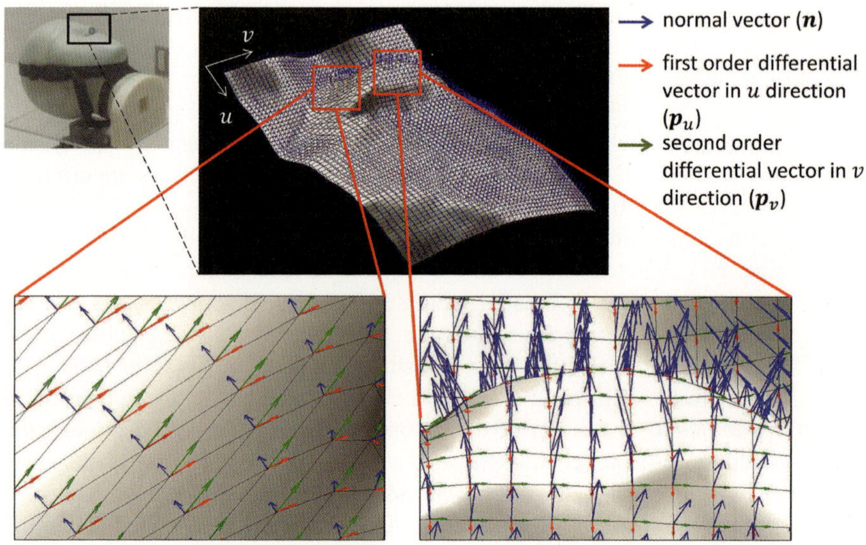

Fig. 10.14 Illustration of first-order differential and normal vectors computed on a surface image of the nose region of a head phantom

10.4.3 Surface Curvature Features

In the process of localizing anatomical landmarks on the analysed surface, it is impractical to use the principal curvatures directly. That is because the relationship between the two curvatures (rather than their values) is what expresses the shape of the region. Therefore, four alternative curvature features, which are the mean and Gaussian curvatures, the curvedness and shape index, are used.

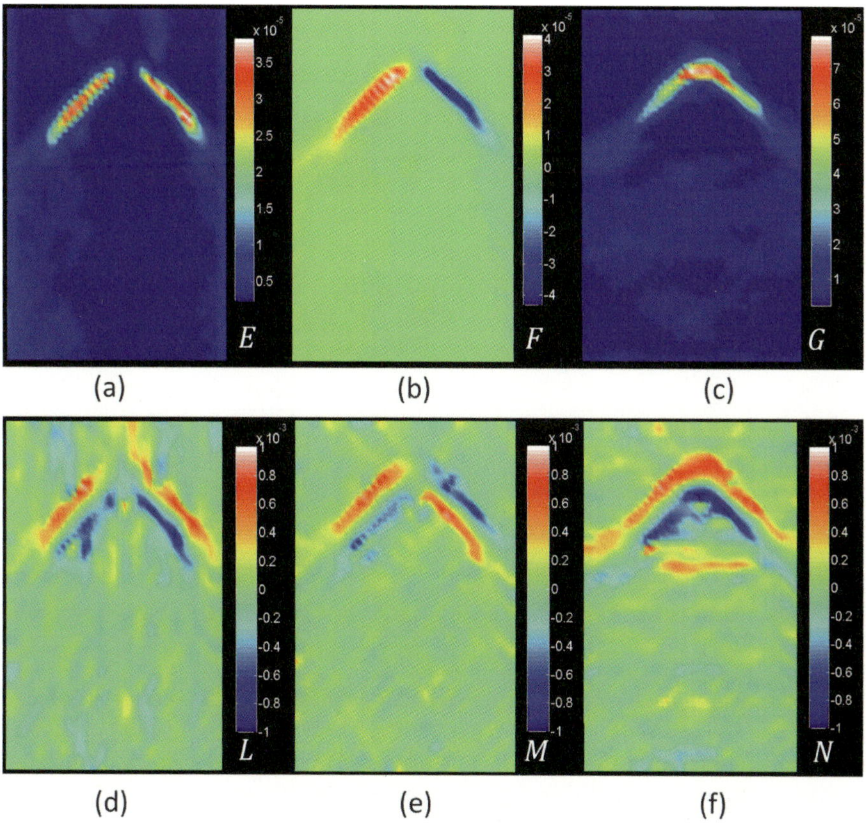

Fig. 10.15 Colour-coded maps of the coefficients of the first and second fundamental forms computed on a surface image of the nose region of a head phantom: (**a**) E, (**b**) F, (**c**) G, (**d**) L, (**e**) M and (**f**) N

The mean and Gaussian curvatures can be estimated using the principal curvatures, as shown in Eqs. (10.25) and (10.26), respectively:

$$H = \frac{1}{2}\mathrm{trace}(\boldsymbol{A}) = \frac{1}{2}(\kappa_1 + \kappa_2), \tag{10.25}$$

$$G = \det(\boldsymbol{A}) = \kappa_1\kappa_2. \tag{10.26}$$

Figure 10.16 illustrates the relationship between the sign of the mean and Gaussian curvatures and the shape of the surface. Based on this relationship, a point classification function can be constructed to localize the points at which the surface has a distinct shape. For example, points located on elliptic-concave regions can be localized by a selection of points that satisfy $H < 0$ and $G > 0$. Similarly, points on elliptic-convex regions can be localized by using the conditions $H > 0$ and

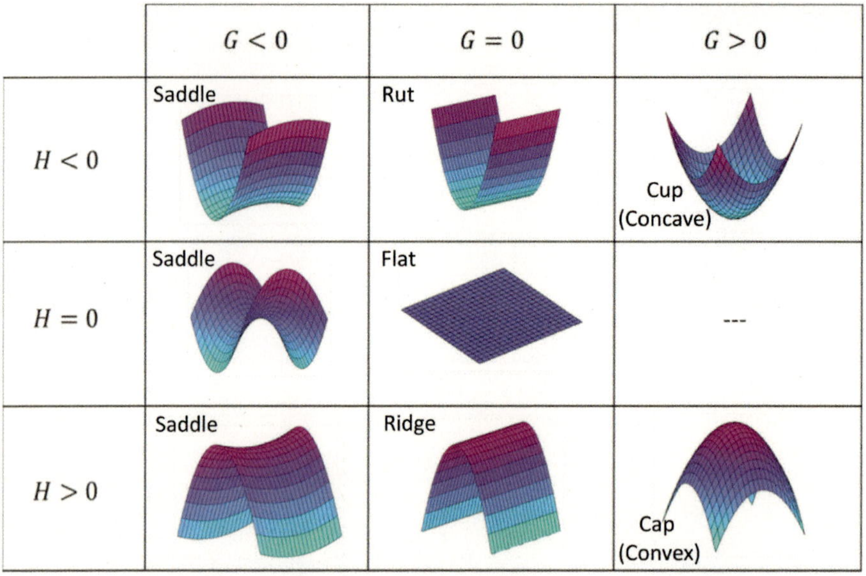

Fig. 10.16 Classification of the surface shape at a point based on mean and Gaussian curvatures

$G > 0$. Points on planar regions can be localized by using the conditions $H \cong 0$ and $G \cong 0$.

As an example, Fig. 10.17 shows colour-coded maps of the mean and Gaussian curvature features computed for a surface image of the nose. The convex regions at the nose, such as the apex and alae, have $G > 0$ and $H > 0$. On the other side, concave regions, such as the nasolabial and nasofacial sulci, have $G > 0$ and $H < 0$.

Thus, the mean and Gaussian curvatures could be utilized for characterizing the local shape of the surface, as shown in Fig. 10.17. However, this method has a limitation of the need for the two curvatures to characterize the shape, where neither the mean nor Gaussian curvature holds the shape type information by its own. A single quantitative measure that characterizes the shape type would be more convenient.

For solving this problem, Koenderink et al. proposed two shape features that are calculated using the principal curvatures (Koenderink and van Doorn 1992). The two measures are the shape index, which is a scale-invariant measure that characterizes the local shape type, and the curvedness, which characterizes the degree of curvature of the surface. The shape index $\gamma \in [-1, 1]$ and curvedness $C \in [0, \infty)$ can be calculated by using the following Eqs. (10.27) and (10.28), respectively:

$$\gamma = \frac{2}{\pi} \tan^{-1}\left(\frac{k_1 + k_2}{k_1 - k_2}\right), \tag{10.27}$$

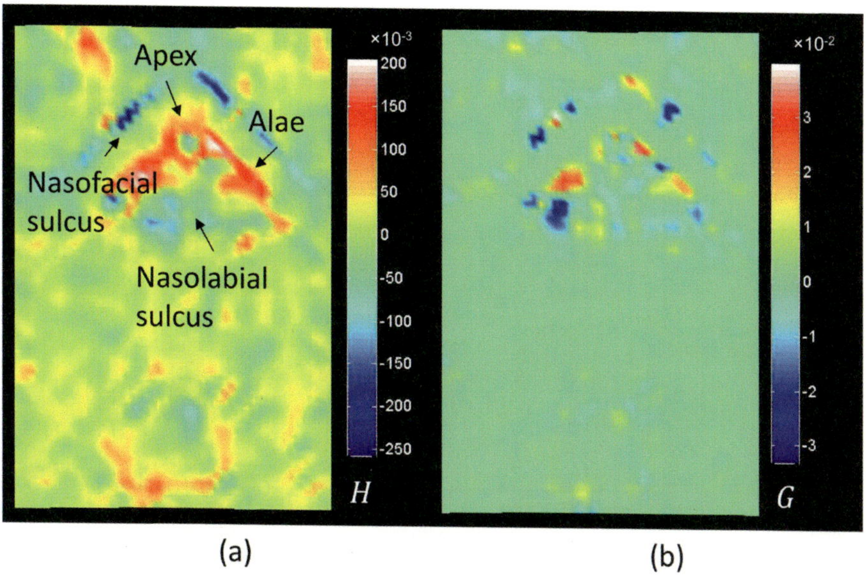

Fig. 10.17 Colour-coded maps of the curvature features computed for a surface image of the nose region of a head phantom: (**a**) mean curvature and (**b**) Gaussian curvature

$$C = \sqrt{\frac{k_1^2 + k_2^2}{2}}. \tag{10.28}$$

Figure 10.18 illustrates the geometrical meaning of the shape index and curvedness features. Figure 10.18a shows the classification of the shape types with respect to the shape index. The end values (i.e. $\gamma = \pm 1$) indicate the surface points that have a spherical concave (cup) or convex (cap) shapes. The points with $0 < |\gamma| < 1$ indicate a cylindrical region, while points with $-0.5 \leq |\gamma| \leq 0.5$ indicate saddle or saddle-like regions. Figure 10.18b shows the curvedness scale, in which larger values indicate larger curvature values. The large curvedness values might result from one of the principal curvatures or both, regardless of the shape type.

Figure 10.19 shows the shape index and curvedness features computed for the surface image of the head phantom. Figure 10.19a shows the shape index feature. The red and white colours indicate the convex regions, whereas the blue colour indicates concave regions. Since the shape index is scale-invariant, regions with large and small curvature degrees take similar values. On the other side, the curvedness feature can distinguish among regions with a large curvature degree, e.g. the apex region, and small curvature regions, as shown in Fig. 10.19b.

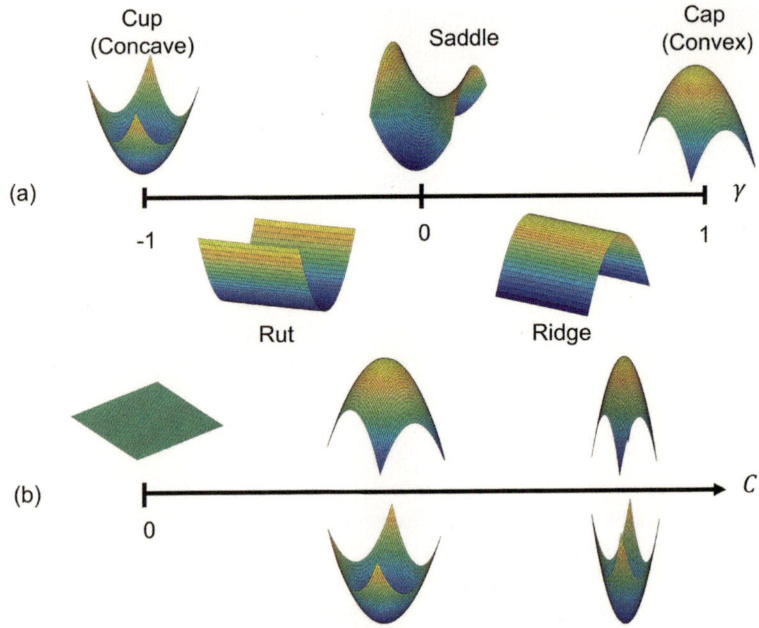

Fig. 10.18 Illustration of local shape types at a point with respect to (**a**) the shape index and (**b**) curvedness features

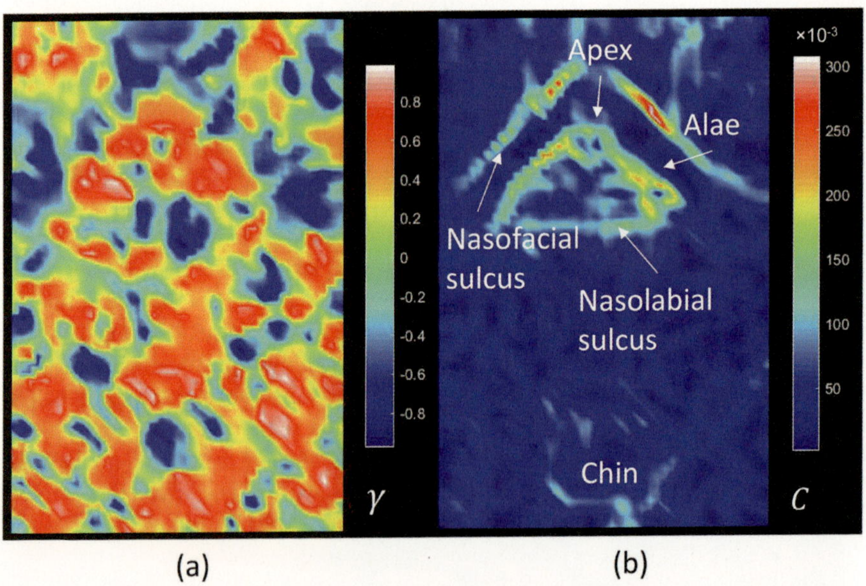

Fig. 10.19 Colour-coded maps of curvature features computed for a surface image of the nose region of a head phantom: (**a**) the shape index and (**b**) curvedness

10.4.4 Computerized Framework for the Localization of Anatomical Feature Points in Infrared Ray-Based Surface Images

10.4.4.1 Overall Scheme

Figure 10.20 shows a flowchart of an automated framework for localization of anatomical feature points in an infrared ray-based surface image by using differential geometry features (Soufi et al. 2016). The basic idea was to reconstruct the patient's surface in the surface image for the computation of the curvature features that characterize the shape of the surface, as explained in the previous sections. The surface image was preprocessed for extracting the region of interest (ROI), which includes the anatomical landmarks, and reducing the noise. Next, a smooth (i.e. continually differentiable) mathematical surface of the patient's body surface was reconstructed by using the NURBS modelling technique. Curvature features, i.e. shape index and curvedness, were computed, and a rule-based function was used for localizing the feature points on the surface.

In the preprocessing step, a template matching technique based on a normalized cross-correlation function was applied on the amplitude images for the extraction of the ROI. The template image was selected so that it included the anatomical landmarks. Next, an edge enhancement Laplacian-of-Gaussian filter was applied on the template and input amplitude images. The ROI was automatically localized by extracting the region with same size of the template at a pixel with the maximum value of the normalized cross-correlation function. Following, temporal filtering techniques (i.e. averaging and Kalman filters) and spatial filter (i.e. bilateral filter) were applied for reducing temporal and spatial noise, respectively.

In the NURBS surface reconstruction, the control points were obtained by using a linear interpolation of the surface image, setting the interval between the points to 1 mm in the X and Y directions in the XY plane. Next, 3rd degree (cubic) B-spline basis functions were used for calculating the reconstructed surface using Eq. (10.4).

The feature points were localized on the reconstructed surface based on the shape index and curvedness features, which were calculated by using Eqs. (10.27) and (10.28), respectively. For localizing the feature points, the following rule-based function was used:

$$p = \begin{cases} \text{feature point on a convex region} \\ \text{if } k_{1,p} < 0, k_{2,p} < 0, \gamma_p > \gamma_{th} \text{ and } C_p \geq C_{th}, \\ \text{feature point on a concave region} \\ \text{if } k_{1,p} > 0, k_{2,p} > 0, \gamma_p < \gamma_{th} \text{ and } C_p \geq C_{th}, \\ \text{not a feature point} \quad \text{otherwise,} \end{cases} \tag{10.29}$$

where γ_{th} and C_{th} are user-defined thresholds, which were set based on the optimization of a similarity measure between a reference (ground-truth) point set and the localized feature point set. The advantages of this method are its simplicity through

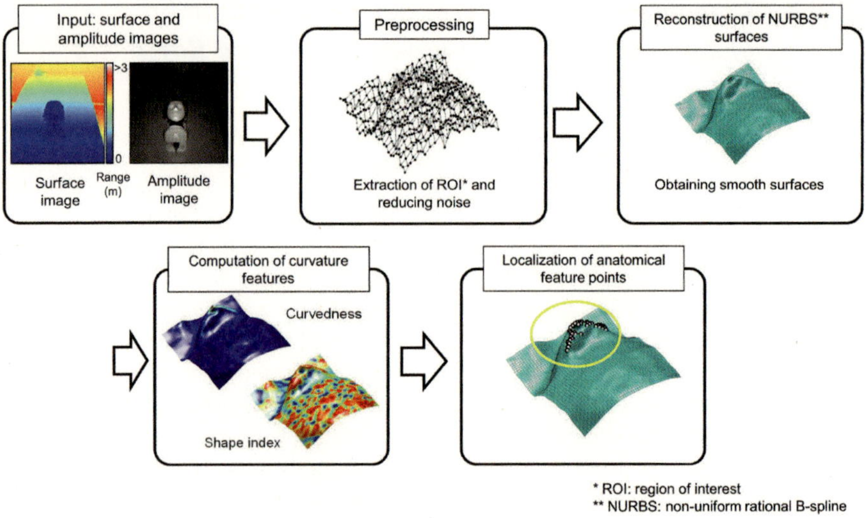

Fig. 10.20 Flowchart of a computerized framework for the localization of anatomical feature points on a surface image based on differential geometry features

the definition of the feature points based on the shape topography. However, a major limitation is the dependence in the localization accuracy on the curvedness and shape index thresholds, which are patient-specific parameters.

For evaluating the localization accuracy, the mean of minimum Euclidean distances (MMED), which is a similarity measure that evaluates the similarity between reference (ground-truth) points and the localized points, was used. The reference points were manually selected by an operator from the anatomical landmark regions from which the feature points are sought to be localized. The similarity was quantified by averaging the Euclidean distances between each reference point and its closest localized point, and similarly the distances between each localized point with its closest reference points (Soufi et al. 2016).

Assume that $\boldsymbol{R} = \{\boldsymbol{r}_j \in \mathbb{R}^3; j = 1, \ldots, U\}$, where U is the number of points, is the set of the reference points and that $\boldsymbol{F} = \{\boldsymbol{f}_i \in \mathbb{R}^3; i = 1, \ldots, T\}$, where T is the number of points, is the set of the feature points localized based on Eq. (10.29). The MMED between the reference points and the localized feature points was measured as shown in Eq. (10.30):

$$\mathrm{MMED} = \frac{\sum_{i=1}^{T} \parallel \boldsymbol{r}_{\min,j} - \boldsymbol{f}_i \parallel + \sum_{j=1}^{U} \parallel \boldsymbol{r}_j - \boldsymbol{f}_{\min,i} \parallel}{T + U}, \tag{10.30}$$

where $\boldsymbol{r}_{\min,j}$ is the closest reference point to the localized feature point $\boldsymbol{f}_i$, and $\boldsymbol{f}_{\min,i}$ is similarly the closest localized feature point to the reference point $\boldsymbol{r}_j$. Thus, the points $\boldsymbol{r}_{\min,j}$ and $\boldsymbol{f}_{\min,i}$ in Eq. (10.30) are obtained by using Eqs. (10.31) and (10.32), respectively:

$$\boldsymbol{r}_{\min,j} = \arg\min_{j} \left\| \boldsymbol{r}_j - \boldsymbol{f}_i \right\|, \tag{10.31}$$

$$\boldsymbol{f}_{\min,i} = \arg\min_{i} \left\| \boldsymbol{r}_j - \boldsymbol{f}_i \right\|. \tag{10.32}$$

10.4.4.2 Experimental Results

Figure 10.21 shows the MMEDs obtained for the localization of convex and concave feature points in surface images of a head phantom, which were acquired by a TOF camera, based on the shape index and curvedness features. The surface images were acquired for the phantom positioned in an initial positioning and displaced positioning for ± 3 mm in right-left (RL), superior-inferior (SI) and anterior-posterior (AP) directions. The convex and concave feature points were localized with MMEDs of 1.79 ± 0.16 and 3.60 ± 0.43 mm, respectively.

Figure 10.22 shows reference and localized feature points on convex and concave anatomical landmarks of the phantom's surface. The concave feature points included points localized at the apex region, where local retractions were present. In addition, less points were localized at the nasofacial sulcus, compared with the reference points, due to the saddle-shaped and deteriorated edges. Therefore, the convex feature points had better localization accuracy compared with the concave feature points.

10.5 Surface Image Registration Algorithms

Image registration is the key step in estimating the positioning errors in surface-imaging-based systems. Image registration refers to the process of estimating a mathematical (geometrical) transformation that optimally aligns two images – i.e. a moving image and a reference (fixed) image based on a similarity measure. In general, image registration algorithms consist of two major steps: (1) the estimation of the correspondence between points in the moving image and points in the reference image and (2) the estimation of the mathematical transformation that minimizes the distance between the corresponding points when applied to the moving image. The positioning errors can thus be estimated from the output parameters of the mathematical transformation. The correspondence step can be performed manually. This requires the user to select certain points on the reference image and define their corresponding points on the moving image. However, such manual definition is time-consuming and prone to uncertainties, such as interobserver variability. Therefore, the correspondence problem is automatically solved by searching through the points of the reference image and determining the point that satisfies a minimum distance criterion with each point in the moving image.

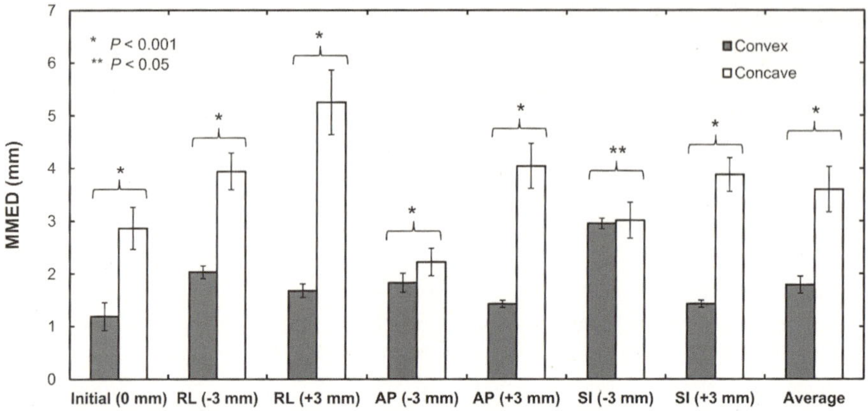

Fig. 10.21 Comparison of the MMED between anatomical feature points on convex (*grey*) and concave (*white*) regions of a phantom imaged with a TOF camera with respect to translation directions

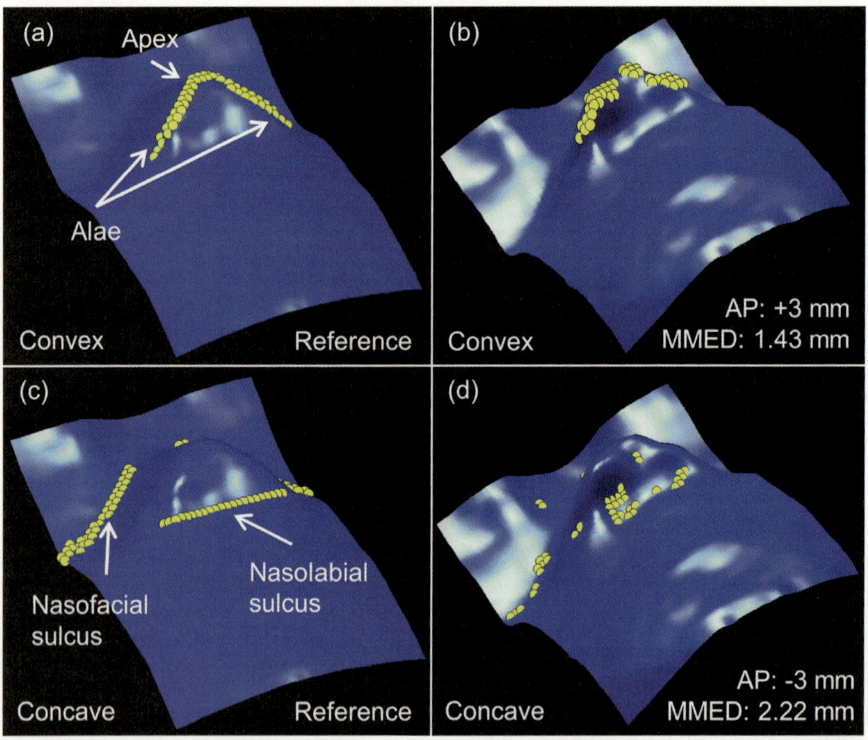

Fig. 10.22 Comparison between reference and localized feature points on the convex regions (i.e. apex and alae of nose) and concave regions (i.e. nasolabial and nasofacial sulci) of a head phantom with a TOF camera: (**a**) reference convex points, (**b**) localized convex feature points, (**c**) reference concave points and (**d**) localized concave feature points

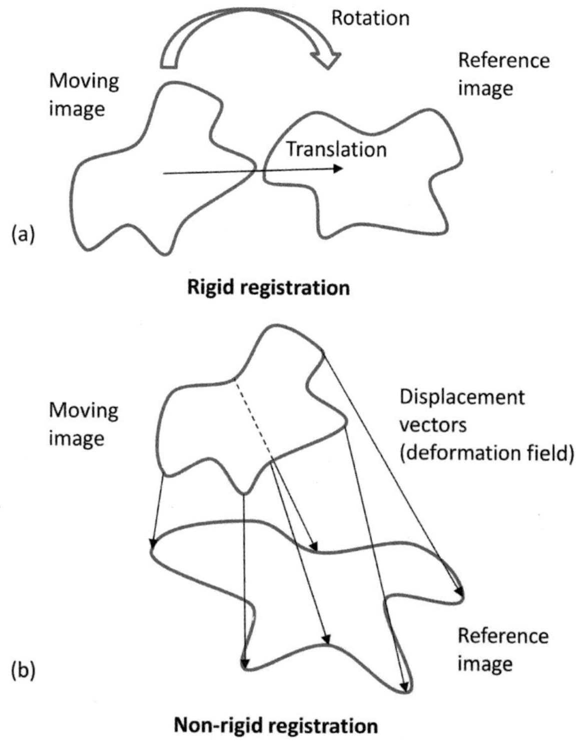

Fig. 10.23 Comparison between rigid and nonrigid registration algorithms based on the utilized mathematical transformations: (**a**) rigid registration including a translation and rotation, (**b**) nonrigid registration including pointwise displacement vectors (deformation field)

Image registration algorithms can be classified based on the utilized mathematical transformation into rigid and nonrigid registration algorithms, as shown in Fig. 10.23. The essential difference between the two types is that in a rigid registration algorithm, the relative distance among the constituent points in a surface image is preserved after the transformation. Therefore, a translation and rotation suffice to align the moving image with the reference image, as shown in Fig. 10.23a. By way of contrast, in nonrigid registration, the relative distance is altered under localized surface deformations. Therefore, pointwise displacement vectors are needed, which compose a deformation field, for aligning the two images, as shown in Fig. 10.23b.

The type of image registration algorithm is selected based on the type of positioning errors to be assessed and the nature of the surface images. Rigid image registration has proved to be useful in verifying the patient positioning after the rotation of the treatment couch during the treatment with non-coplanar beams (Placht et al. 2012). The most widely used algorithm for such an application is the iterative closest point (ICP) algorithm (Besl and McKay 1992), which we discuss in this section in detail.

10.5.1 Iterative Closest Point (ICP) Algorithm

The ICP algorithm was proposed for the rigid registration of 3D rigid shapes (Besl and McKay 1992) and has been used to estimate the positioning errors in surface-imaging-based systems (Bert et al. 2005, Placht et al. 2012, Pallotta et al. 2013). The algorithm assumes that the correspondences between the points $M = \{\boldsymbol{m}_i \in \mathbb{R}^3; i = 1, \ldots, N_M\}$, where N_M is the number of points, in the moving image and the points $F = \{\boldsymbol{r}_j \in \mathbb{R}^3; j = 1, \ldots, N_F\}$, where N_F is the number of points, in the reference image are unknown. Therefore, the basic idea of the algorithm is to find the optimal registration parameters iteratively, with two key steps performed at each iteration. The first step is to estimate the points $Y_k = \{\boldsymbol{y}_i \in F; i = 1, \ldots, N_M\}$ in the reference point set F, where k is the iteration number, that correspond to the point set M. The second step is to estimate rigid transformation parameters – i.e. a translation vector $\boldsymbol{t} = [t_x, t_y, t_z]$ and a rotation matrix $\boldsymbol{R}$ that is calculated based on the rotation angles $\boldsymbol{\theta} = [\alpha, \beta, \gamma]$ around the $x-$, $y-$ and $z-$ axes, respectively, as shown in Eq. (10.33):

$$\boldsymbol{R} = \begin{bmatrix} \cos(\beta)\cos(\gamma) & \cos(\gamma)\sin(\alpha)\sin(\beta) - \sin(\gamma)\cos(\alpha) & \sin(a)\sin(\gamma) + \cos(\alpha)\sin(\beta)\cos(\gamma) \\ \cos(\beta)\sin(\gamma) & \cos(\alpha)\cos(\gamma) + \sin(\alpha)\sin(\beta)\sin(\gamma) & -\cos(\gamma)\sin(\alpha) + \sin(\gamma)\sin(\beta)\cos(\alpha) \\ -\sin(\beta) & \sin(\alpha)\cos(\beta) & \cos(\alpha)\cos(\beta) \end{bmatrix}. \tag{10.33}$$

The optimal transformation parameters are estimated by minimizing a distance (error) function among the points in M and their closest reference points Y_k. The procedure – i.e. the calculation of the correspondence and optimal transformation parameters – is repeated until the error function is minimized. The detailed steps of the algorithm can be explained as follows:

Step 1: Set initial transformation parameters $\boldsymbol{t}_0$ and $\boldsymbol{R}_0$.

Step 2 (Correspondence Step): For each point $\boldsymbol{m}_{i,k}$ in the moving image, find the closest point $\boldsymbol{y}_i$ (i.e. the corresponding point) in F that minimizes the following error function:

$$d_k(\boldsymbol{m}_i, Q) = \min_{y_{i,k} \in F} \left\| \boldsymbol{y}_{i,k} - \boldsymbol{m}_{i,k} \right\|, \tag{10.34}$$

where d denotes the Euclidean distance function, k denotes the iteration number and $\|\cdot\|$ denotes the L_2 norm.

Step 3: Estimate the transformation parameters – i.e. the translation vector $\boldsymbol{t}_k$ and the rotation matrix $\boldsymbol{R}_k$ that minimize the following error function:

$$J_k(\boldsymbol{t}_k, \boldsymbol{R}_k) = \frac{1}{N_M} \sum_{i=1}^{N_M} \| \boldsymbol{y}_{i,k} - \boldsymbol{R}_k \boldsymbol{m}_{i,k} - \boldsymbol{t}_k \|^2. \tag{10.35}$$

Step 4: Transform the points in the moving image by using the estimated transformation parameters:

$$\boldsymbol{m}_{i,k+1} = \boldsymbol{R}_k \boldsymbol{m}_{i,k} + \boldsymbol{t}_k. \tag{10.36}$$

Step 5: Terminate if $|J_{k-1} - J_k| < \epsilon$, where ϵ is a threshold value. Otherwise, repeat **Steps 2–5.**

Notice that the transformed points in Eq. (10.36) are iteratively reinserted as moving points into Eq. (10.34).

The minimization of the function in Eq. (10.35) is a least squares problem. In order to estimate the optimal transformation parameters that satisfy the minimal error value, a singular value decomposition (SVD) technique can be used as follows (Bergström 2011). We start by calculating the derivative of the function $J(\boldsymbol{t}, \boldsymbol{R})$ with respect to $\boldsymbol{t}$, assuming a fixed $\boldsymbol{R}$ and setting the derivative equal to zero:

$$\frac{\partial J(\boldsymbol{t},\boldsymbol{R})}{\partial \boldsymbol{t}} = \frac{-2}{N_M}\left(\sum_{i=1}^{N_M}(\boldsymbol{y}_i - \boldsymbol{R}\boldsymbol{m}_i - \boldsymbol{t})\right) = \frac{2}{N_M}\left(N_M \boldsymbol{t} + \boldsymbol{R}\sum_{i=1}^{N_M}\boldsymbol{m}_i - \sum_{i=1}^{N_M}\boldsymbol{y}_i\right) = 0. \tag{10.37}$$

Now, let $\bar{\boldsymbol{m}}$ and $\bar{\boldsymbol{y}}$ be the centroids of the point sets M and Y, respectively, which can be calculated as

$$\bar{\boldsymbol{m}} = \frac{1}{N_M}\sum_{i=1}^{N_M}\boldsymbol{m}_i, \bar{\boldsymbol{y}} = \frac{1}{N_M}\sum_{i=1}^{N_M}\boldsymbol{y}_i. \tag{10.38}$$

By rearranging the terms of Eq. (10.37), the optimal translation vector can be expressed as follows:

$$\hat{\boldsymbol{t}} = \bar{\boldsymbol{y}} - \boldsymbol{R}\bar{\boldsymbol{m}}. \tag{10.39}$$

At this stage, by substituting the optimal translation vector back into the error function, we obtain

$$\sum_{i=1}^{N_M} \| \boldsymbol{y}_i - \boldsymbol{R}\boldsymbol{m}_i - \widehat{\boldsymbol{t}} \|^2 = \sum_{i=1}^{N_M} \| \boldsymbol{y}_i - \boldsymbol{R}\boldsymbol{m}_i + \boldsymbol{R}\bar{\boldsymbol{m}} - \bar{\boldsymbol{y}} \|^2$$
$$= \sum_{i=1}^{N_M} \| \boldsymbol{R}(\bar{\boldsymbol{m}} - \boldsymbol{m}_i) - (\bar{\boldsymbol{y}} - \boldsymbol{y}_i) \|^2. \tag{10.40}$$

Then, we apply the following substitution into Eq. (10.40):

$$\boldsymbol{p}_i = \bar{\boldsymbol{m}} - \boldsymbol{m}_i, \boldsymbol{q}_i = \bar{\boldsymbol{y}} - \boldsymbol{y}_i. \tag{10.41}$$

In this manner, the problem can be formalized as finding the optimal rotation matrix $\boldsymbol{R}$ such that

$$\widehat{\boldsymbol{R}} = \underset{\boldsymbol{R}}{\operatorname{argmin}} \sum_{i=1}^{N_M} \| \boldsymbol{R}\boldsymbol{p}_i - \boldsymbol{q}_i \|^2. \tag{10.42}$$

Now we expand the expression to be minimized within the summation as follows:

$$\| \boldsymbol{R}\boldsymbol{p}_i - \boldsymbol{q}_i \|^2 = (\boldsymbol{R}\boldsymbol{p}_i - \boldsymbol{q}_i)^T (\boldsymbol{R}\boldsymbol{p}_i - \boldsymbol{q}_i) = (\boldsymbol{p}_i{}^T \boldsymbol{R}^T - \boldsymbol{q}_i{}^T)(\boldsymbol{R}\boldsymbol{p}_i - \boldsymbol{q}_i)$$
$$= \boldsymbol{p}_i{}^T \boldsymbol{p}_i - 2\boldsymbol{q}_i{}^T \boldsymbol{R}\boldsymbol{p}_i + \boldsymbol{q}_i{}^T \boldsymbol{q}_i. \tag{10.43}$$

Therefore, Equation (10.42) can be reduced to

$$\widehat{\boldsymbol{R}} = \underset{\boldsymbol{R}}{\operatorname{argmin}} \sum_{i=1}^{N_M} (-2\boldsymbol{q}_i{}^T \boldsymbol{R}\boldsymbol{p}_i) = \underset{\boldsymbol{R}}{\operatorname{argmax}} \sum_{i=1}^{N_M} (\boldsymbol{q}_i{}^T \boldsymbol{R}\boldsymbol{p}_i). \tag{10.44}$$

The summation term on the right-hand side of Eq. (10.44) can be expressed using matrix notation as follows:

$$\sum_{i=1}^{N_M} (\boldsymbol{q}_i{}^T \boldsymbol{R}\boldsymbol{p}_i) = \operatorname{trace}(\boldsymbol{Q}^T \boldsymbol{R}\boldsymbol{P}), \tag{10.45}$$

where $\boldsymbol{Q}$ is the $3 \times N_M$ matrix of the corresponding points, $\boldsymbol{P}$ is the $3 \times N_M$ matrix of the moving points and *trace* denotes the trace operator, which sums up the diagonal elements of a matrix. Thus, Eq. (10.41) can be rewritten as

$$\widehat{\boldsymbol{R}} = \underset{\boldsymbol{R}}{\operatorname{argmax}} \operatorname{trace}(\boldsymbol{Q}^T \boldsymbol{R}\boldsymbol{P}). \tag{10.46}$$

By using the commutative property of the tracer operator, Eq. (10.46) can be rewritten as

$$\widehat{\boldsymbol{R}} = \underset{\boldsymbol{R}}{\operatorname{argmax}} \operatorname{trace}(\boldsymbol{R}\boldsymbol{P}\boldsymbol{Q}^T). \tag{10.47}$$

The matrix $\boldsymbol{PQ}^T$ is a 3×3 matrix, which can be decomposed using SVD as follows:

$$\boldsymbol{P}\boldsymbol{Q}^T = \boldsymbol{U}\boldsymbol{\Lambda}\boldsymbol{V}^T, \tag{10.48}$$

where $\boldsymbol{U}$ and $\boldsymbol{V}$ are orthogonal matrices whose columns are the eigenvectors of the matrices $\boldsymbol{W}\boldsymbol{W}^T$ ($\boldsymbol{W}=\boldsymbol{P}\boldsymbol{Q}^T$) and $\boldsymbol{W}^T\boldsymbol{W}$, respectively, and $\boldsymbol{\Lambda}$ is a diagonal matrix with the nonnegative singular values σ_1, σ_2 and σ_3 on its diagonal. By substituting Eq. (10.48) into Eq. (10.47), we obtain

$$\widehat{\boldsymbol{R}} = \underset{\boldsymbol{R}}{\operatorname{argmax}} \operatorname{trace}(\boldsymbol{\Lambda}\boldsymbol{V}^T\boldsymbol{R}\boldsymbol{U}) = \underset{\boldsymbol{R}}{\operatorname{argmax}} \operatorname{trace}(\boldsymbol{\Lambda}\boldsymbol{B}). \tag{10.49}$$

Because the matrices $\boldsymbol{R}$, $\boldsymbol{U}$ and $\boldsymbol{V}$ are all orthogonal matrices, the matrix $\boldsymbol{B}$ is also orthogonal. When the column vectors of $\boldsymbol{B}$ are unit vectors, then $b_{ij} < 1$. Therefore, the trace to be maximized can be written as

$$\operatorname{trace}(\boldsymbol{\Lambda}\boldsymbol{B}) = \sum_{i=1}^{3} \sigma_i b_{ii} \le \sum_{i=1}^{3} \sigma_i. \tag{10.50}$$

Equation (10.50) indicates that the maximum trace value can be obtained when $b_{ii} = 1$, which means that $\boldsymbol{B} = \boldsymbol{I}$, where $\boldsymbol{I}$ is the identity matrix. Therefore, we have the following:

$$\begin{gathered} \boldsymbol{I} = \boldsymbol{B} = \boldsymbol{V}^T\widehat{\boldsymbol{R}}\boldsymbol{U} \\ \boldsymbol{V} = \widehat{\boldsymbol{R}}\boldsymbol{U} \\ \widehat{\boldsymbol{R}} = \boldsymbol{V}\boldsymbol{U}^T \end{gathered} . \tag{10.51}$$

Equation (10.51) holds true because both $\boldsymbol{V}$ and $\boldsymbol{U}$ are orthogonal matrices. However, the matrix $\widehat{\boldsymbol{R}}$ computed with this procedure might include a reflection in addition to the rotation. Therefore, the following modification upon Eq. (10.51) ensures that we obtain the desired rotation matrix $\boldsymbol{R}_{\text{opt}}$ without a reflection:

$$\boldsymbol{R}_{\text{opt}} = \boldsymbol{V}\begin{pmatrix} 1 & 0 & 0 \\ 0 & 1 & 0 \\ 0 & 0 & \det(\boldsymbol{V}\boldsymbol{U}^T) \end{pmatrix}\boldsymbol{U}^T. \tag{10.52}$$

Finally, the optimal translation vector $\boldsymbol{t}_{\text{opt}}$ is obtained by substituting $\boldsymbol{R}_{\text{opt}}$ into Eq. (10.39), which we rewrite here for consistency:

$$\boldsymbol{t}_{\text{opt}} = \bar{\boldsymbol{y}} - \boldsymbol{R}_{\text{opt}}\bar{\boldsymbol{m}}. \tag{10.53}$$

The advantages of using the ICP algorithm for patient positioning are as follows:

- It is independent of the shape representation of the surface image, which means that it can be applied on point distributions represented as scattered points, triangulated surfaces or surface patches.
- It is feasible for point distributions without outliers, such as patient surface images acquired with a laser scanner.
- The output of the last iteration can be used directly as the patient positioning errors.

However, the algorithm has the following disadvantages:

- It is sensitive to outliers in the surface image. Therefore, when registering images with significant outliers, it might require a prior preprocessing (filtering) step or a modification that excludes outliers from the registration procedure.
- When the reference image includes a dense point distribution (e.g. if it is derived from a planning CT image), the ICP algorithm becomes computationally expensive. As a result, real-time performance might not be obtained from the monitoring system. In order to overcome this problem, algorithms for a faster search for the closest points – e.g. the space partitioning or downsampling of the reference image – can be used to accelerate the search process.

Next, we introduce a simple example of registration by applying the ICP algorithm to a surface image. The input images are acquired for a head phantom using a TOF camera and consist of an initial positioning image (with no translation or rotation) and a treatment image (with a simulated positioning error). The positioning error was simulated by displacing the initial positioning image by 20 mm in the left-right (LR) direction and rotating it by 15° about the anterior-posterior (AP) direction. Figure 10.24 shows the initial positioning and treatment images without registration (Fig. 10.24a) and with registration (Fig. 10.24b).

10.5.2 Evaluation of Registration Accuracy

In order to evaluate the registration accuracy, two criteria are used. The first criterion is called the fiducial registration error (FRE) (Fitzpatrick et al. 1998). This criterion estimates the accuracy with which the corresponding points were aligned after the registration. However, because the FRE might not reflect the accuracy of the registration in terms of positioning error, the target registration error (TRE) is also used (Fitzpatrick et al. 1998, Placht et al. 2012). The TRE estimates the difference between a reference (ground-truth) positioning error and the error estimated by the registration algorithm. Let $\boldsymbol{t}_{\text{ref}}$ and $\boldsymbol{\theta}_{\text{ref}}$ be the reference translation and rotation angle vectors, respectively, and let $\boldsymbol{t}_{\text{est}}$ and $\boldsymbol{\theta}_{\text{est}}$ be the

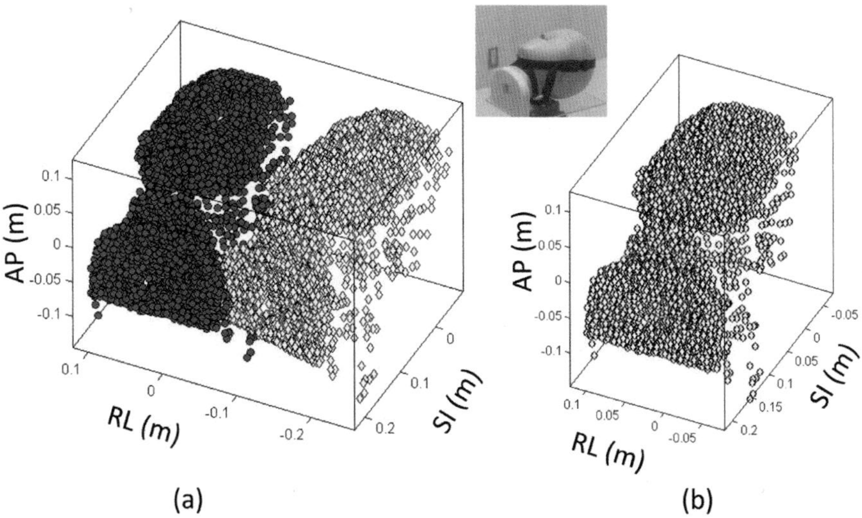

Fig. 10.24 Registration of surface images using the ICP algorithm. (**a**) Reference (initial positioning) surface image with a treatment surface image (including positioning error) without registration. (**b**) The surface images registered using the ICP algorithm

translation and rotation angles vectors estimated by the ICP registration algorithm, respectively. Then, the TRE of the estimated translation vector ($\mathrm{TRE}_{\mathrm{trans}}$) and rotation angle vector ($\mathrm{TRE}_{\mathrm{rot}}$) can be calculated as follows:

$$\mathrm{TRE}_{\mathrm{trans}} = \| \boldsymbol{t}_{ref} - \boldsymbol{t}_{est} \| , \quad (10.54)$$

$$\mathrm{TRE}_{\mathrm{rot}} = \| \boldsymbol{\theta}_{ref} - \boldsymbol{\theta}_{est} \| . \quad (10.55)$$

References

Agam G, Tang X (2005) A sampling framework for accurate curvature estimation in discrete surfaces. IEEE Trans Vis Comput Graph 11(5):573–583

Bauer S, Seitel S, Hoffman H et al (2013) Real-time range imaging in health care: a survey. In: Time-of-Flight and depth imaging. Sensors, algorithms, and applications, LNCS, vol 8200, pp 228–254

Bergström P (2011) Computational methods for shape verification of free form surfaces. Doctoral Thesis, Luleå University of Technology, Sweden

Bert C, Metheaney KG, Doppke K et al (2005) A phantom evaluation of a stereo-vision surface imaging system for radiotherapy patient setup. Med Phys 32(9):2753–2762

Besl PJ, McKay ND (1992) A method for registration of 3-D shapes. Pattern Anal Mach 14 (2):239–256

Brahme A, Nyman P, Skatt B (2008) 4D laser camera for accurate patient positioning, collision avoidance, image fusion and adaptive approaches during diagnostic and therapeutic procedures. Med Phys 35(5):1670–1681. doi:10.1118/1.2889720

Büttgen B, Seitz P (2008) Robust optical time-of-flight range imaging based on smart pixel structures. IEEE Trans Circuits Syst Regul Pap 55(6):1512–1525. doi:10.1109/TCSI.2008.916679

Colombo A, Cusano C, Schettini R (2006) 3D face detection using curvature analysis. Pattern Recogn 39(3):444–455. doi: 10.1016/j.patcog.2005.09.009

Cox MG (1972) The numerical evaluation of B-splines. IMA J Appl Math 10(2):134–149. doi:10.1093/imamat/10.2.134

de Boor C (1972) On calculation with B-splines. J Approx Theory 6:50–62

Fitzpatrick J, West J, Maurer C Jr (1998) Predicting error in rigid-body point based registration. IEEE Trans Med Imaging 17:694–702

Koenderink JJ, van Doorn AJ (1992) Surface shape and curvature scales. Image Vis Comput 10 (8):557–565. doi:10.1016/0262-8856(92)90076-F

Meeks SL, Tomé WA, Willoughby TR et al (2005) Optically guided patient positioning techniques. Semin Radiat Oncol 15:192–201. doi:10.1016/j.semradonc.2005.01.004

Pallotta S, Simontacchi G, Marrazzo L et al (2013) Accuracy of a 3D laser/camera surface imaging system for setup verification of the pelvic and thoracic regions in radiotherapy treatments. Med Phys 40(1):011710-1–011710-8

Piegl L, Tiller W (1997) The NURBS book, 2nd edn. Springer, Berlin/Heidelberg

Placht S, Stancanello J, Schaller C et al (2012) Fast time-of-flight camera based surface registration for radiotherapy patient positioning. Med Phys 39(1):4–17

Pressley A (2010) Elementary differential geometry, 2nd edn. Springer, London

Soufi M, Arimura H, Nakamura K et al (2016) Feasibility of differential geometry-based features in detection of anatomical feature points on patient surfaces in range image-guided radiation therapy. Int J Comput Assist Radiol Surg 11:1993. doi:10.1007/s11548-016-1436-x

Timmerman RD, Xing L (2009) Image-guided and adaptive radiation therapy. Wolters Kluwer, London

Wagner TH, Meeks SL, Bova FJ et al (2007) Optical tracking technology in stereotactic radiation therapy. Med Dosim 32:111–120. doi:10.1016/j.meddos.2007.01.008

Wang LT, Solberg TD, Medin PM et al (2001) Infrared patient positioning for stereotactic radiosurgery of extracranial tumors. Comput Biol Med 31(2):101–111. doi:10.1016/S0010-4825(00)00026-3

Willoughby T, Lehmann J, Bencomo J et al (2012) Quality assurance for nonradiographic radiotherapy localization and positioning systems: report of Task Group 147. Med Phys 39 (4):1728–1747. doi:10.1118/1.3681967

Yoshitake T, Nakamura K, Shioyama Y et al (2008) Breath-hold monitoring and visual feedback for radiotherapy using a charge-coupled device camera and a head-mounted display: system development and feasibility. Radiat Med 26:50–55. doi:10.1007/s11604-007-0189-4

Part IV
Intelligent Radiation Treatment Approaches

Chapter 11
Tumor Tracking Approach

Masayori Ishikawa and Shubhechha J. Shrestha

Abstract In radiotherapy practice, the planning target volume (PTV) must include larger margin for moving tumor compared to tumors at rest with same clinical target volume (CTV). In order to avoid normal tissue complications, organ motion should either be freezed relative to treatment beam or the tumor must be tracked in a real time. The real-time tracking of the tumor can reduce the tumor motion margin in the dose distribution, sparing the healthy tissues near the tumor. Several methods have been proposed for tracking the tumor in a real time. The most widely used method is external surrogate system, where the tumor position is based on external surrogates, such as the abdomen that expands and contracts as the patient breathes. Gold fiducials are also used as a surrogate marker because it is easily detectable in the fluoroscopic image allowing the continuous monitoring of the tumor. In this chapter, recent techniques will be introduced with their benefits and limitations.

Keywords Tumor tracking • Radiotherapy • SBRT • IGRT

11.1 Introduction

Image-guided radiotherapy (IGRT) has been widely used for patient setup with bony structures or fiducial markers, enabling high-accuracy external radiotherapy. For even higher accurate radiotherapy, organ motion has been the main issue in external radiotherapy for extracranial diseases. The conventional way to account for organ motion and setup error is to add a safety margin to the clinical target volume (CTV) to get the planning target volume (PTV), which is recommended by ICRU Report 50 and 62 (Wambersie and Landgerg 1999). But we must also keep in mind that increasing the margin exposes a larger volume of healthy normal tissues to radiation dose. Efforts have been made to "cut corners" in the sense of keeping the irradiated volume as close to the CTV as possible (Goitein 2004). Past studies have also shown a correlation between organ motion and respiration (Keall et al.

M. Ishikawa (✉) • S.J. Shrestha
Department of Biomedical Science and Engineering, Graduate School of Health Science, Hokkaido University, N-12 W-5 Kitaku, Sapporo 060-0812, Japan
e-mail: masayori@med.hokudai.ac.jp

H. Arimura (ed.), *Image-Based Computer-Assisted Radiation Therapy*,
DOI 10.1007/978-981-10-2945-5_11

2006b). Furthermore, for lung tumors, it has been reported that lung tumors may move up to 40 mm in superior-inferior (SI), 15 mm in anterior-posterior (AP), and 10 mm in left-right (LR) direction during normal breathing and follow complicated 3D tracks (Plathow et al. 2004) (Shirato et al. 2007). The maximum movement of liver tumors was found to be 2.1 cm in the SI direction and about 0.8 cm in the AP direction (Shimizu et al. 1999). Such motion presents significant limitations during the entire radiotherapy process: imaging, planning, and delivery. Similarly, another important source of uncertainty in external radiotherapy is setup error (Shirato et al. 2000b). Setup error comprises of both random and systematic errors. In particular, the motion of skin with respect to the internal anatomy degrades the reproducibility of the patient setup on the CT scanner, thereby introducing a systematic setup error (Van Herk 2004). For lungs, setup errors of the order of 2–4 mm have been reported (De Boer et al. 2001). Random errors blur the dose distribution (Leong 1987), whereas systematic errors cause a shift of the cumulative dose distribution relative to the target (Van Herk 2004).

Several methods have been proposed for tracking the tumor in a real time. The tumor tracking approach can be grouped into the following categories: [I] internal surrogate tracking, (1) implanted fiducials, (2) electromagnetic tracking, and (3) combined MV/kV imaging; [II] external surrogate tracking; [III] internal and external surrogate tracking, (1) direct tumor tracking (DTT) and (2) respiratory tracking system (RTS); and [IV] markerless tracking, (1) direct fluoroscopic tumor tracking and (2) MRI tracking. The most widely used method is the external surrogate system, where the tumor position is based on external surrogates, such as on the abdomen that expands and contracts as the patient breathes. Under this approach, the most common technique is the placement of a pressure sensor belt (Li et al. 2006) and infrared reflector (Berbeco et al. 2005b; Berbeco et al. 2006) on the patient's abdomen that are tracked with an infrared camera. Another approach is internal surrogate tracking, where high-electron-density metal (gold) markers or transponders are implanted in the tumor site. Chen, Murphy, and Shirato have used gold fiducials for tumor tracking (Chen et al. 2001; Murphy et al. 2002; Shirato et al. 2000b). Gold fiducials are easily detectable in fluoroscopic images allowing the continuous monitoring of the tumor. One such system that is used clinically for tumor tracking is the Mitsubishi/Hokkaido RTRT system (Shirato et al. 2000b). For this purpose, organ motion should either be frozen relative to the treatment beam or the tumor must be tracked in real time. The former technique is referred as the breath-hold technique (Hanley et al. 1999; Wong et al. 1999), and the latter is known as real-time tumor tracking (Chen et al. 2001; Shirato et al. 2000b). Both techniques transform the problem of targeting a moving tumor into a more easily manageable static treatment case. The Japanese Society of Therapeutic Radiology and Oncology (JASTRO) defines real-time tumor tracking (RTRT) as external radiotherapy which utilizes real-time tracking technology during therapy. Generally, RTRT can be classified into two divisions; one is interrupted irradiation and the other pursuing irradiation (Shirato et al. 2007). In the former, the therapeutic beam is irradiated only when the tumor is within the irradiation field. In the latter, the therapeutic beam is continuously delivered to a moving target. A 5-mm motion-limit criterion is generally chosen, because this level of motion can cause significant artifacts and systematic errors during imaging procedures.

Another method of internal surrogate tracking is based on nonionizing electromagnetic fields, using a small wireless transponder implanted in the tumor region (Balter et al. 2003). A combined MV/kV system has also been explored with a marker tracking approach (Wiersma et al. 2008). The main advantage of the MV/kV system is that the same treatment beam can be used for therapy and imaging. Similarly, another approach toward tumor tracking is fluoroscopic tracking of the tumor without implanted fiducial markers which is also referred to as markerless tracking (Berbeco et al. 2005a; Cui et al. 2008; Xu et al. 2007; Lin et al. 2009). In addition, fluoroscopy is an ionizing imaging technique. When acquired throughout the entire treatment, it adds a considerable dose to the patient. Recently, several groups are integrating radiotherapy treatment units with magnetic resonance imaging (MRI) (Fallone et al. 2009; Dempsey et al. 2005). The main advantages of using MRI for treatment guidance purposes is that it does not involve any additional dose to the patient and has better soft tissue contrast than that of X-rays. In the following sections, we describe the abovementioned tumor tracking approaches in detail along with their accuracy and clinical implementation.

11.2 Internal Surrogate Tracking System

11.2.1 Implanted Fiducial Tracking

The fluoroscopic real-time tumor tracking system synchronized with a linear accelerator was developed by Hokkaido University and Mitsubishi Electronics in 1999. The system gates a linear accelerator such that the beam can be turned on and off without shutting down the entire linac. It consists of four sets of diagnostic X-ray fluoroscope systems. Each set consists of an X-ray tube with a fixed collimator embedded under the floor and an image intensifier mounted on the ceiling (Fig. 11.1). The beam axis of two diagnostic X-ray units will meet at the isocenter of the linear accelerator (Shirato et al. 2000b). In this technique, a gold marker with a diameter of 1.5–2 mm is implanted in or near the tumor which can be detected in fluoroscopic images. Generally, three or more fiducial markers are inserted, and one is selected at treatment time for tracking. Multiple fiducial markers may also help measure tumor translation, rotation, and even marker migration which can be determined by monitoring the distance between markers (Keall et al. 2006b).

Among the four X-ray fluoroscopy systems, two sets are selected to view the gold marker in the patient body. The marker is first located within each digital image via a template matching (TM) algorithm. The image processor compares the digitized image and the template image of the marker by using a correlation function. The marker position is assumed to be the location with the maximum pattern recognition score (PRS). If the PRS is less than a predefined value, the

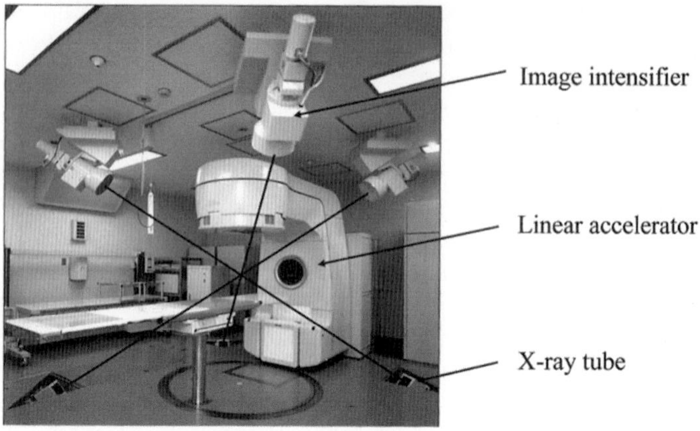

Fig. 11.1 The Hokkaido fluoroscopic real-time tumor tracking system with motion-gated linear accelerator and X-ray tubes (Shirato et al. 2000a, b)

fluoroscopic RTRT system halts the linac operation. If the PRS is above the predefined value and the position is within the gating window, the linac is triggered to irradiate the tumor. When the marker moves outside the gating window, the beam is turned off. The PRS between the search area and template are displayed on the CRT every 0.03 s (Shirato et al. 2000a).

Shirato et al. (2000a, b) showed in a phantom experiment that the coordinates of the marker were detected with an accuracy of +/− 1 mm (Shirato et al. 2007). Similarly, in the moving targets, the geometric accuracy of the tumor tracking system was found to be better than 1.5 mm up to a speed of 40 mm/s, which is much better than the external surrogate approach. The RTRT system significantly improves the accuracy of irradiation of the target in motion at the expense of an acceptable amount of diagnostic X-ray exposure (Shimizu et al. 2001).

Shimizu et al. (2001) treated four lung cancer patients with the RTRT system and found that the range of the marker during the beam on period was reduced to within 5.3 mm in all directions (Shimizu et al. 2001). Kitamura et al. (2002) suggested that the RTRT system was useful in prostate cancer for reducing uncertainty due to the effects of the respiratory cycle, especially with the patient in the prone position (Kitamura et al. 2002). Yamamoto et al. (2004) used the RTRT system for patients with gynecology malignancies. The PTV margin with three gold marker setup reduced by 3.3 mm, 6.1 mm, and 4.6 mm with respect to manual setup, which indicated that RTRT was useful to reduce the PTV margin and to perform 3DCB (Yamamoto et al. 2004). Similarly, in RTRT-based head and neck treatment, Oita et al. (2006) concluded that the setup error in RL, CC, and AP directions was reduced by 1.6 mm, 1.3 mm, and 0.8 mm, respectively, with respect to manual setup (Oita et al. 2006). Ahn et al. (2004) applied the RTRT system for unresectable pancreatic cancer. The average movements of markers in RL, CC, and AP directions were 3.0 mm (range 1.7–5.2 mm), 5.2 mm (range 3.5–6.8 mm), and 3.5 mm (range 2.7–5.1 mm), respectively (Ahn et al. 2004).

As there are limitations in any system, the present RTRT system also has shortcomings. First, the major uncertainty of the system is the migration of the implanted markers. Second, as the tracking method requires invasive marker implantation, there is a risk of pneumothorax (Abdefg et al. 2002; Geraghty et al. 2003). Finally, the system irradiates only when the tumor is within the gating window, thus a duty cycle of no more than 20–30 % leads to long treatment time (Depuydt et al. 2011).

11.2.2 Electromagnetic Tracking

Electromagnetic tracking is another real-time tumor tracking modality and has many benefits over the use of simple gold markers (Balter et al. 2003; Balter et al. 2005). The main advantages are (1) no requirement of ionizing radiation during localization, (2) the target isocenter may be monitored continuously at the frequency of 10 Hz during radiation delivery rather than once at the beginning of each fraction, and (3) real-time feedback is provided so that action may be taken to limit the influence of intrafraction motion (Litzenberg et al. 2007). Research shows that the complication rates of gold marker and transponder implantation are similar (Willoughby et al. 2004; Pouliot et al. 2004). The use of electromagnetic technology was first elaborated for stereotactic radiotherapy localization utilizing a wired transponder sensor (PV et al. 1992). Position tracking systems used in image-guided surgery using a wired transponder are Aurora and microBird (Hummel et al. 2002). Similarly, a miniature implantable radiofrequency (RF) coil (8 mm x 0.8 mm) was proposed by Seiler et al. (2000). The coil can be tracked magnetically in 3D in real time (Seiler et al. 2000). Currently, a novel wireless electromagnetic localization system, Calypso 4D Localization System (Calypso Medical, Seattle, WA) has been developed for real-time tracking in radiotherapy (Balter et al. 2003).

The major components of the Calypso 4D Localization System are shown in Fig. 11.2, which include (1) a mobile AC electromagnetic console; (2) a receiver array; (3) three ceiling-mounted infrared optical cameras and a hub, all located in the treatment room; (4) wireless transponders (8 mm × 2 mm) (Beacons); and (5) a tracking station in the control area (Balter et al. 2005). The array contains four source coils and 32 receiver coils. The source coil generates an electromagnetic field in the 300 to 500 kHz frequency range which induces a resonance in the transponder. The spatial coordinates of the transponder are determined from the treatment-planning CT scan and the offset between the transponder centroid, and the intended isocenter is updated at a rate of 10 Hz.

The Calypso system can be used in two ways: localization and tracking. When a patient is planned for radiotherapy, no fewer than two transponders are first implanted into the tumor region. The patient then undergoes thin CT simulation after 4–14 days. Transponder coordinates on the CT scan relative to the treatment plan isocenter are calculated and entered into the Calypso system. The Calypso receiver is placed over the patient, and its position relative to the isocenter, as well

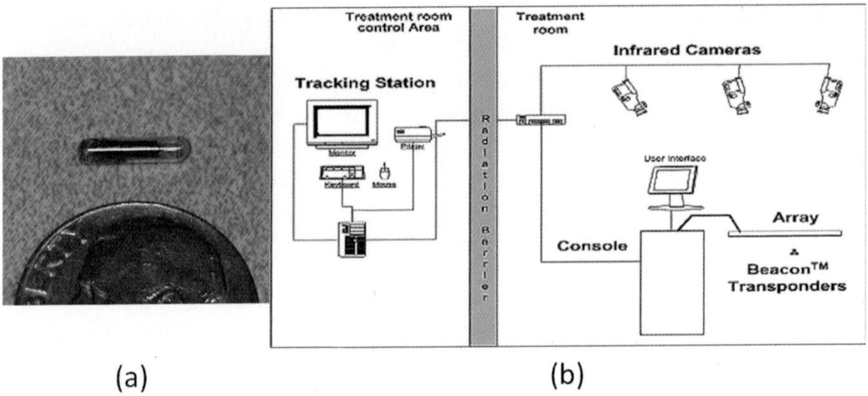

Fig. 11.2 (**a**) Transponder (Mayse et al. 2008). (**b**) Diagram showing the localization process of electromagnetic tracking system (Balter et al. 2005)

as the transponder position relative to the array, is determined. Transponders are excited by an external field generated by the array and emit an electromagnetic signal at one of the three unique resonance frequencies which is detected and localized by an electromagnetic array placed above the patient (Mayse et al. 2008). Several sensors are placed inside the array which measures the strength and orientation of the resonant signal from the transponders. The data is then transferred to a manufacturer-provided software to determine and continuously monitor the target position with respect to the array. For continuous tracking, the transponder must be placed 23 cm or less from the detection array above the patient (Quigley et al. 2009). Infrared cameras continuously monitor the array's position relative to the linear accelerator which helps to calculate the position of the target with respect to the linear accelerator's isocenter. In this way, the electromagnetic system serves as a kind of Global Positioning System (GPS), and hence this system is often referred to as "GPS for Body."

A phantom experiment showed that submillimeter accuracy was maintained using the electromagnetic tracking technique (Balter et al. 2005). A clinical evaluation showed a comparable localization accuracy to the isocenter (within 1.5 mm) compared with X-ray localization (Burch et al. 2005; Kupelian et al. 2005; Willoughby et al. 2006). Similarly, the root mean square (RMS) accuracy of this system for real-time verification of 4DCT data has been shown to be 0.28 mm (maximum error 1.2 mm) (Parikh et al. 2005). Similarly, the time lapse between the Calypso readout and X-ray imaging was approximately 8 min, and the patient localization accuracy (difference between the Calypso system-predicted transponder location and the radiographic system-predicted transponder position location) was within 1.5+/− 0.9 mm in research carried out by multiple institutions (Santanam et al. 2008).

The initial US Food and Drug Administration (FDA) approval in July 2006 allows for the Calypso system to be used in the treatment of prostate cancer only. Kupelian et al. reported that the difference between the skin marker and Calypso alignment was greater than 5 mm in more than 75 % of all fractions (Kupelian et al. 2007). Similarly, Quigley et al. showed the patient positioned with conventional tattoos and laser to have alignment error exceeding 5 mm when compared with the Calypso positioning and monitoring system (Quigley et al. 2009). Litzenberg et al. showed that the margins required to account for intrafraction motion were around 2 mm in all directions considering that 90 % of patients received 95 % of the prescribed dose using the Calypso system, but in the absence of this system, the margins are 10 mm (Litzenberg et al. 2007). This shows that a significant reduction in margin is possible using the Calypso system.

11.2.3 Combined MV/kV Imaging System

The feasibility of using electronic portal image devices (EPIDs) for real-time tumor tracking has recently been explored (Keall et al. 2004). However, since only a single in-line MV is used, this approach suffers from insufficient information to completely determine the 3D coordinates of the implanted fiducials. The combined use of MV treatment beams with kV projection images has recently been proposed (Wiersma et al. 2008). Unlike other fluoroscopy tracking systems which require two or more additional kV X-ray imaging sources for obtaining spatial information, the system uses the treatment beam and only one kV X-ray imaging source as shown in Fig. 11.3.

Wiersma et al. demonstrated a real-time 3D internal fiducial tracking system based on the combined use of MV and kV imaging systems. The Varian Trilogy system (Varian Medical Systems, Palo Alto, CA) with kV and MV imagers operating in the 6 MV photon mode was used for this study. MV beam images were obtained using an *a*SI EPID (Portal Vision MV AS-500, Varian Medical Systems, Palo Alto, CA), and the kV imaging was acquired using an onboard kV imaging system located perpendicular to the treatment beam. Two channels of a four-channel PCI video grabber (Pro Video 149P, ProVideo Co., Taipei, Taiwan) were used to grab the kV and MV video streams at 30 fps per channel with a resolution of 640 × 480 pixels. To analyze the video, software was used with a sequence of filters for detecting the fiducials.

The geometrical accuracy of the system was found to be on the order of 1 mm in all three spatial directions. With this tracking system, the MV trace lags behind the kV trace by approximately 70 msec. Moreover, the system is intensity based in nature; thus, when the fiducial moves in the vicinity of high-density objects such as the bone that can have similar intensity values as the fiducial, the tracking becomes difficult or even impossible.

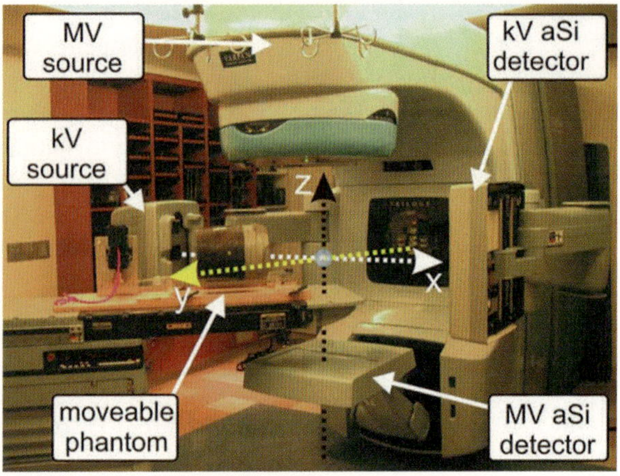

Fig. 11.3 Varian Trilogy with KV and MV imager, with KV beam and MV beam perpendicular to each other (Modified from Wiersma et al. 2008)

11.3 External Surrogate Tracking System

The external surrogate tracking system is a respiratory gating technology which is based on the correlation between the tumor position and the patient's respiratory cycle. The most available and widely discussed respiratory gating system utilizing external respiration signal is the Real-time Position Management (RPM) system (Varian Medical Systems, Palo Alto, CA). By measuring the patient's respiratory pattern and range of motion, the system software creates a graphical sinusoidal form (waveform) as a function of time. The major components of the RPM system are a marker block, an infrared tracking camera, and a predictive filter. The marker block is a plastic box with two or six reflective dots on one side and serves as the external fiducial marker. The marker is placed on the patient's anterior abdominal surface, usually between the umbilicus and the xiphoid because this region has been shown to yield the largest amplitude in maker motion (typically 1–2 cm) (Fig. 11.4) (Mageras et al. 2001). It should be placed nearly horizontal and at the same location during imaging for planning, simulation, and treatment. The camera is a charge-coupled device (CCD) with an array of LEDs that emits infrared light. Dots on the marker block reflect the infrared light back to the camera, which captures the signal. The system software then utilizes this signal to track and analyze the motion of the dots, which corresponds to the motion of the chest or abdomen. The predictive filter is a vital part of the RPM software which detects and predicts the patient's breathing pattern. After recognizing the pattern, the predictive filter makes sure that this pattern is being followed. If there is any interruption in the breathing pattern, the predictive filter detects the interruption, and RPM instantly turns the beam off.

Berson et al. from September 2000 to January 2002 evaluated RPM on 108 patients (lung, liver, breast, mediastinum) and concluded that the system is a practical and achievable solution for minimizing respiratory-induced target motion during both simulation and treatment (Berson et al. 2004). Ford et al. found that the residual intra- and interfraction movements measured by fluoroscopic and portal

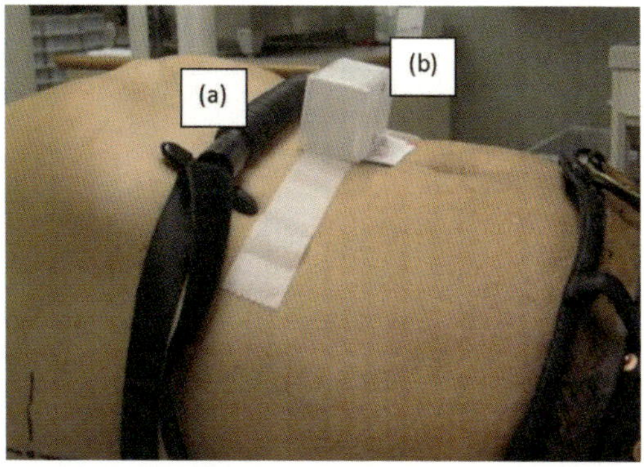

Fig. 11.4 The external surrogate system (**a**) pressure belt (**b**) RPM block (Glide-Hurst and Chetty 2014)

imaging using this technique were 2.6+/− 1.7 mm and 2.8 +/−1.0 mm, respectively. With no gating, the intrafraction excursion became 6.9+/−2.1 mm (Ford et al. 2002). In research carried out by Wagman et al., ten patients with liver tumors were treated using the RPM system. Average superior-to-inferior (SI) diaphragm motion on initial fluoroscopy was reduced from 22.7 mm without gating to 5.1 mm with gating (Wagman et al. 2003). Similarly, reproducible decrease in liver motion with gating reduced the GTV-to-PTV margin from 2 cm to 1 cm and resulted in a dose increase of 7–27 % (median 21.3 %) in six patients. Underberg et al. evaluated 4D CT scans on 31 lung tumor patients; the mean mobility vector decreased from 8.5 +/− 6.5 mm for the entire breathing cycle to 1.4 mm +/− 0.7 mm in the tidal-expiration gated window (Underberg et al. 2005).

Other gating devices have also been used for external surrogate tracking, such as pressure-sensitive belts (Li et al. 2006). Similar to the positioning of the RPM marker block (Fig. 11.4), a pressure sensor is placed on the abdomen. The belt detects the abdominal motion (both amplitude and phase) by measuring pressure variation and then transfers the motion signal to the monitoring station. The software records the patient's respiratory data and controls the irradiation beam accordingly. However, as in the external surrogate systems, the relationship between the external surrogate and the internal tumor motion seems to vary, even during treatment on the same day (Lin et al. 2009). This approach is therefore often considered to suffer from lack of accuracy.

11.4 Internal and External Surrogate Tracking System

11.4.1 Direct Tumor Tracking System

An RTRT system in which the beam is continuously delivered pursuing the position of the tumor is known as non-gated RTRT or dynamic tracking radiotherapy (DTT). Mitsubishi Heavy Industries in collaboration with Kyoto University and Brain LAB (Feld Kirichen, Germany) developed the DTT system, also referred to as Vero

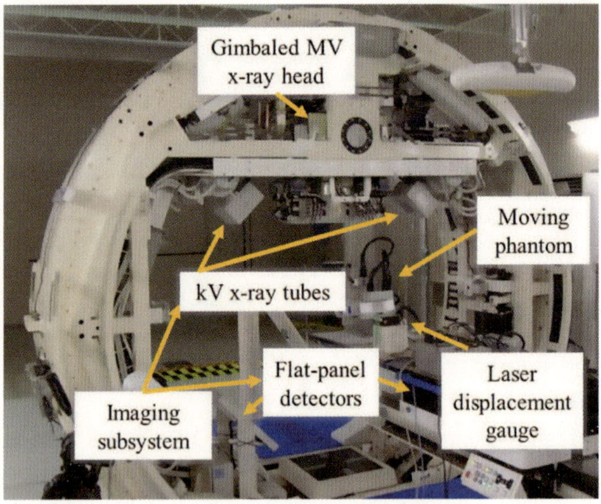

Fig. 11.5 Dynamic tumor tracking DTT system (Vero system) with gimbaled MV X-ray head and KV X-ray tubes (Mukumoto et al. 2012)

(Fig. 11.5) (Mukumoto et al. 2012). It is composed of a small and light 6MV C-band linac mounted on a gimbaled X-ray head with MLC. The entire system is installed on an O-ring gantry (Takayama et al. 2009). The X-ray head can rotate in both horizontal and vertical axes relative to the O-ring direction to track a moving target. The imaging system, which is fixed in the gantry, consists of two types of imaging systems, each consisting of a kV X-ray tube and a flat panel detector (FPD) with an infrared IR camera mounted on the ceiling of the treatment room.

IR markers are placed on the surface of patient's abdominal wall for detecting respiratory signal, and fiducial markers are implanted in the tumor and are continuously and simultaneously monitored using the IR camera and the orthogonal kV X-ray imaging system. After tracking, a correlation model (4D) is developed using the detected respiratory signals and the position of the moving marker (Suzuki et al. 2014). In the 4D model, the peak-to-peak amplitude of the detected target motion, mean, and the standard deviation between the moving position and the IR marker are calculated automatically (Mukumoto et al. 2013). Then using the gimbal mechanism, the therapeutic X-ray beam tracks and follows the real-time position of the tumor and delivers therapeutic X-rays continuously, while the beam is tracking the moving tumor until the prescribed dose is completely delivered. According to Tom Depuydt et al., the systematic tracking error of the Vero system was found to be below 0.14 mm. Similarly, the sinusoidal motion tracking was found to be accurate with a tracking error of 90 % percentile $E_{90\%}$ <0.82 mm (Depuydt et al. 2011).

In 2011, the world's first DTT was performed on a lung cancer patient using Vero 4DRT at Kyoto University Hospital (Suzuki et al. 2014). Matsuo et al. (2014) performed DTT on a lung cancer patient using a gimbal-mounted linac. The tracking plan showed PTV volume reduction from 56.2 cm^3 to 39.6 cm^3 covering 95 % of the GTV. Dose to the normal lung and liver were also reduced (Matsuo et al. 2014).

11.4.2 Respiratory Tracking System (RTS)

The Synchrony™ Respiratory Tracking System (RTS) is a subsystem of the CyberKnife robotic treatment device (Accuray Inc., Sunnyvale, CA). It is used to irradiate extracranial tumors that move due to respiration and is considered to be an external-internal tumor tracking modality. The main advantages of RTS are that the patients can breathe normally, and there is no loss of duty cycle such as with gated therapy systems. The duty cycle is generally 100 % (Seppenwoolde et al. 2007). Tracking is based on a measured correspondence model (linear or polynomial) between internal tumor motion and external (chest/abdominal) marker motion. The radiation beam follows the tumor movement via the continuously measured marker motion. The RTS uses computer simulation based upon the recorded external and internal marker positions which allow the robot to accurately follow tumor motion even in the case of irregular respiration signal. The correspondence model predicts tumor position and sends feedback to the robotic linear accelerator, and the robot realigns the beam with the tumor (Glide-Hurst and Chetty 2014).

The imaging system consists of two kV X-ray tubes and a pair of orthogonal positioned flat panel imagers. The internal marker (implanted at or near the tumor position) is determined via X-ray images. Similarly, three external markers, i.e., optical markers, are tracked using a light-emitting diode (LED) fixed on the chest or abdomen of the patient. A stereo camera system measures the 3D position of the markers continuously at 30 Hz (Hoogeman et al. 2009).

For the correlation mode, first the position of the internal marker is determined by X-ray fluoroscopy and is related to the external signal. Functions that are considered for establishing a correspondence model are linear model and polynomial model. The linear model is applied for the AP and LR directions and the polynomial model for the CC direction and for the phase shift and hysteresis in the trajectory (Hoogeman et al. 2009).

Misha et al. calculated residual error of the correlation model using the Synchrony treatment log file from 44 patients with 158 treatment fractions. The analysis included four log files. The files are comprised of image data, the time stamp of image acquisition, the center of mass (CoM) of the internal marker, and the correlation model for each component of motion and external marker separately. The correlation model error (e) was calculated for each X-ray image acquisition. If the value of e is greater than 5 mm, the system operation is halted, and a new model is generated by removing all existing data points and obtaining new sets of X-ray images. The operator takes X-ray images until the entire respiration cycle is included. Usually 6–8 images are needed for analysis.

The accuracy of the RTS calculated using the average and 95th percentile of 3D residual motion over each fraction phantom experiment showed that Synchrony performs real-time respiration motion tracking with an accuracy of 0.7 +/− 0.3 mm^3 and suggested that irregular breathing, varying the phase relationship between internal and external markers and rapid baseline shifts, might reduce the clinical accuracy of respiratory motion tracking (Hoogeman et al. 2009). In the RTS, as the imaging is performed before each treatment, setup errors are virtually absent.

Research conducted by Seppenwoolde et al. showed eight lung cancer patients treated with the RTS (Seppenwoolde et al. 2007). The study found that the treatment errors due to breathing motion were reduced in all patients. The polynomial model was better for the patients having time delay between internal and external motion. Similarly, the residual treatment error was greater for fractions with more tumor motion.

The DTT and RT systems are both real-time beam-positioning methods, i.e., the treatment beam directly follows the tumor. Another method used for the same purpose is dynamic multi-leaf collimator (DMLC) tracking (Keall et al. 2005; Papiez et al. 2005; Rangaraj and Papiez 2005). In this system, once tumor motion is detected, the motion signal is transferred to the computer, and the software calculates the required leaf position to track the target based on the incoming signal (Keall et al. 2006a). The DMLC leaf travel speed can safely reach 2.5 cm/s, which is comparable with breathing-induced tumor motion speed (Giraud and Houle 2013).

Recently, positron emission tomography (PET) incorporated with linac has been proposed as one of the dynamic tumor tracking approaches (Darwish et al. 2010; Yamaya et al. 2011; Tashima et al. 2012). Tong Xu et al. implanted positron emission marker (PeTrack) and detected in real time using positron-sensitive detectors which is similar to PET (Xu et al. 2006). The computation time was less than 20 ms with less than 10 mm initial estimation error. Yamaguchi et al. studied m-IGRT by comparing the PET-based digitally reconstructed planar image (PDRI) registration with radiographic registration (Yamaguchi et al. 2011) and suggested that it is feasible for clinical use. Yang et al. proposed a center of mass (CoM) tumor tracking algorithm using gated PET images combined with respiratory monitor (Yang et al. 2014). The algorithm determines the target position information through the CoM of the segmented target volume on gated PET images reconstructed from accumulated coincidence events, which is continuously updated throughout a scan (Yang et al. 2014). The overall tracking error in phantom studies was found to be less than 2 mm.

11.5 Tumor Tracking Without Implanted Fiducials (Markerless Tracking)

11.5.1 Fluoroscopic Tracking

The fiducial implantation method involves the risk of pneumothorax as percutaneous marker implantation is involved and markers may also migrate (Jiang 2006). Many clinicians are thus reluctant to use this method. In order to overcome such effects, fluoroscopic tracking of the tumor without implanted fiducial markers has been developed (Berbeco et al. 2005a; Cui et al. 2008; Xu et al. 2007). Direct fluoroscopic tumor tracking is possible in the case of lung tumors since the density difference between the tumor mass and normal lung tissues may be large enough to provide a good visualization in radiographic images (Giraud and Houle 2013). The direct detection of a lung tumor in the kV X-ray image is possible if the tumor mass is small, well defined, and has a high-contrast edge (Berbeco et al. 2005a). However, it is extremely difficult to track tumors in the abdomen using this tracking procedure.

The markerless tracking technique can be divided into two groups: one is classification algorithms and the other direct tracking algorithms. In classification algorithms, a training data set is used to identify possible tumor locations in subsequent images. In direct tracking algorithms, a set of features is extracted and localized on each image frame (Rottmann et al. 2010).

Tong Lin et al. (2009) proposed a markerless method based on the correlation between the tumor position and surrogate anatomic features in the image (Lin et al. 2009). The algorithm consists of four steps: (1) position of the surrogate features are tracked using principal component analysis (PCA) of a region of interest (ROI) (which implies that a surrogate ROI is not tracked directly); (2) obtaining parametric representation of the motion pattern from the surrogate ROI; (3) building a regression model between the tumor position and the motion pattern; and (4) predicting the tumor location using the established regression model. The following regression methods were used: linear and two-degree polynomial regression, artificial neural network (ANN), and support vector machine (SVM). The above algorithm was used to treat ten lung cancer patients showing a mean tracking error of 2.1 pixels and a maximum error at a 95 % confidence level of 4.6 pixels (pixel size is about 0.5 mm). However, the presented method lacks the ability to adapt to change in the breathing pattern that cannot be described with the motion observed during the training session (extrapolation) (Rottmann et al. 2010).

In direct tracking algorithms, a set of features is extracted and localized on each image frame. Rottmann et al. described a direct tracking algorithm which can be implemented in real time and is independent of prior information of the exact tumor motion range during treatment (Rottmann et al. 2010). Arimura et al. proposed markerless lung tumor tracking on cine EPID images, which uses cross correlation to match a single tumor template defined in the center of the treatment aperture to each portal images (Arimura et al. 2009). The average tracking error ranged from 0.58 mm to 2.53 mm, calculated by comparing with a manually defined gold standard (Rottmann et al. 2010).

11.5.2 MRI-Guided Tumor Tracking

MRI has become attractive for tumor and organ motion monitoring because it is noninvasive and nonionizing and provides excellent soft tissue contrast (Korin et al. 1992; Plathow et al. 2004; Doyle et al. 2000). Several research groups are integrating radiotherapy with MRI (Fallone et al. 2009; Raaymakers et al. 2009; Dempsey et al. 2005). Similarly, various algorithms have been proposed for tumor motion tracking using MRI images. Ries et al. demonstrated 3D tracking in 2D MRI by continuous shifts of the 2D image plane to follow the through-plane target motion, which was estimated by a perpendicular pencil beam navigator (Ries et al. 2010).

In research carried out by Cervino et al., two prediction models were suggested for tumor tracking (Cervino et al. 2011). They are (1) ANN model and (2) template matching (TM) algorithm. The ANN model is based on biological neural networks. For the model to focus on the target motion, an ROI around the target is used rather than the whole image, which contains the target and its expected motion through the sequence. The ROI is defined only once and is fixed for all the sequence. The TM algorithm defines a template and determines the best location of the template in the image by searching various locations within the search image. But in the TM algorithm, two problems arise during tracking. One is related to the size of the search window, and the other is the target moving out of plane. The first issue can be solved by performing a multi-grid search and limiting the search window. The second issue can be handled by using a diaphragm as a surrogate for the position of the target when it moves outside the imaged 2D plane. The performance of the ANN model was found to be good for regular breathing, but its performance diminishes when breathing becomes irregular. The TM algorithm, on the other hand, proved to be good in both regular and irregular breathing. For the TM algorithm, an average prediction error of 0.6 mm at 95 % confidence level of 1.0 mm was achieved.

Similarly, Lau Brix et al. suggested three-dimensional liver motion tracking using real-time 2D MRI (Brix et al. 2014). The proposed 3D tracking method has three steps. First, a 3D volumetric scan of the structure to be tracked is recorded. Second, the 3D volume is resliced for 2D series orientation, and a library of 2D templates with well-defined 3D position relative to the tracked structure is defined. Third, template-based 3D target localization is performed with real-time 2D MRI series. The template and 2D position that yields the highest cross correlation coefficient is selected.

11.6 Summary

There are several commercially available devices to track organ motion, especially respiratory-induced tumor motion. These devices enable gated stereotactic body radiotherapy. The tumor tracking approaches are summarized in Table 11.1 along with each system's benefits and limitations.

Although correlation between external surrogate maker and respiratory phase is generally high, correlation between respiratory phase and tumor motion due to phase shift, so that the tracking is based on a measured correspondence model between internal tumor motion and external marker motion, is less well established.

Table 11.1 Benefits and limitations of recent techniques for tumor tracking approach

Tracking method	Benefits	Limitations
I. Internal surrogate		
Implanted gold fiducials	Real time, high accuracy	Invasive, additional dose on patient from fluoroscope, possibility of migration of the implanted marker
Implanted transponder	Real time, high accuracy, no additional radiation dose to patient	Invasive, clinically available only for prostate cancer treatment
Combined MV/kV	Real time, MV treatment beam used for imaging, use of only one kV X-ray imaging system	Intensity-based tracking, the fiducial may be not possible to track in the vicinity of high-density matter like bone
II. External surrogate		
Pressure sensor belt	Noninvasive, real time, no additional radiation dose to patient	Limited dimensionality, variable correlation between tumor position and external surrogate, accuracy less than implanted fiducial tracking
Infrared reflector		
III. Internal and external surrogate		
RTS	Radiation beam dynamically tracks the tumor, no loss of duty cycle	System has limited beam output and beam size; treatment time can be lengthy for large tumors
DTT	Radiation beam dynamically tracks the tumor, no loss of duty cycle	Dependence on 4D modeling and fiducial insertion. If no appropriate 4D model is acquired DTT, tracking cannot be performed
IV. Markerless tracking		
Direct fluoroscopic tracking	Noninvasive, real time	Additional dose to the patient from fluoroscope, applicable only in the region where there exists a density difference between tumor mass and normal tissue and with high-contrast edge
MRI tracking	Noninvasive, real time, large dimensionality, excellent soft tissue contrast	MRI is confounded by distortion resulting from nonuniformity in the magnetic susceptibility artifacts, patient motion

Internal fiducial marker tracking can accurately indicate tumor motion. However, it requires invasive marker implantation.

Several additional tumor tracking approaches have been reported using molecular imaging device such as positron emission tomography (PET). New tumor tracking approaches are expected to be commercially available in the near future. Users who attempt to irradiate moving tumors using a tumor tracking device must understand the characteristics of the device and apply adequate margin for treatment planning.

References

Abdefg SA, Abcdeg AY, Bdf BB, Özlem Uzman B, Edhem Ünver B, Esen Akkaya D (2002) CT-guided transthoracic fine needle aspiration of pulmonary lesions: accuracy and complications in 294 patients. Signature 8:497

Ahn YC, Shimizu S, Shirato H, Hashimoto T, Osaka Y, Zhang XQ, Abe T, Hosokawa M, Miyasaka K (2004) Application of real-time tumor-tracking and gated radiotherapy system for unresectable pancreatic cancer. Yonsei Med J 45:584–590

Arimura H, Egashira Y, Shioyama Y, Nakamura K, Yoshidome S, Anai S, Nomoto S, Honda H, Toyofuku F, Higashida Y (2009) Computerized method for estimation of the location of a lung tumor on EPID cine images without implanted markers in stereotactic body radiotherapy. Phys Med Biol 54:665

Balter J, Wright N, Dimmer S, Friemel B, Newell J, Cheng Y, Mate T (2003) Demonstration of accurate localization and continuous tracking of implantable wireless electromagnetic transponders. Int J Radiat Oncol Biol Phys 57:S264–S265

Balter JM, Wright JN, Newell LJ, Friemel B, Dimmer S, Cheng Y, Wong J, Vertatschitsch E, Mate TP (2005) Accuracy of a wireless localization system for radiotherapy. Int J Radiat Oncol Biol Phys 61:933–937

Berbeco RI, Mostafavi H, Sharp GC, Jiang SB (2005a) Towards fluoroscopic respiratory gating for lung tumours without radiopaque markers. Phys Med Biol 50:4481

Berbeco RI, Nishioka S, Shirato H, Chen GT, Jiang SB (2005b) Residual motion of lung tumours in gated radiotherapy with external respiratory surrogates. Phys Med Biol 50:3655

Berbeco RI, Nishioka S, Shirato H, Jiang SB (2006) Residual motion of lung tumors in end-of-inhale respiratory gated radiotherapy based on external surrogates. Med Phys 33:4149–4156

Berson AM, Emery R, Rodriguez L, Richards GM, Ng T, Sanghavi S, Barsa J (2004) Clinical experience using respiratory gated radiation therapy: comparison of free-breathing and breath-hold techniques. Int J Radiat Oncol Biol Phys 60:419–426

Brix L, Ringgaard S, Sørensen TS, Poulsen PR (2014) Three-dimensional liver motion tracking using real-time two-dimensional MRI. Med Phys 41:042302

Burch D, Willoughby T, Meeks S, Kupelian P, Litzenberg D, Sandler H, Levine L, Vertatschitsch D, Vertatschitsch E (2005) Real Time Prostate Translation, Rotation, Deformation Evaluated with Calypso Beacon™ Transponders. Int J Radiat Oncol Biol Phys 63:S195

Cervino LI, Du J, Jiang SB (2011) MRI-guided tumor tracking in lung cancer radiotherapy. Phys Med Biol 56:3773

Chen Q-S, Weinhous MS, Deibel FC, Ciezki JP, Macklis RM (2001) Fluoroscopic study of tumor motion due to breathing: facilitating precise radiation therapy for lung cancer patients. Med Phys 28:1850–1856

Cui Y, Dy JG, Alexander B, Jiang SB (2008) Fluoroscopic gating without implanted fiducial markers for lung cancer radiotherapy based on support vector machines. Phys Med Biol 53: N315

Darwish N, Mackie T, Thomadsen B, Kao C (2010) MO-E-204C-03: On the Development of On-Board PET with Tomotherapy Using Open Dual Ring Geometry. Med Phys 37:3357–3357

De Boer HC, De Koste JRVS, Senan S, Visser AG, Heijmen BJ (2001) Analysis and reduction of 3D systematic and random setup errors during the simulation and treatment of lung cancer patients with CT-based external beam radiotherapy dose planning. Int J Radiat Oncol Biol Phys 49:857–868

Dempsey J, Benoit D, Fitzsimmons J, Haghighat A, Li J, Low D, Mutic S, Palta J, Romeijn H, Sjoden G (2005) A device for realtime 3D image-guided IMRT. Int J Radiat Oncol Biol Phys 63:S202

Depuydt T, Verellen D, Haas O, Gevaert T, Linthout N, Duchateau M, Tournel K, Reynders T, Leysen K, Hoogeman M (2011) Geometric accuracy of a novel gimbals based radiation therapy tumor tracking system. Radiother Oncol 98:365–372

Doyle V, Howe F, Griffiths J (2000) The effect of respiratory motion on CSI localized MRS. Phys Med Biol 45:2093

Fallone B, Murray B, Rathee S, Stanescu T, Steciw S, Vidakovic S, Blosser E, Tymofichuk D (2009) First MR images obtained during megavoltage photon irradiation from a prototype integrated linac-MR system. Med Phys 36:2084–2088

Ford E, Mageras G, Yorke E, Rosenzweig K, Wagman R, Ling C (2002) Evaluation of respiratory movement during gated radiotherapy using film and electronic portal imaging. Int J Radiat Oncol Biol Phys 52:522–531

Geraghty PR, Kee ST, Mcfarlane G, Razavi MK, Sze DY, Dake MD (2003) CT-guided transthoracic needle aspiration biopsy of pulmonary nodules: Needle size and pneumothorax rate 1. Radiology 229:475–481

Giraud P, Houle A (2013) Respiratory gating for radiotherapy: main technical aspects and clinical benefits. ISRN Pulmonology

Glide-Hurst CK, Chetty IJ (2014) Improving radiotherapy planning, delivery accuracy, and normal tissue sparing using cutting edge technologies. J Thorac Dis 6:303

Goitein M (2004) Organ and tumor motion: an overview. Seminars in radiation oncology. Elsevier, pp 2–9

Hanley J, Debois MM, Mah D, Mageras GS, Raben A, Rosenzweig K, Mychalczak B, Schwartz LH, Gloeggler PJ, Lutz W (1999) Deep inspiration breath-hold technique for lung tumors: the potential value of target immobilization and reduced lung density in dose escalation. Int J Radiat Oncol Biol Phys 45:603–611

Hoogeman M, Prévost J-B, Nuyttens J, Pöll J, Levendag P, Heijmen B (2009) Clinical accuracy of the respiratory tumor tracking system of the cyberknife: assessment by analysis of log files. Int J Radiat Oncol Biol Phys 74:297–303

Houdek PV, Schwade JG, Landy HJ, Ginsberg MS (1992) Computer controlled stereotaxic radiotherapy system and method. Google Patents

Hummel J, Figl M, Kollmann C, Bergmann H, Birkfellner W (2002) Evaluation of a miniature electromagnetic position tracker. Med Phys 29:2205–2212

Jiang SB (2006) Technical aspects of image-guided respiration-gated radiation therapy. Med Dosim 31:141–151

Keall P, Todor A, Vedam S, Bartee C, Siebers J, Kini V, Mohan R (2004) On the use of EPID-based implanted marker tracking for 4D radiotherapy. Med Phys 31:3492–3499

Keall PJ, Joshi S, Vedam SS, Siebers JV, Kini VR, Mohan R (2005) Four-dimensional radiotherapy planning for DMLC-based respiratory motion tracking. Med Phys 32:942–951

Keall PJ, Cattell H, Pokhrel D, Dieterich S, Wong KH, Murphy MJ, Vedam SS, Wijesooriya K, Mohan R (2006a) Geometric accuracy of a real-time target tracking system with dynamic multileaf collimator tracking system. Int J Radiat Oncol Biol Phys 65:1579–1584

Keall PJ, Mageras GS, Balter JM, Emery RS, Forster KM, Jiang SB, Kapatoes JM, Low DA, Murphy MJ, Murray BR (2006b) The management of respiratory motion in radiation oncology report of AAPM Task Group 76 a. Med Phys 33:3874–3900

Kitamura K, Shirato H, Seppenwoolde Y, Onimaru R, Oda M, Fujita K, Shimizu S, Shinohara N, Harabayashi T, Miyasaka K (2002) Three-dimensional intrafractional movement of prostate measured during real-time tumor-tracking radiotherapy in supine and prone treatment positions. Int J Radiat Oncol Biol Phys 53:1117–1123

Korin HW, Ehman RL, Riederer SJ, Felmlee JP, Grimm RC (1992) Respiratory kinematics of the upper abdominal organs: a quantitative study. Magn Reson Med 23:172–178

Kupelian PA, Willoughby TR, Meeks SL, Forbes A, Wagner T, Maach M, Langen KM (2005) Intraprostatic fiducials for localization of the prostate gland: monitoring intermarker distances during radiation therapy to test for marker stability. Int J Radiat Oncol Biol Phys 62:1291–1296

Kupelian P, Willoughby T, Mahadevan A, Djemil T, Weinstein G, Jani S, Enke C, Solberg T, Flores N, Liu D (2007) Multi-institutional clinical experience with the Calypso System in localization and continuous, real-time monitoring of the prostate gland during external radiotherapy. Int J Radiat Oncol Biol Phys 67:1088–1098

Leong J (1987) Implementation of random positioning error in computerised radiation treatment planning systems as a result of fractionation. Phys Med Biol 32:327

Li XA, Stepaniak C, Gore E (2006) Technical and dosimetric aspects of respiratory gating using a pressure-sensor motion monitoring system. Med Phys 33:145–154

Lin T, Cervino LI, Tang X, Vasconcelos N, Jiang SB (2009) Fluoroscopic tumor tracking for image-guided lung cancer radiotherapy. Phys Med Biol 54:981

Litzenberg DW, Willoughby TR, Balter JM, Sandler HM, Wei J, Kupelian PA, Cunningham AA, Bock A, Aubin M, Roach M (2007) Positional stability of electromagnetic transponders used for prostate localization and continuous, real-time tracking. Int J Radiat Oncol Biol Phys 68:1199–1206

Mageras GS, Yorke E, Rosenzweig K, Braban L, Keatley E, Ford E, Leibel SA, Ling CC (2001) Fluoroscopic evaluation of diaphragmatic motion reduction with a respiratory gated radiotherapy system. J Appl Clin Med Phys 2:191–200

Matsuo Y, Ueki N, Takayama K, Nakamura M, Miyabe Y, Ishihara Y, Mukumoto N, Yano S, Tanabe H, Kaneko S (2014) Evaluation of dynamic tumour tracking radiotherapy with real-time monitoring for lung tumours using a gimbal mounted linac. Radiother Oncol 112:360–364

Mayse ML, Parikh PJ, Lechleiter KM, Dimmer S, Park M, Chaudhari A, Talcott M, Low DA, Bradley JD (2008) Bronchoscopic implantation of a novel wireless electromagnetic transponder in the canine lung: a feasibility study. Int J Radiat Oncol Biol Phys 72:93–98

Mukumoto N, Nakamura M, Sawada A, Takahashi K, Miyabe Y, Takayama K, Mizowaki T, Kokubo M, Hiraoka M (2012) Positional accuracy of novel x-ray-image-based dynamic tumor-tracking irradiation using a gimbaled MV x-ray head of a Vero4DRT (MHI-TM2000). Med Phys 39:6287–6296

Mukumoto N, Nakamura M, Sawada A, Suzuki Y, Takahashi K, Miyabe Y, Kaneko S, Mizowaki T, Kokubo M, Hiraoka M (2013) Accuracy verification of infrared marker-based dynamic tumor-tracking irradiation using the gimbaled x-ray head of the Vero4DRT (MHI-TM2000) a. Med Phys 40:041706

Murphy MJ, Isaakson M, Jalden J (2002) Adaptive filtering to predict lung tumor motion during free breathing. CARS 2002 Computer Assisted Radiology and Surgery. Springer

Oita M, Ohmori K, Obinata K, Kinoshita R, Onimaru R, Tsuchiya K, Suzuki K, Nishioka T, Ohsaka H, Fujita K (2006) Uncertainty in treatment of head-and-neck tumors by use of intraoral mouthpiece and embedded fiducials. Int J Radiat Oncol Biol Phys 64:1581–1588

Papiez L, Rangaraj D, Keall P (2005) Real-time DMLC IMRT delivery for mobile and deforming targets. Med Phys 32:3037–3048

Parikh P, Hubenschmidt J, Dimmer S, Vertatschitsch E, Eidens R, Wright J, Low D (2005) 4D verification of real-time accuracy of the Calypso system with lung cancer patient trajectory data. Int J Radiat Oncol Biol Phys 63:S26–S27

Plathow C, Ley S, Fink C, Puderbach M, Hosch W, Schmähl A, Debus J, Kauczor H-U (2004) Analysis of intrathoracic tumor mobility during whole breathing cycle by dynamic MRI. Int J Radiat Oncol Biol Phys 59:952–959

Pouliot J, Roach M, Shinohara K, Willoughby T, Kupelian P, Skrumeda L, Balter J, Litzenberg D, Wei J, Sandler H (2004) Positional stability and implant experience of AC magnetic Beacon (TM) transponders used to localize patients for external beam radiation therapy. Medical Physics, (2004). Amer Assoc Physicists Medicine Amer Inst Physics Ste 1 No 1, 2 Huntington Quadrangle, Melville, NY 11747–4502 USA, 1847–1847

Quigley MM, Mate TP, Sylvester JE (2009) Prostate tumor alignment and continuous, real-time adaptive radiation therapy using electromagnetic fiducials: Clinical and cost-utility analyses. Urol oncology: seminars and original investigations. Elsevier, pp 473–482

Raaymakers B, Lagendijk J, Overweg J, Kok J, Raaijmakers A, Kerkhof E, Van Der Put R, Meijsing I, Crijns S, Benedosso F (2009) Integrating a 1.5 T MRI scanner with a 6 MV accelerator: proof of concept. Physics in medicine and biology 54:N229

Rangaraj D, Papiez L (2005) Synchronized delivery of DMLC intensity modulated radiation therapy for stationary and moving targets. Med Phys 32:1802–1817

Ries M, De Senneville BD, Roujol S, Berber Y, Quesson B, Moonen C (2010) Real-time 3D target tracking in MRI guided focused ultrasound ablations in moving tissues. Magn Reson Med 64:1704–1712

Rottmann J, Aristophanous M, Chen A, Berbeco R (2010) A multi-region algorithm for markerless beam's-eye view lung tumor tracking. Phys Med Biol 55:5585

Santanam L, Malinowski K, Hubenshmidt J, Dimmer S, Mayse ML, Bradley J, Chaudhari A, Lechleiter K, Goddu SKM, Esthappan J (2008) Fiducial-based translational localization accuracy of electromagnetic tracking system and on-board kilovoltage imaging system. Int J Radiat Oncol Biol Phys 70:892–899

Seiler P, Blattmann H, Kirsch S, Muench R, Schilling C (2000) A novel tracking technique for the continuous precise measurement of tumour positions in conformal radiotherapy. Phys Med Biol 45:N103

Seppenwoolde Y, Berbeco RI, Nishioka S, Shirato H, Heijmen B (2007) Accuracy of tumor motion compensation algorithm from a robotic respiratory tracking system: a simulation study. Med Phys 34:2774–2784

Shimizu S, Shirato H, Xo B, Kagei K, Nishioka T, Hashimoto S, Tsuchiya K, Aoyama H, Miyasaka K (1999) Three-dimensional movement of a liver tumor detected by high-speed magnetic resonance imaging. Radiother Oncol 50:367–370

Shimizu S, Shirato H, Ogura S, Akita-Dosaka H, Kitamura K, Nishioka T, Kagei K, Nishimura M, Miyasaka K (2001) Detection of lung tumor movement in real-time tumor-tracking radiotherapy. Int J Radiat Oncol Biol Phys 51:304–310

Shirato H, Shimizu S, Kitamura K, Nishioka T, Kagei K, Hashimoto S, Aoyama H, Kunieda T, Shinohara N, Dosaka-Akita H (2000a) Four-dimensional treatment planning and fluoroscopic real-time tumor tracking radiotherapy for moving tumor. Int J Radiat Oncol Biol Phys 48:435–442

Shirato H, Shimizu S, Kunieda T, Kitamura K, Van Herk M, Kagei K, Nishioka T, Hashimoto S, Fujita K, Aoyama H (2000b) Physical aspects of a real-time tumor-tracking system for gated radiotherapy. Int J Radiat Oncol Biol Phys 48:1187–1195

Shirato H, Shimizu S, Kitamura K, Onimaru R (2007) Organ motion in image-guided radiotherapy: lessons from real-time tumor-tracking radiotherapy. Int J Clin Oncol 12:8–16

Suzuki Y, Takahashi K, Yamada M, Kaneko S, Yoshida M, Toyama K (2014) The challenge of innovative cancer treatments enabled by Vero4DRT-development of high-precision dose delivery features for reducing radiation exposure of healthy tissue. Mitsubishi Heavy Ind Tech Rev 51:76

Takayama K, Mizowaki T, Kokubo M, Kawada N, Nakayama H, Narita Y, Nagano K, Kamino Y, Hiraoka M (2009) Initial validations for pursuing irradiation using a gimbals tracking system. Radiother Oncol 93:45–49

Tashima H, Yamaya T, Yoshida E, Kinouchi S, Watanabe M, Tanaka E (2012) A single-ring OpenPET enabling PET imaging during radiotherapy. Phys Med Biol 57:4705

Underberg RW, Lagerwaard FJ, Slotman BJ, Cuijpers JP, Senan S (2005) Benefit of respiration-gated stereotactic radiotherapy for stage I lung cancer: an analysis of 4DCT datasets. Int J Radiat Oncol Biol Phys 62:554–560

Van Herk M (2004) Errors and margins in radiotherapy. Seminars in radiation oncology. Elsevier, pp 52–64

Wagman R, Yorke E, Ford E, Giraud P, Mageras G, Minsky B, Rosenzweig K (2003) Respiratory gating for liver tumors: use in dose escalation. Int J Radiat Oncol Biol Phys 55:659–668

Wambersie A, Landgerg T (1999) ICRU report 62: prescribing, recording and reporting photon beam therapy. ICRU Publ Bethesda MD

Wiersma R, Mao W, Xing L (2008) Combined kV and MV imaging for real-time tracking of implanted fiducial markers a. Med Phys 35:1191–1198

Willoughby T, Kupelian P, Pouliot J, Shinohara K, Aubin M, Roach Iii M, Skrumeda L, Balter J, Litzenberg D, Hadley S (2004) Implant experience and positional stability of AC Magnetic

Beacon™ Transponders used to localize patients for external beam radiation therapy of the prostate. Int J Radiat Oncol Biol Phys 60:S267–S268

Willoughby TR, Kupelian PA, Pouliot J, Shinohara K, Aubin M, Roach M, Skrumeda LL, Balter JM, Litzenberg DW, Hadley SW (2006) Target localization and real-time tracking using the Calypso 4D localization system in patients with localized prostate cancer. Int J Radiat Oncol Biol Phys 65:528–534

Wong JW, Sharpe MB, Jaffray DA, Kini VR, Robertson JM, Stromberg JS, Martinez AA (1999) The use of active breathing control (ABC) to reduce margin for breathing motion. Int J Radiat Oncol Biol Phys 44:911–919

Xu T, Wong JT, Shikhaliev PM, Ducote JL, Al-Ghazi MS, Molloi S (2006) Real-time tumor tracking using implanted positron emission markers: concept and simulation study. Med Phys 33:2598–2609

Xu Q, Hamilton RJ, Schowengerdt RA, Jiang SB (2007) A deformable lung tumor tracking method in fluoroscopic video using active shape models: a feasibility study. Phys Med Biol 52:5277

Yamaguchi S, Ishikawa M, Bengua G, Sutherland K, Nishio T, Tanabe S, Miyamoto N, Suzuki R, Shirato H (2011) A feasibility study of a molecular-based patient setup verification method using a parallel-plane PET system. Phys Med Biol 56:965

Yamamoto R, Yonesaka A, Nishioka S, Watari H, Hashimoto T, Uchida D, Taguchi H, Nishioka T, Miyasaka K, Sakuragi N (2004) High dose three-dimensional conformal boost (3DCB) using an orthogonal diagnostic X-ray set-up for patients with gynecological malignancy: a new application of real-time tumor-tracking system. Radiother Oncol 73:219–222

Yamaya T, Yoshida E, Inaniwa T, Sato S, Nakajima Y, Wakizaka H, Kokuryo D, Tsuji A, Mitsuhashi T, Kawai H (2011) Development of a small prototype for a proof-of-concept of OpenPET imaging. Phys Med Biol 56:1123

Yang J, Yamamoto T, Mazin SR, Graves EE, Keall PJ (2014) The potential of positron emission tomography for intratreatment dynamic lung tumor tracking: a phantom study. Med Phys 41:021718

Chapter 12
Visualization of Dose Distributions for Photon Beam Radiation Therapy During Treatment Delivery

Takahiro Nakamoto and Hidetaka Arimura

Abstract In radiation treatment planning, dose distributions within patients' bodies are designed so that high doses can be delivered to target volumes while minimizing exposure to normal tissues. The dose distributions are delivered in accordance with those designed in the treatment plans. However, certain discrepancies inevitably exist between the designed and delivered dose distributions because of systematic and random errors during the actual treatment. Therefore, it is necessary to visualize dose distributions during treatment delivery in order to ensure the quality of the radiation therapy by comparing the actual distributions against the designed dose distributions. In this chapter, we describe the fundamental principles involved in visualizing the dose distributions for photon beam radiation therapy during treatment delivery.

Keywords Dose distributions during treatment delivery • Dose calculation algorithm • Electronic portal imaging device (EPID) • Portal dose image (PDI)

12.1 Introduction

The principle of radiation therapy is to prescribe high doses to tumors while reducing the doses to normal tissues (organs at risk (OAR)). Therefore, dose distributions should be designed based on contours of tumor targets and OAR by changing various parameters (e.g., number of beams, beam angles, voltages, shapes of irradiation fields, multi-leaf collimator (MLC) motions, etc.) in a radiation treatment plan. Several algorithms (Mackie et al. 1985; Boyer and Mok 1985; Mohan et al. 1986; Ahnesjö et al. 1987; Ahnesjö 1989; Battista and Sharpe 1992; Sharpe and Battista 1993; McNutt et al. 1996a, b; Liu et al. 1997; Verhaegen and Seuntiens 2003; Chetty et al. 2007; Vassiliev et al. 2010; Kan et al. 2013) enable us

T. Nakamoto (✉) • H. Arimura
Computer-aided Diagnosis and Radiotherapy Laboratory, Graduate School of Medical Sciences, Kyushu University, 3-1-1, Maidashi, Higashi-ku, Fukuoka 812-8582, Japan
e-mail: takahiro.nakamoto321@gmail.com

H. Arimura (ed.), *Image-Based Computer-Assisted Radiation Therapy*,
DOI 10.1007/978-981-10-2945-5_12

to produce the dose distributions in computed tomography (CT) images. In intensity-modulated radiation therapy (IMRT), the dose distributions are designed so that high-dose regions can be fitted to targets by optimizing fluence maps (Lan et al. 2012; Dias et al. 2016; Gao 2016). Although the doses are delivered during treatment based on the treatment plan, there are differences between the designed and delivered dose distributions owing to mechanical errors in the linear accelerators (linacs), patients' setup (positioning) errors, and physiological motions, despite efforts that are made to minimize these errors during treatment (McNutt et al. 1996a, b, 1997; Mizoguchi et al. 2013; Nakamoto et al. 2015). This results in uncertainties in the delivered dose distributions, which might lead to dose deficiencies with respect to the targets and complications with respect to normal tissues. Consequently, it is crucial to visualize the dose distributions during treatment delivery in order to ensure the quality of the radiation therapy.

The authors present a methodology for visualizing the dose distributions for photon beam radiation therapy during treatment delivery. The methodology consists of the following steps:

- Model-based dose calculation algorithm for visualizing dose distributions
- Estimation of the delivered dose distributions based on electronic portal imaging device images
- Prediction of the delivered three-dimensional dose distributions using portal dose images
- Estimation of four-dimensional dose distributions during treatment delivery

In this chapter, the key technologies and theories are described.

12.2 Model-Based Dose Calculation Algorithm for Visualizing Dose Distributions

12.2.1 Pencil Beam Convolution Method

The pencil beam convolution (PBC) method is a dose calculation algorithm that can consider scattered doses by modeling all interactions of photons and electrons in water (Mackie et al. 1985; Boyer and Mok 1985; Mohan et al. 1986; Ahnesjö et al. 1987; Ahnesjö 1989; Battista and Sharpe 1992; Sharpe and Battista 1993).

Figure 12.1 shows a conceptual illustration of dose calculation using a PBC method. The absorbed dose at a position is deposited by incident primary and scattered photons at that position and can be calculated using the following equation:

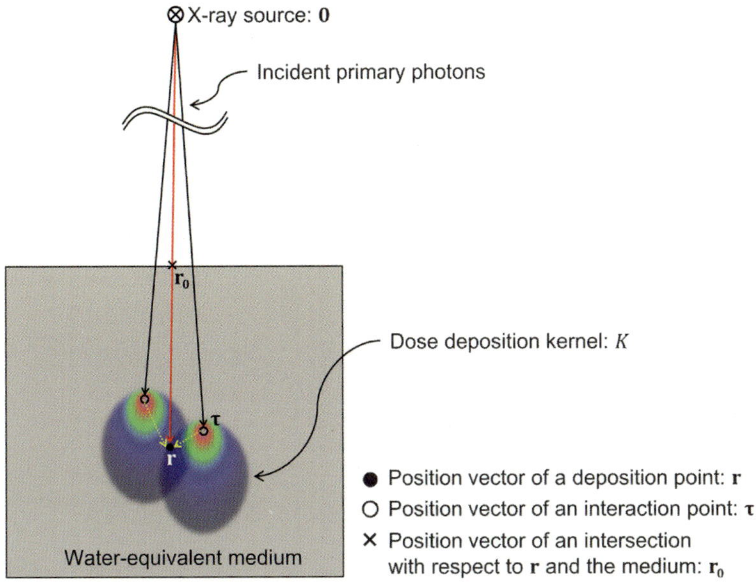

Fig. 12.1 A conceptual illustration of a dose calculation using a pencil beam convolution (PBC) method

$$D(\mathbf{r}) = \iiint T(\boldsymbol{\tau}) \cdot K(\mathbf{r} - \boldsymbol{\tau}) d\boldsymbol{\tau} = T(\mathbf{r}) * K(\mathbf{r}), \tag{12.1}$$

where **r** is the three-dimensional (3D) position vector, D is the dose, T is the total energy released per unit mass (TERMA), and K is the dose deposition kernel (DDK). $\boldsymbol{\tau}$ is the position vector of an interaction point (described later). The dose distributions are calculated by convolving the DDK with the TERMA for all positions.

The TERMA is the total released radiant energy per unit mass that results from interactions of the primary photons with the medium (Ahnesjö et al. 1987; Ahnesjö 1989). The TERMA at a position is calculated by using the following equation:

$$T(\mathbf{r}) = \int \Phi(E, \mathbf{r}) \cdot E \cdot \frac{\mu}{\rho}(E, \mathbf{r}) dE, \tag{12.2}$$

where E is the energy (often measured in mega-electron volts (MeV)), Φ is the fluence ($\mathrm{MeV}^{-1} \cdot \mathrm{m}^{-2}$), and (μ/ρ) is the mass attenuation coefficient ($\mathrm{m}^2 \cdot \mathrm{kg}^{-1}$). The TERMA at any arbitrary position, **r** for the PBC method can be described by

$$T(\mathbf{r}) = \frac{1}{\| \mathbf{r} \|^2} \int \Phi(E, \mathbf{0}) \cdot E \cdot \exp\Big(- \mu_w(E) \cdot W(\mathbf{r}) \Big) \cdot \left(\frac{\mu}{\rho} \right)_w (E, \mathbf{r}) dE, \quad (12.3)$$

where $\mathbf{0}$ is the position vector of the linac source (origin), μ_w is the linear attenuation coefficient of the water (m^{-1}), W is the water-equivalent path length (WEPL) (m), and $(\mu/\rho)_w$ is the mass attenuation coefficient of the water ($m^2 \cdot kg^{-1}$). $1/\|\mathbf{r}\|^2$ is a correction term for beam divergence (Ahnesjö 1989). Equation (12.3) is rewritten by

$$T(\mathbf{r}) = \frac{\| \mathbf{r}_0 \|^2}{\| \mathbf{r} \|^2} \int \Phi(E, \mathbf{r}_0) \cdot E \cdot \exp\Big(- \mu_w(E) \cdot W(\mathbf{r} - \mathbf{r}_0) \Big) \cdot \left(\frac{\mu}{\rho} \right)_w (E, \mathbf{r}) dE, \quad (12.4)$$

where

$$\Phi(E, \mathbf{r}_0) = \frac{1}{\| \mathbf{r}_0 \|^2} \cdot \Phi(E, \mathbf{0}) \cdot \exp\Big(- \mu_w(E) \cdot W(\mathbf{r}_0) \Big), \quad (12.5)$$

$\mathbf{r}_0$ is the position vector of an intersection with respect to $\boldsymbol{r}$ and the body or phantom surface (Mackie et al. 1985; Boyer and Mok 1985, 1986; Mohan et al. 1986; Ahnesjö et al. 1987; Ahnesjö 1989; Battista and Sharpe 1992; Papanikolaou et al. 1993; Sharpe and Battista 1993). The WEPL at each position can be calculated by using the following equation:

$$W(\mathbf{r}) = \sum_{i=0}^{S-1} \rho_{e,re}(\mathbf{r}_i) \cdot d\mathbf{r}, \quad (12.6)$$

where $\rho_{e,re}(\mathbf{r}_i)$ is the relative electron density at the ith sampling position vector $\mathbf{r}_i$ and $d\mathbf{r}$ is the sampling interval on a ray (Seco and Evans 2006). The TERMA distributions within the irradiation field are calculated from the WEPL distributions, the energy spectrum of the fluence, and the mass attenuation coefficients of the water by using Eq. (12.6).

Figure 12.2 shows a diagram chart for calculating the TERMA distributions. The planning CT images are converted into relative electron density maps between the medium and the water using a conversion curve between Hounsfield unit (HU) and the relative electron density between the medium and the water. The electron density of a medium, $\rho_{e,med}$, can be calculated by

$$\rho_{e,med} = \frac{N_A \cdot Z_{med}}{A_{med}} \cdot \rho_{med}, \quad (12.7)$$

where N_A is the Avogadro constant (mol^{-1}), Z_{med} is the atomic number of a medium, A_{med} is the atomic weight of the medium ($kg \cdot mol^{-1}$), and ρ_{med} is the mass density of the medium ($kg \cdot m^{-3}$) (Seco and Evans 2006; Yang et al. 2008).

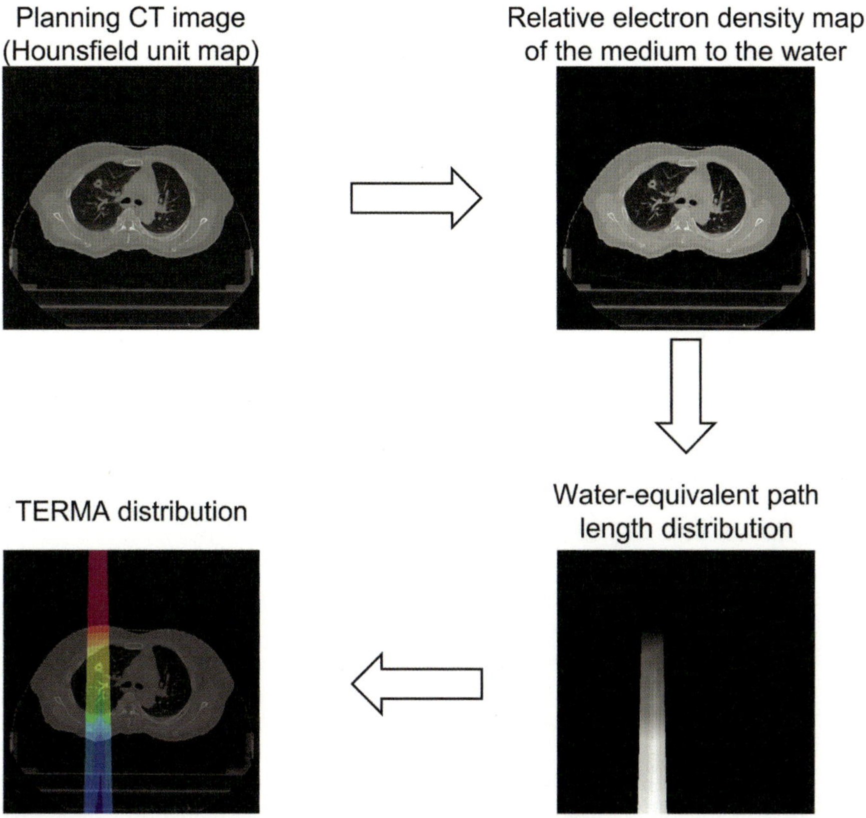

Fig. 12.2 A diagram chart for calculating total energy released per unit mass (TERMA) distributions

According to the PBC method, the relative electron density of the medium to the water is required for calculating the WEPL distributions. In particular, the relative electron density of the medium to the water, $\rho_{e,re}$, can be calculated by

$$\rho_{e,re} = \frac{\rho_{e,med}}{\rho_{e,water}}, \tag{12.8}$$

where $\rho_{e,water}$ is the electron density of the water (Seco and Evans 2006; Yang et al. 2008). Figure 12.3 shows an example of the conversion curve between HU and the relative electron density. It is worth noting that the conversion curve should be produced and calibrated using an electron density phantom in each institution because the HU depends on X-ray spectra produced by CT scanners. The WEPLs for all positions within the irradiation field are calculated based on an electron density scaling method (Seco and Evans 2006).

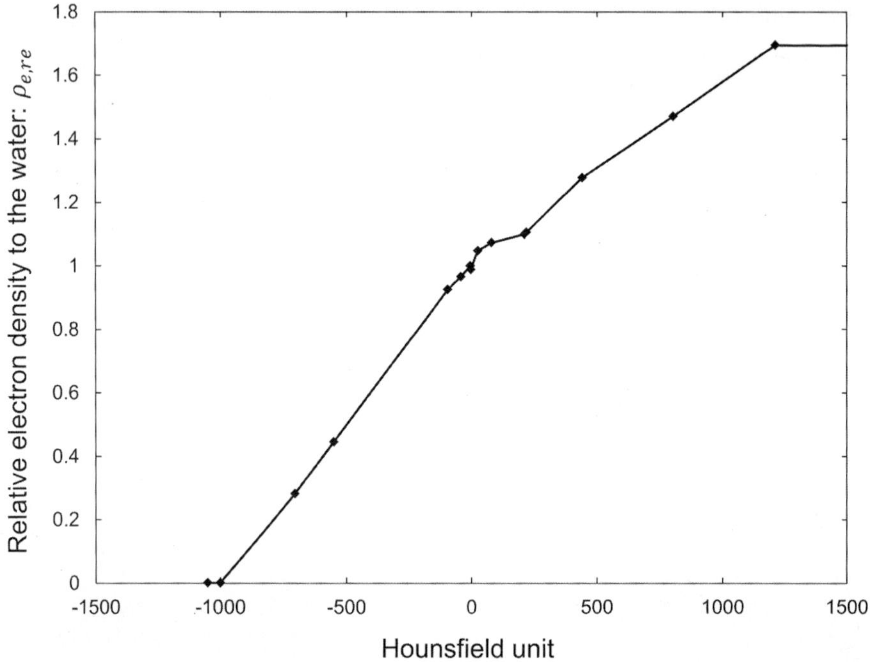

Fig. 12.3 An example of a conversion curve between Hounsfield unit (HU) and the relative electron density between the medium and the water

The X-ray spectra depend on the linacs and accelerating voltages. Since it could be very difficult to measure the high-energy X-ray spectra, the spectra should be estimated by using Monte Carlo simulations so that the estimated percent depth dose (PDD) curves can be similar to the measured PDD curves. Mohan et al. (1985) calculated the energy spectra of the fluence for each voltage in the range of 4–24 MV using Monte Carlo simulations. Sheikh-Bagheri and Rogers (2002) also modeled the energy spectra of the fluence for each voltage in the range of 4–25 MV for a variety of manufacturers (Varian, Elekta, and Siemens) using Monte Carlo simulations. Figure 12.4 shows the relative fluence spectra of the X-rays estimated by using Monte Carlo simulations for 4, 6, and 10 MV in a linac manufactured by Varian derived from the original data of Sheikh-Bagheri and Rogers (2002).

According to the PBC method, the DDK is required in order to calculate the energy deposited by scattered photons. The DDK describes the spatial distribution of total released energy from the interaction point in the water (Mackie et al. 1985, 1988; Boyer and Mok 1985; Mohan et al. 1986; Ahnesjö et al. 1987; Ahnesjö 1989; Battista and Sharpe 1992; Sharpe and Battista 1993). Ahnesjö (1989) modeled the DDK using Monte Carlo simulations based on the following equation:

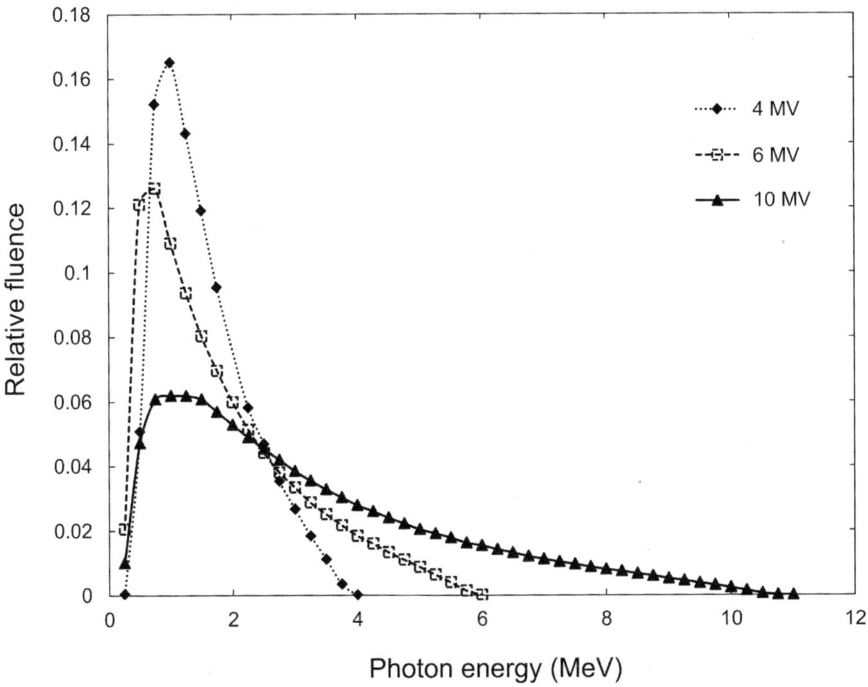

Fig. 12.4 Relative fluence spectra of X-rays estimated by using Monte Carlo simulations for 4, 6, and 10 MV in a linac manufactured by Varian derived from the original data of Sheikh-Bagheri and Rogers (2002)

$$K(\mathbf{r}-\boldsymbol{\tau}) = \frac{A_\theta e^{-a_\theta l} + B_\theta e^{-b_\theta l}}{l^2}, \tag{12.9}$$

where the following equation holds:

$$l = \|\mathbf{r}-\boldsymbol{\tau}\|, \tag{12.10}$$

where $\boldsymbol{\tau}$ is the position vector of the interaction point, θ is the scattering angle between $\boldsymbol{\tau}$ and $\mathbf{r}-\boldsymbol{\tau}$ (Fig. 12.5), A_θ and a_θ are parameters of the energy deposited by primary photons, and B_θ and b_θ are parameters of the energy deposited by scattered photons (Ahnesjö 1989).

These parameters for 4–24 MV were provided in Ahnesjö's (1989) paper. We produced the DDKs as image data based on Ahnesjö's (1989) paper. Figure 12.6 shows DDKs for 4, 6, and 10 MV based on Ahnesjö's (1989) model. The lateral scattering decreases as the voltages of the linac increase. In addition, the forward scattering increases, and the shape of the DDKs becomes narrow for high voltages.

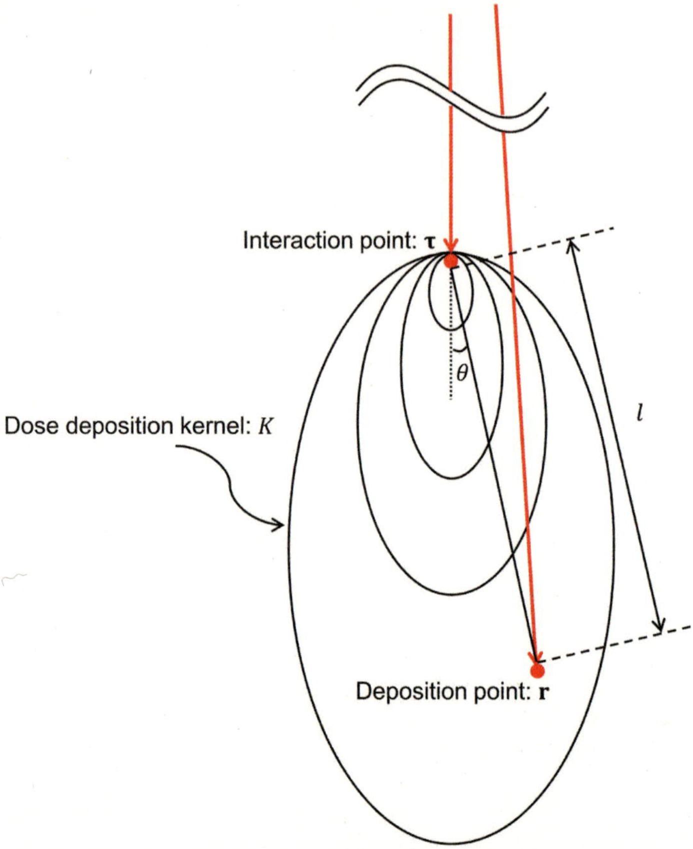

Fig. 12.5 The geometry used for calculating the dose deposition kernel (DDK)

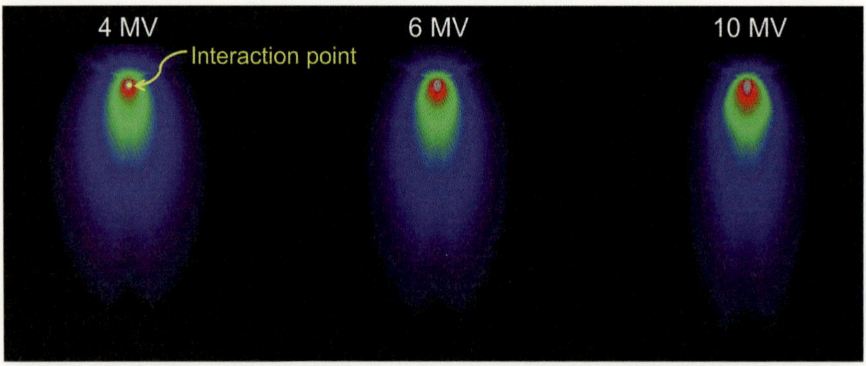

Fig. 12.6 Dose deposition kernels (DDKs) for 4, 6, and 10 MV based on an Ahnesjö's model

12.2.2 Convolution/Superposition Method

According to the PBC method, the heterogeneity of tissues in the directions of primary photons can be calculated using the WEPLs for all points based on the electron density scaling method. However, the heterogeneity of tissues in the other directions can be ignored because of the fact that the homogeneity DDKs in the water, as expressed by Eqs. (12.9) and (12.10), are convolved in Eq. (12.1). Therefore, according to the convolution/superposition method, the DDK is modeled by considering the heterogeneity based on the electron density scaling method (Sharpe and Battista 1993; McNutt et al. 1996a, b; Liu et al. 1997). Figure 12.7 shows an illustration of the dose calculation differences between the PBC and convolution/superposition methods. The basic concept used in calculating the dose distributions for the convolution/superposition method is equal to that of the PBC method, except the modeling of the DDK. More specifically, the DDK used in the convolution/superposition method can be expressed by

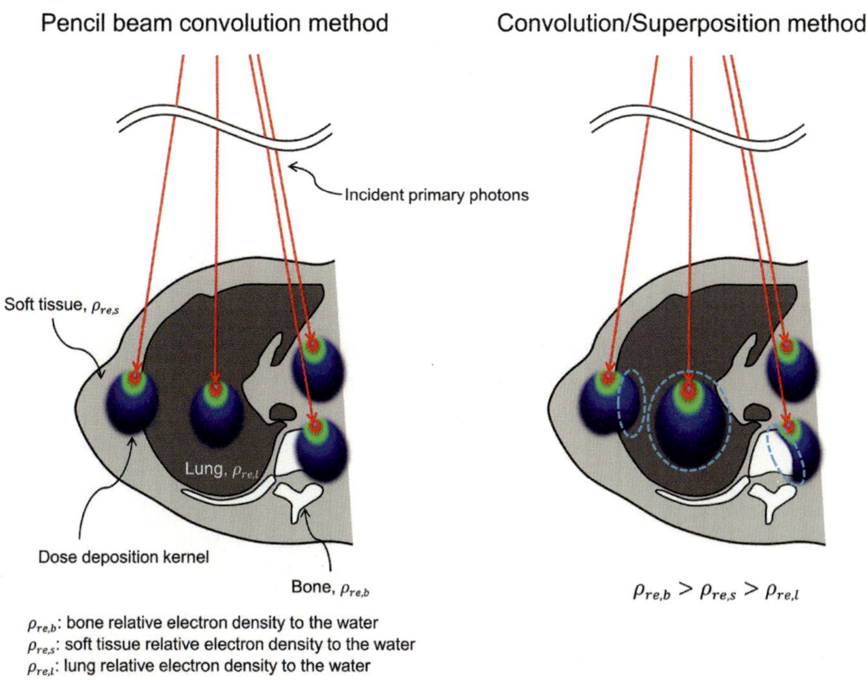

Fig. 12.7 An illustration of the dose calculation differences between the pencil beam convolution (PBC) method and the convolution/superposition method

$$K'(\mathbf{r}-\boldsymbol{\tau}) = \frac{A_\theta e^{-a_\theta l_w} + B_\theta e^{-b_\theta l_w}}{l_w^2}, \tag{12.11}$$

where

$$l_w = W(\mathbf{r}-\boldsymbol{\tau}). \tag{12.12}$$

In order to model the DDK in the convolution/superposition method, the WEPL between the interaction point and the deposition point is required (instead of the physical distance); that is because the heterogeneity (i.e., variation in the relative electron density) must be considered. Although the dose distributions calculated by considering the heterogeneity in all directions are more accurate (as compared to the PBC method), it should be noted that the dose calculation is time-consuming because of the fact that the DDK must be modeled for each point.

12.3 Estimation of Delivered Dose Distributions Based on Electronic Portal Imaging Device Images

Electronic portal imaging device (EPID) images are taken before the actual dose delivery in order to verify whether the patients are appropriately positioned on a treatment couch in the radiation therapy based on the treatment plan. More specifically, these images are compared with digitally reconstructed radiograph (DRR) images that are derived from planning CT images. Since the EPID detector can also acquire dynamic portal images acquired using therapeutic beams during treatment delivery, tumor motions can be monitored on the EPID during the treatment delivery.

Certain studies have estimated 2D dose distributions on the EPID detector plane based on the portal images (Heijmen et al. 1995; Pasma et al. 1998; de Boer et al. 2000; Greer and Popescu 2003; Chen et al. 2006; Mizoguchi et al. 2013). Chen et al. (2006) proposed two main clinical applications for estimating the 2D dose distributions on the EPID detector planes, which were verification of the delivered energy fluence in IMRT, and monitoring the exit-beam dose distribution from the patient during the treatment time. In this section, an effective method for estimating the delivered 2D dose distributions using the EPID images based on previous studies (and in particular the approach of Chen et al. (2006)) is introduced.

The basic approach of the method is to convert the EPID images into images that represent the 2D dose distributions in a water-equivalent phantom at the same level of the EPID detector planes (hereafter referred to as the portal dose images (PDIs)). Figure 12.8 shows a conceptual diagram for calculating PDIs based on the method of Chen et al. The EPID images include signals of laterally scattered photons in the EPID. Therefore, an EPID signal can be formulated by

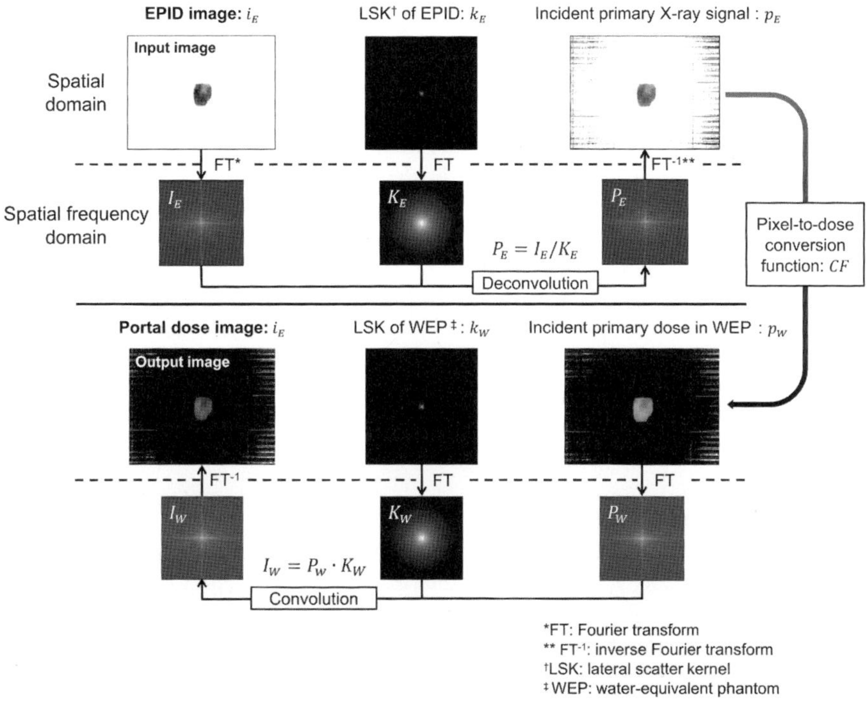

Fig. 12.8 A conceptual diagram for calculating portal dose images (PDIs) based on the method of Chen et al. (2006)

$$i_E(\mathbf{r}) = \iint p_E(\mathbf{r}') \cdot k_E(\mathbf{r} - \mathbf{r}')d\mathbf{r}' = p_E(\mathbf{r}) * k_E(\mathbf{r}), \tag{12.13}$$

where i_E is the EPID signal, p_E is the incident primary X-ray signal, k_E is the lateral scatter kernel (LSK) of the EPID, $\mathbf{r}$ is the position vector in the spatial domain, and $\mathbf{r}'$ is a shift vector in the spatial domain. The incident primary X-ray signals are extracted by deconvolving the EPID signals from the LSK of the EPID. The deconvolution can be performed in the spatial frequency domain, as follows:

$$P_E(\mathbf{u}) = \frac{I_E(\mathbf{u})}{K_E(\mathbf{u})}, \tag{12.14}$$

where I_E, P_E, and K_E are the Fourier transforms of i_E, p_E, and k_E, respectively, and $\mathbf{u}$ is the position vector in the spatial frequency domain. The incident primary X-ray signals are converted to incident primary doses in the water using a pixel-to-dose conversion function, as expressed by the following equation:

$$p_W(\mathbf{r}) = CF(p_E(\mathbf{r})), \tag{12.15}$$

where p_W is the incident primary dose in the water-equivalent phantom and CF is the conversion function. After converting the incident primary X-ray signal to the incident primary dose in the water-equivalent phantom, the PDI is calculated by convolving the incident primary dose in the water-equivalent phantom with the LSK of the water by using the following equation:

$$i_W(\mathbf{r}) = \iint p_W(\mathbf{r}') \cdot k_W(\mathbf{r} - \mathbf{r}')d\mathbf{r}' = p_W(\mathbf{r}) * k_W(\mathbf{r}), \tag{12.16}$$

where i_W is the PDI and k_W is the LSK of the water-equivalent phantom. Consequently, the following equation holds:

$$I_W(\mathbf{u}) = P_W(\mathbf{u}) \cdot k_W(\mathbf{u}), \tag{12.17}$$

where I_W, P_W, and K_W are the Fourier transforms of i_E, p_E, and k_E, respectively.

The LSK is a model that represents the spread of the laterally scattered X-rays caused by interaction with incident primary X-rays (Heijmen et al. 1995, Steciw et al. 2005, Chen et al. 2006, van Elmpt et al. 2006, Mizoguchi et al. 2013). The LSK is a point spread function (PSF) for describing the blurring effect caused by the scattered X-rays. The LSKs of the EPID and water-equivalent phantom were experimentally determined in the approach of Chen et al. (2006). The LSKs were obtained using Monte Carlo simulations (Mizoguchi et al. 2013). The LSKs of the EPID and water-equivalent phantom obtained by Monte Carlo simulations at 6 and 10 MV are shown in Fig. 12.9.

The pixel-to-dose conversion function was measured experimentally (Chen et al. 2006). We also measured the pixel-to-dose conversion function at 6 MV based on the method of Chen et al. (2006) (Mizoguchi et al. 2013). Figure 12.10 shows an experimental geometry for measuring the pixel-to-dose conversion function at our institution.

The field size was 5×5 cm^2 at an isocenter plane, and an ion chamber was located in the water-equivalent phantom at the same level of the EPID detector plane. The EPID signal and dose were measured at the level of the detector plane with off-axis distances at the detector plane of 0, 7.2, and 14.4 cm while changing the thickness of the water-equivalent phantom on the treatment couch. Then, the pixel-to-dose conversion function was produced by approximating measured values using a first-order polynomial. Figure 12.11 shows the pixel-to-dose conversion function at 6 MV at our institution.

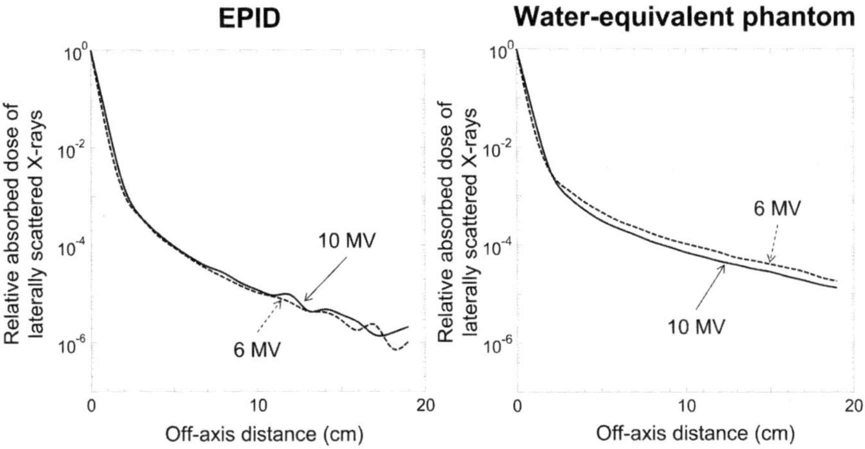

Fig. 12.9 Lateral scatter kernels (LSKs) of an electronic portal imaging device (EPID) and water-equivalent phantom obtained by Monte Carlo simulations at 6 and 10 MV

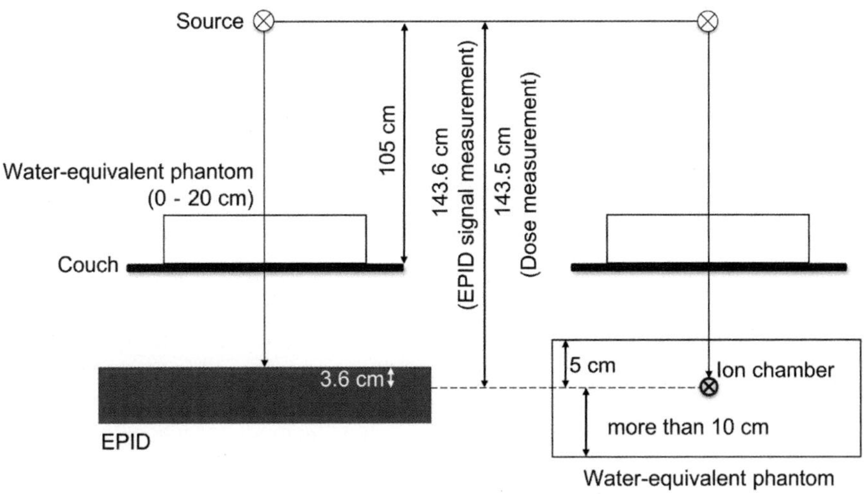

Fig. 12.10 Experimental geometry for measuring the pixel-to-dose conversion function at our institution

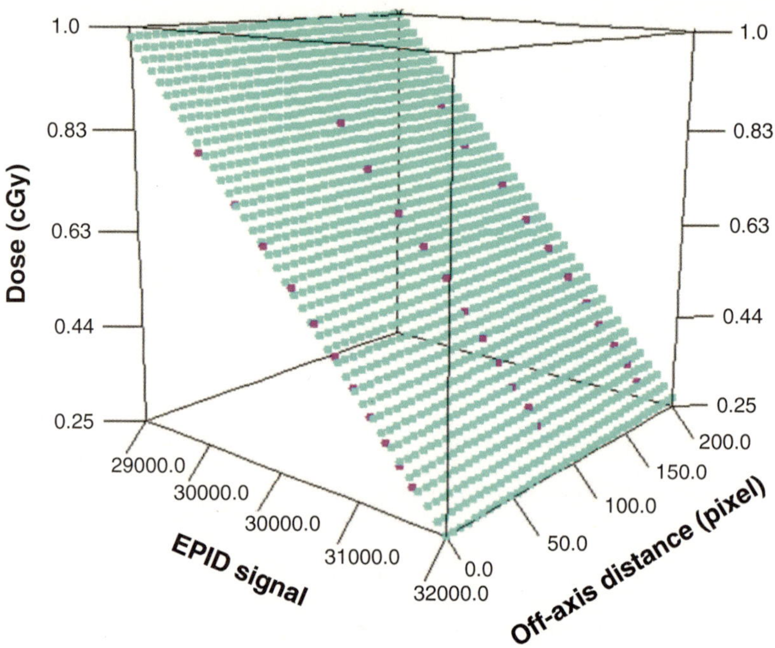

Fig. 12.11 Pixel-to-dose conversion function at 6 MV at our institution. *Pink dots* indicate experimentally measured points with off-axis distances of 0, 7.2, and 14.4 cm. *Blue dots* indicate approximated points using a first-order polynomial

12.4 Prediction of the Delivered Three-Dimensional Dose Distributions Using the Portal Dose Images

The delivered 3D dose distributions within patients' bodies should be verified during treatment time. That is because there exist discrepancies between the designed and delivered dose distributions due to uncertainties associated with several factors (machine, delineation, organ motion, patient setup errors, etc.) (McNutt et al. 1996a, b, 1997). Therefore, various methods for reconstructing the delivered 3D dose distributions within phantoms and patients' bodies based on PDIs have been proposed (McNutt et al. 1996a, b, 1997, Hansen et al. 1996; Partridge et al. 2002; Louwe et al. 2003; Renner et al. 2003, Steciw et al. 2005; Wendling et al. 2006; van Elmpt et al. 2006). The basic idea in predicting delivered 3D dose distributions during treatment is that the primary energy fluences in patients' bodies should be determined iteratively in such a way that 2D dose distributions calculated on the imaging detector planes (i.e., computed PDIs) are rendered equal to the 2D dose distributions on the EPID detector planes during treatment (i.e., measured PDIs) estimated using the method described in Sect. 12.3. The 3D dose distributions delivered during treatment time are calculated using the determined primary energy fluences. McNutt et al. (1996a, b , 1997) proposed an approach for predicting the 3D dose distribution delivered during treatment time, which was called "back projection." In this section, the back-projected procedure for predicting the 3D dose distributions during treatment delivery is reviewed based on McNutt et al. (1996b).

Algorithm 12.1 A pseudo-code of a back-projected iterative algorithm for predicting the 3D dose distributions during treatment delivery proposed by McNutt et al. (1996b)

//Comments
/*D_m: measured PDI, D_c: computed PDI, D: dose distribution, Ψ: primary energy fluence
K: dose deposition kernel, I_{CT}: CT volume, T: TERMA
n: iteration number, ε: small number
$\mathbf{r}$: position vector in image detector plane coordinate
$\mathbf{u}$: position vector in dose calculation coordinate*/
Input D_m, K, I_{CT};
Output D, Ψ;
Initialization $n \leftarrow 0, \Psi^n(\mathbf{r}) \leftarrow D_m(\mathbf{r})$;
while do
    $\Psi^n(\mathbf{u}) \leftarrow$ Back projection$(\Psi^n(\mathbf{r}))$;
    $T^n(\mathbf{u}) \leftarrow$ TERMA$(I_{CT}(\mathbf{u}), \Psi^n(\mathbf{u}))$;
    $D^n(\mathbf{u}) \leftarrow T^n(\mathbf{u}) * K(\mathbf{u})$;
    $D_c^n(\mathbf{r}) \leftarrow$ Extraction of the dose distribution at image detector plane$(D^n(\mathbf{u}))$;
    if $\sum_i |D_m(\mathbf{r}_i) - D_c^n(\mathbf{r}_i)| \leq \varepsilon$ **then**
        $D(\mathbf{u}) \leftarrow D^n(\mathbf{u})$;
        $\Psi(\mathbf{u}) \leftarrow \Psi^n(\mathbf{u})$;
        break
    else
        $\Psi^{n+1}(\mathbf{r}) \leftarrow (D_m(\mathbf{r})/D_c^n(\mathbf{r})) \cdot \Psi^n(\mathbf{r})$;
        $n \leftarrow n + 1$;
    end if
end while

Algorithm 12.1 shows a pseudo-code of the back-projected iterative algorithm for predicting the 3D dose distributions during treatment delivery proposed by McNutt et al. (1996b). The primary goal for predicting the 3D dose distributions delivered during treatment time is to determine the primary energy fluences in 3D dose calculation volumes by back-projecting the primary energy fluences at the detector planes to the calculation volumes, which renders the computed PDIs equal to the measured PDIs. An initial primary energy fluence at the detector plane should be determined in order to perform the iterative procedure, and the initial primary energy fluence is equal to the measured PDI. At this stage, the primary energy fluence at the detector plane is back-projected through the dose calculation volume by considering the radiological distance (e.g., the WEPL, as described in Sect. 12.2) between a point at the detector plane and one in the dose calculation volume. The computed PDI is produced by extracting the calculated dose distribution on the detector plane derived from the primary energy fluence. If the computed PDI is converged to the measured PDI, the back-projected primary energy fluence is then used for calculating the 3D dose distribution in the volume, and the calculated 3D dose distribution is regarded as the delivered 3D dose distribution during treatment delivery. Otherwise, the primary energy fluence at the detector plane is updated by

$$\Psi^{n+1}(\mathbf{r}) = \frac{D_m(\boldsymbol{r})}{D_c^n(\boldsymbol{r})} \cdot \Psi^n(\mathbf{r}) \tag{12.18}$$

where $\mathbf{r}$ is the position vector in the detector plane, Ψ is the primary energy fluence, D_m is the measured PDI, D_c is the computed PDI, and n is the iteration number. After updating the primary energy fluence, the procedure returns to the back-projection step.

12.5 Estimation of Four-Dimensional Dose Distributions During Treatment Delivery

12.5.1 Background

Discrepancies between the treatment plan and the actual delivery should ideally be removed in order to administer exact dose distributions. However, discrepancies can occur as a result of the patients' setup (positioning) errors and internal errors caused by the patients' physiological motions during treatment delivery. If the dose distributions are delivered without considering these discrepancies, this can lead to a low tumor control probability and a high normal tissue complication probability. Therefore, the discrepancies should be monitored during treatment delivery in order to check whether or not they fall certain within tolerances. In clinical situations (especially stereotactic body radiation therapy (SBRT) for lung cancer), the patients' motions within irradiation fields are monitored by acquiring the EPID dynamic images in order to verify location errors during treatment delivery. By contrast, the errors between the designed and delivered doses are not investigated because the tolerances of the location errors are considered those of the dose errors in the clinical situations. However, there might be no correspondence between the location and dose errors. In such cases, there would be uncertainties in the dose distributions during treatment delivery. Consequently, it is essential to estimate the 4D dose distributions during treatment delivery in order to ensure the quality of the radiation therapy.

In response to these considerations, the authors have developed an automated framework for estimating the 4D dose distributions during treatment delivery based on the EPID dynamic images (Nakamoto et al. 2015). In this section, we introduce the basic framework for estimating the 4D dose distributions during treatment delivery.

12.5.2 *Overall Scheme of the Framework*

Figure 12.12 shows a schematic illustration of the procedure for estimating the 4D dose distributions during treatment delivery based on the EPID dynamic images. The 4D dose distributions during treatment delivery were estimated by applying the PBC method to simulated 4D-CT images during treatment delivery (hereafter referred to as "treatment" 4D-CT images). The "treatment" 4D-CT images were simulated by transforming the planning CT images using a nonrigid registration technique so that the planning PDIs (described as computed PDIs in Sect. 12.4) could be similar to the dynamic clinical PDIs (described as measured PDIs in Sect. 12.4) for all frames. The parameters of the nonrigid registration for transforming the planning CT images were optimized in each frame. The planning PDIs were calculated by applying the PBC method to the planning CT images and a virtual water phantom (described in Sect. 12.4). The dynamic clinical PDIs were also estimated from the EPID dynamic images by applying the method to all frames (described in Sect. 12.3).

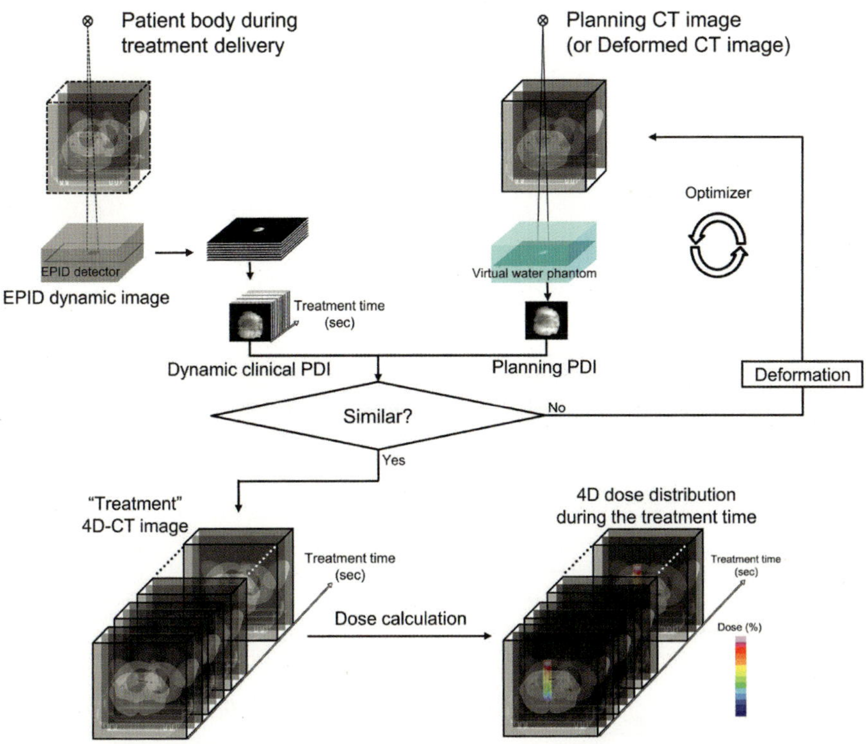

Fig. 12.12 A schematic illustration of the procedure for estimating four-dimensional (4D) dose distributions during treatment delivery based on electronic portal imaging device (EPID) dynamic images

12.5.3 Calculation of the "Treatment" 4D-CT Images

Figure 12.13 shows a flow chart for calculating the "treatment" 4D-CT images at each frame. The basic idea is that the planning CT images should be transformed so that the planning PDIs are rendered similar to the dynamic clinical PDIs for all frames of the EPID dynamic images. In this manner, the "treatment" 4D-CT images are constructed from the aggregate data of the transformed planning CT images for all frames.

The planning CT images were transformed by using an affine transformation (Burger and Burge 2009). The parameters of the affine transformation matrix (transformation parameters) were described as a nine-dimensional vector, which represented a rotation, translation, and scaling in a CT coordinate system, as expressed by the following vector:

$$\mathbf{s} = [\theta_x, \theta_y, \theta_z, \tau_x, \tau_y, \tau_z, \mu_x, \mu_y, \mu_z]^{\mathrm{T}}, \tag{12.19}$$

where θ, τ, and μ are the rotation, translation, and scaling parameters, respectively. (x, y, z) are the CT coordinates, and T indicates transpose. The affine transformation matrix, **A**, was produced by using the following equation:

$$\mathbf{A} = \mathbf{RS} + \mathbf{T}, \tag{12.20}$$

where the following equations hold:

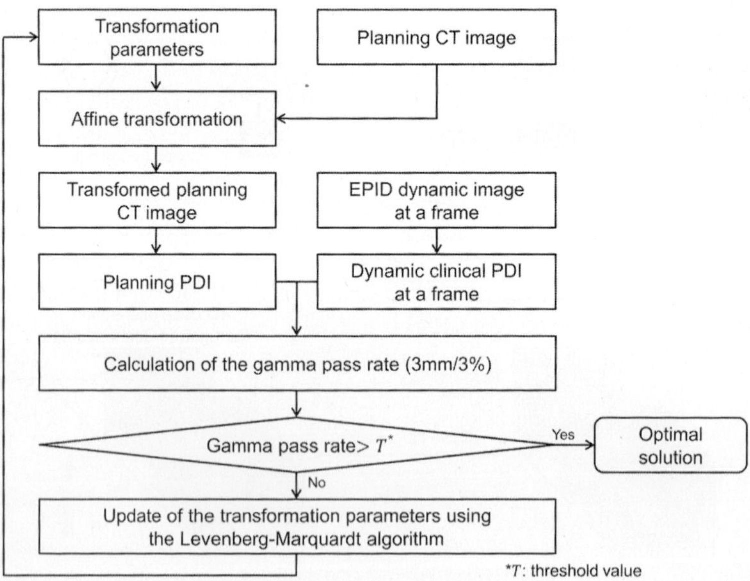

Fig. 12.13 A flow chart for calculating "treatment" 4D-CT images at each frame

$$\mathbf{R} = \begin{bmatrix} C\theta_y C\theta_z & C\theta_x S\theta_z + S\theta_x S\theta_y C\theta_z & S\theta_x S\theta_z - C\theta_x S\theta_y C\theta_z & 0 \\ -C\theta_y S\theta_z & C\theta_x C\theta_z - S\theta_x S\theta_y S\theta_z & S\theta_x C\theta_z + C\theta_x S\theta_y S\theta_z & 0 \\ S\theta_y & S\theta_x C\theta_y & C\theta_x C\theta_y & 0 \\ 0 & 0 & 0 & 1 \end{bmatrix}, \tag{12.21}$$

$$\mathbf{S} = \begin{bmatrix} \mu_x & 0 & 0 & 0 \\ 0 & \mu_y & 0 & 0 \\ 0 & 0 & \mu_z & 0 \\ 0 & 0 & 0 & 1 \end{bmatrix}, \tag{12.22}$$

and

$$\mathbf{T} = \begin{bmatrix} 0 & 0 & 0 & \tau_x \\ 0 & 0 & 0 & \tau_y \\ 0 & 0 & 0 & \tau_z \\ 0 & 0 & 0 & 0 \end{bmatrix}. \tag{12.23}$$

R, **S**, and **T** are the rotation, scaling, and translation matrices, respectively. S and C in the rotation matrix indicate sine and cosine, respectively. The planning PDI was calculated from the transformed planning CT image. After calculating the planning PDI, the similarity between the planning PDI and dynamic clinical PDI at each frame was calculated, which constituted the main criterion of the procedure. A gamma pass rate (3 mm/3 %), which will be described in Sect. 12.5.5, was adopted as a similarity index. If the gamma pass rate reached a threshold value (described in Sect. 12.5.4), then the transformation parameters were regarded as an optimal solution and the transformed planning CT image was regarded as the "treatment" 4D-CT image at each frame. Otherwise, the transformation parameters were optimized using a Levenberg-Marquardt (LM) algorithm until meeting the criterion. The "treatment" 4D-CT images can be produced by applying the procedure to all frames.

12.5.4 Optimization of the Transformation Parameters Using the Levenberg-Marquardt Algorithm

The LM algorithm is a gradient-based method for solving nonlinear least squares problems (Levenberg 1944; Marquardt 1963; Press et al. 1986; Nielsen 1999). The LM algorithm can solve such problems more efficiently and accurately than other gradient-based methods by changing the damping factor (Press et al. 1986; Nielsen 1999).

In this study, the problem is to minimize the objective function expressed by the following equation:

$$J_{\mathbf{s}} = \frac{1}{2}\sum_{i,j}\{\Phi(\mathbf{s})_{i,j} - I^{c}_{i,j}\}^{2}, \tag{12.24}$$

where (i, j) are the pixel coordinates, Φ (**s**) is the planning PDI calculated from the transformed planning CT images using **s**, and I^c is the dynamic clinical PDI at each frame; this function should be minimized while meeting the gamma pass rate criterion. The transformation parameters, *s*, were optimized by solving the above problem. Figure 12.14 shows the overall procedure for optimizing the transformation parameters using the LM algorithm. In this study, the transformation parameter vector as an initial searching point for optimization, $\mathbf{s}_{ini}$, was defined as

$$\mathbf{s}_{ini} = [0, 0, 0, 0, 0, 0, 1, 1, 1]^{\mathrm{T}}. \tag{12.25}$$

The affine transformation matrix derived from $\mathbf{s}_{ini}$ was the identity matrix. The transformation parameter vector, $\mathbf{s}'$, was updated by

$$\mathbf{s}' = \mathbf{s} + \Delta\mathbf{s}, \tag{12.26}$$

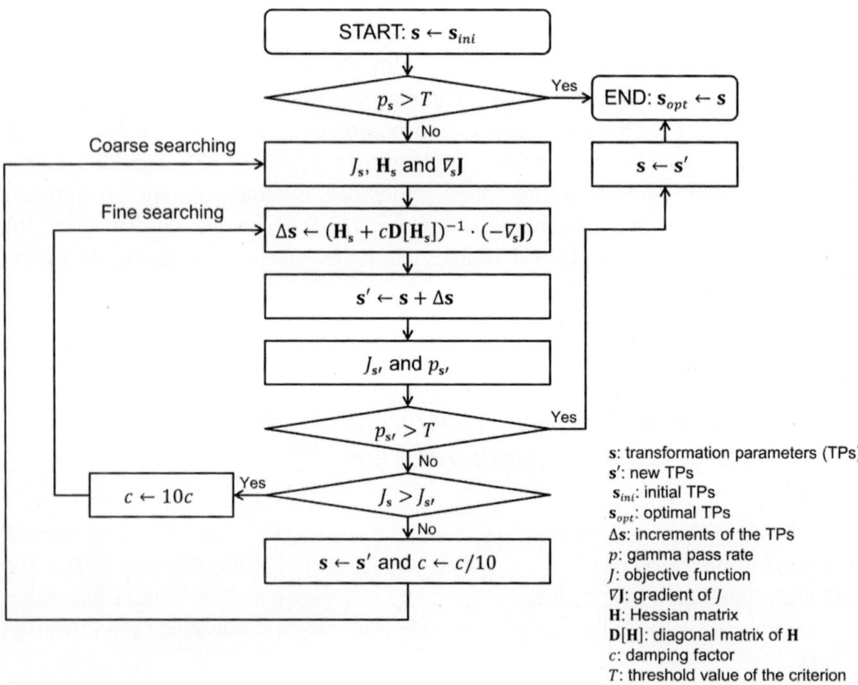

Fig. 12.14 The overall procedure for optimizing the transformation parameters using a Levenberg-Marquardt algorithm

where $\Delta\mathbf{s}$ is the increment vector of the transformation parameters, which was calculated according to the following equation:

$$\Delta\mathbf{s} = (\mathbf{H}_\mathbf{s} + c\mathbf{D}[\mathbf{H}_\mathbf{s}])^{-1} \cdot (-\nabla_\mathbf{s}\mathbf{J}), \tag{12.27}$$

where $\mathbf{H}_\mathbf{s}$ is the Hessian matrix, $\mathbf{D}[\mathbf{H}_\mathbf{s}]$ is the diagonal matrix of the Hessian matrix, $\nabla_\mathbf{s}\mathbf{J}$ is the gradient of the objective function, and c is the damping factor. Adjusting the damping factors results in altering the value of the increment $\Delta\mathbf{s}$ in each iteration. The initial damping factor was 10^{-4} in this study. $\nabla_\mathbf{s}\mathbf{J}$ and $\mathbf{H}_\mathbf{s}$ were calculated by

$$\begin{aligned} \nabla_\mathbf{s}\mathbf{J} &= \sum_{i,j} \{\Phi(\mathbf{s})_{i,j} - I^c_{i,j}\} \cdot \{\nabla_\mathbf{s}\{\Phi(\mathbf{s})_{i,j} - I^c_{i,j}\}\} \\ &= \sum_{i,j} \{\Phi(\mathbf{s})_{i,j} - I^c_{i,j}\} \cdot \{\nabla_\mathbf{s}\Phi(\mathbf{s})_{i,j}\}, \end{aligned} \tag{12.28}$$

and

$$\begin{aligned} \mathbf{H}_\mathbf{s} &= \sum_{i,j} \begin{pmatrix} \frac{\partial^2 \Phi(\mathbf{s})_{i,j}}{\partial \theta_x^2} & \cdots & \frac{\partial^2 \Phi(\mathbf{s})_{i,j}}{\partial \theta_x \partial \mu_z} \\ \vdots & \ddots & \vdots \\ \frac{\partial^2 \Phi(\mathbf{s})_{i,j}}{\partial \mu_z \partial \theta_x} & \cdots & \frac{\partial^2 \Phi(\mathbf{s})_{i,j}}{\partial \mu_z^2} \end{pmatrix} \\ &\approx \sum_{i,j} \{\nabla_\mathbf{s}\Phi(\mathbf{s})_{i,j}\} \cdot \{\nabla_\mathbf{s}\Phi(\mathbf{s})_{i,j}\}^\mathrm{T}, \end{aligned} \tag{12.29}$$

respectively, where $\nabla_\mathbf{s}\Phi(\mathbf{s})$ is the gradient vector of the planning PDI:

$$\nabla_\mathbf{s}\Phi(\mathbf{s}) = \left[\frac{\partial\Phi(\mathbf{s})}{\partial\theta_x}, \frac{\partial\Phi(\mathbf{s})}{\partial\theta_y}, \frac{\partial\Phi(\mathbf{s})}{\partial\theta_z}, \frac{\partial\Phi(\mathbf{s})}{\partial\tau_x}, \frac{\partial\Phi(\mathbf{s})}{\partial\tau_y}, \frac{\partial\Phi(\mathbf{s})}{\partial\tau_z}, \frac{\partial\Phi(\mathbf{s})}{\partial\mu_x}, \frac{\partial\Phi(\mathbf{s})}{\partial\mu_y}, \frac{\partial\Phi(\mathbf{s})}{\partial\mu_z}\right]^\mathrm{T}. \tag{12.30}$$

All elements of the gradient vector were the partial derivatives of the planning PDI with respect to each of the parameters; and these were approximated by a finite-difference method (Xu and Wan 2008). After calculating the new transformation parameters, a gamma pass rate, $p_{\mathbf{s}'}$, was calculated in order to investigate whether or not $p_{\mathbf{s}'}$ met the criterion; the threshold value of the gamma pass rate was 98 % in the study. If the gamma pass rate did not exceed 98 %, the transformation parameters were updated by comparing $J_\mathbf{s}$ with $J_{\mathbf{s}'}$. If $J_{\mathbf{s}'}$ was smaller than $J_\mathbf{s}$, then $\mathbf{s}$ and c were updated to $\mathbf{s}'$ and $c/10$, respectively, and the procedure returned to the step of calculating $\nabla_\mathbf{s}\mathbf{J}$ and $\mathbf{H}_\mathbf{s}$. This schema was referred to as "coarse searching".

Otherwise, c was updated to $10c$ and the procedure returned to the step of calculating $\Delta\mathbf{s}$. This schema was referred to as "fine searching". Although the procedure was iterated until meeting the criterion, if the gamma pass rate did not wholly exceed 98 %, the procedure was forced to stop based on the number of iterations. In such cases, the transformation parameters with the maximum gamma pass rate in the iterations were regarded as the optimal transformation parameter vector, $\mathbf{s}_{opt}$.

12.5.5 Gamma Analysis

Gamma analysis is a method for evaluating the similarity between two dose distributions (Low et al. 1998; Low and Dempsey 2003). Gamma analysis is a combination of the dose difference (DD) and distance-to-agreement (DTA) methods, and it is widely used for verifying dose distributions in IMRT. Figure 12.15 shows a conceptual illustration of verifying the similarity of two dose distributions using gamma analysis. The ellipsoid which states the acceptable criteria of the DD and DTA is determined for all reference points on a reference dose distribution. The boundary of the ellipsoid can be described by the following equation:

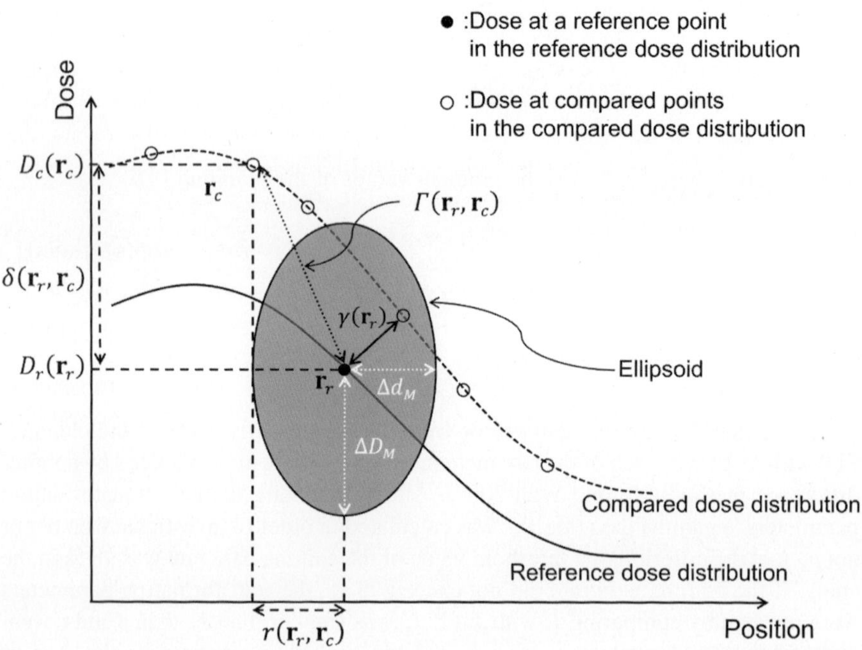

Fig. 12.15 A conceptual illustration for verifying the similarity of two dose distributions using gamma analysis

$$\sqrt{\frac{r^2(\mathbf{r}_r,\mathbf{r})}{\Delta d_M^2}+\frac{\delta^2(\mathbf{r}_r,\mathbf{r})}{\Delta D_M^2}}=1, \tag{12.31}$$

where

$$r(\mathbf{r}_r,\mathbf{r})=\|\mathbf{r}-\mathbf{r}_r\|, \tag{12.32}$$

is the spatial distance between the reference point on the reference dose distribution, $\mathbf{r}_r$, and the arbitrary point on the dose distribution, $\mathbf{r}$. Furthermore, the dose difference between $\mathbf{r}_r$ and $\mathbf{r}$ is expressed by

$$\delta(\mathbf{r}_r,\mathbf{r})=D(\mathbf{r})-D_r(\mathbf{r}_r). \tag{12.33}$$

Δd_M and ΔD_M are the criteria of the DTA and DD, respectively. The 3 mm/3 % quantity that appears in Sect. 12.5.3 indicates that Δd_M and ΔD_M are 3 mm and 3 %, respectively. After setting the ellipsoid in the reference point, the Γ $(\mathbf{r}_r,\mathbf{r}_c)$ values are calculated at each compared point using the following equation:

$$\Gamma(\mathbf{r}_r,\mathbf{r}_c)=\sqrt{\frac{r^2(\mathbf{r}_r,\mathbf{r}_c)}{\Delta d_M^2}+\frac{\delta^2(\mathbf{r}_r,\mathbf{r}_c)}{\Delta D_M^2}}, \tag{12.34}$$

where $\mathbf{r}_c$ is the compared point on the compared dose distribution. The gamma value at the reference point, $\gamma(\mathbf{r}_r)$, is defined by the following equation:

$$\gamma(\mathbf{r}_r)=\min\{\Gamma(\mathbf{r}_r,\mathbf{r}_c)\}\forall\{\mathbf{r}_c\}. \tag{12.35}$$

Therefore, the gamma value at the reference point is a minimum $\Gamma(\mathbf{r}_r,\mathbf{r}_c)$ for all compared points. The conditions of agreement and disagreement of the dose similarity at the reference point are shown below:

$$\gamma(\mathbf{r}_r)\leq 1;\text{agreement},\quad \gamma(\mathbf{r}_r)>1;\text{disagreement}, \tag{12.36}$$

based on the ellipsoid expressed in Eq. (12.31). Consequently, the agreement (disagreement) of the dose at the reference point indicates that a compared point on the compared dose distribution that minimizes $\Gamma(\mathbf{r}_r,\mathbf{r}_c)$ exists in the boundary and interior (exterior) region of the ellipsoid. The gamma pass rate is calculated by investigating the agreement for all reference points, and that is defined as follows:

$$\text{Gamma passrate}(\%)=\frac{\text{Number of agreement points}}{\text{Number of all reference points}}\cdot 100. \tag{12.37}$$

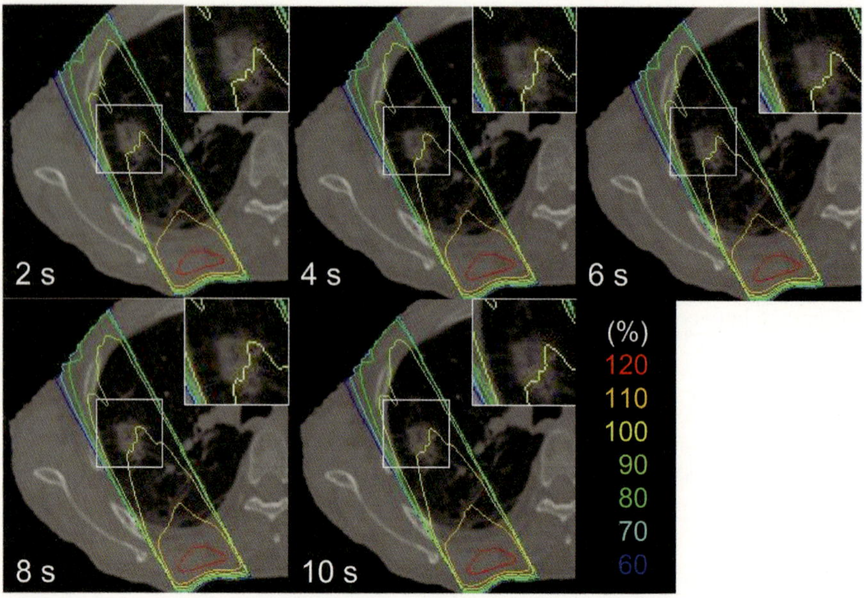

Fig. 12.16 Four-dimensional dose distribution on an isocenter plane of the transversal section at treatment times of 2, 4, 6, 8, and 10 s during stereotactic body radiation therapy (SBRT) at a gantry angle of 150°

12.5.6 Estimation of the Four-Dimensional Dose Distributions During Treatment Delivery

The 4D dose distributions during treatment delivery were estimated by applying the convolution method to the "treatment" 4D-CT images for all frames. Figure 12.16 shows the 4D dose distribution on an isocenter plane of the transversal section at treatment times of 2, 4, 6, 8, and 10 s during SBRT at a gantry angle of 150°.

Acknowledgements This work was supported by a Grant-in-Aid for Japan Society for the Promotion of Science (JSPS) Fellows and KAKENHI (Grants-in-Aid for Scientific Research) Grant Number 15J03603.

References

Ahnesjö A (1989) Collapsed cone convolution of radiant energy for photon dose calculation in heterogeneous media. Med Phys 16(4):577–592

Ahnesjö A, Andreo P, Brahme A (1987) Calculation and application of point spread functions for treatment planning with high energy photon beams. Acta Oncol 26(1):49–56

Battista JJ, Sharpe MB (1992) True three-dimensional dose computations for megavoltage x-ray therapy: a role for the superposition principle. Australas Phys Eng Sci Med 15(4):159–178

Boyer AL, Mok EC (1985) A photon dose distribution model employing convolution calculations. Med Phys 12(2):169–177

Boyer AL, Mok EC (1986) Calculation of photon dose distributions in an inhomogeneous medium using convolutions. Med Phys 13(4):503–509

Burger W, Burge MJ (2009) Principles of digital image processing. Springer, Heidelberg

Chen J, Chuang CF, Morin O, Aubin M, Pouliot J (2006) Calibration of an amorphous-silicon flat panel portal imager for exit-beam dosimetry. Med Phys 33(3):584–594

Chetty IJ, Curran B, Cygler JE, DeMarco JJ, Ezzell G, Faddegon BA, Kawrakow I, Keall PJ, Liu H, Ma CM, Rogers DW, Seuntjens J, Sheikh-Bagheri D, Siebers JV (2007) Report of the AAPM Task Group No. 105: issues associated with clinical implementation of Monte Carlo-based photon and electron external beam treatment planning. Med Phys 34(12):4818–4853

de Boer JC, Heijmen BJ, Pasma KL, Visser AG (2000) Characterization of a high-elbow, fluoroscopic electronic portal imaging device for portal dosimetry. Phys Med Biol 45 (1):197–216

Dias J, Rocha H, Ventura T, Ferreira B, Lopes Mdo C (2016) Automated fluences map optimization based on fuzzy inference systems. Med Phys 43(3):1083–1095

Gao H (2016) Robust fluence map optimization via alternating direction method of multipliers with empirical parameter optimization. Phys Med Biol 61(7):2838–2850

Greer PB, Popescu CC (2003) Dosimetric properties of an amorphous silicon electronic portal imaging device for verification of dynamic intensity modulated radiation therapy. Med Phys 30 (7):1618–1627

Hansen VN, Evans PM, Swindell W (1996) The application of transit dosimetry to precision radiotherapy. Med Phys 23(5):713–721

Heijmen BJ, Pasma KL, Kroonwijk M, Althof VG, de Boer JC, Visser AG, Huizenga H (1995) Portal dose measurement in radiotherapy using an electronic portal imaging device (EPID). Phys Med Biol 40(11):1943–1955

Kan MW, Yu PK, LH L (2013) A review on the use of grid-based Boltzmann equation solvers for dose calculation in external photon beam treatment planning. Biomed Res Int 2013 (2013):692874. doi:10.1155/2013/692874

Lan Y, Li C, Ren H, Zhang Y, Min Z (2012) Fluence map optimization (FMO) with dose-volume constraints in IMRT using the geometric distance sorting method. Phys Med Biol 57 (20):6407–6426

Levenberg K (1944) A method for the solution of certain non-linear problems in least squares. Q Appl Math 2(2):164–168

Liu HH, Mackie TR, McCullough EC (1997) Correcting kernel tilting and hardening in convolution/superposition dose calculations for clinical divergent and polychromatic photon beams. Med Phys 24(11):1729–1741

Louwe RJ, Damen EM, van Herk M, Minken AW, Törzsök O, Mijnheer BJ (2003) Three-dimensional dose reconstruction of breast cancer treatment using portal imaging. Med Phys 30(9):2376–2389

Low DA, Dempsey JF (2003) Evaluation of the gamma dose distribution comparison method. Med Phys 30(9):2455–2464

Low DA, Harms WB, Mutic S, Purdy JA (1998) A technique for the quantitative evaluation of dose distributions. Med Phys 25(5):656–661

Mackie TR, Scrimger JW, Battista JJ (1985) A convolution method of calculating dose for 15-MV x rays. Med Phys 12(2):188–196

Mackie TR, Bielajew AF, Rogers DW, Battista JJ (1988) Generation of photon energy deposition kernels using the EGS Monte Carlo code. Phys Med Biol 33(1):1–20

Marquardt DW (1963) An algorithm for least-squares estimation of nonlinear parameters. J Soc Ind Appl Math 11(2):431–441

McNutt TR, Mackie TR, Reckwerdt P, Papanikolaou N, Paliwal BR (1996a) Calculation of portal dose using the convolution/superposition method. Med Phys 23(4):527–535

McNutt TR, Mackie TR, Reckwerdt P, Paliwal BR (1996b) Modeling dose distributions from portal dose images using the convolution/superposition method. Med Phys 23(8):1381–1392

McNutt TR, Mackie TR, Paliwal BR (1997) Analysis and convergence of the iterative convolution/superposition dose reconstruction technique for multiple treatment beams and tomotherapy. Med Phys 24(9):1465–1476

Mizoguchi A, Arimura H, Shioyama Y, Nakamoto T, Yoshidome S, Hirose TA, Anai S, Honda H, Umezu Y, Hirata H, Ohki M, Nakamura K, Toyofuku F (2013) Estimation of four-dimensional dose distribution using electronic portal imaging device in radiation therapy. IEICE Trans D J96-D(4):813–823 (Japanese edition)

Mohan R, Chui C, Lidofsky L (1985) Energy and angular distributions of pho-tons from medical linear accelerators. Med Phys 12(5):592–597

Mohan R, Chui C, Lidofsky L (1986) Differential pencil beam dose computation model for photons. Med Phys 13(1):64–73

Nakamoto T, Arimura H, Nakamura K, Shioyama Y, Mizoguchi A, Hirose TA, Honda H, Umezu Y, Nakamura Y, Hirata H (2015) A computerized framework for monitoring four-dimensional dose distributions during stereotactic body radiation therapy using a portal dose image-based 2D/3D registration approach. Comput Med Imaging Graph 40:1–12

Nielsen HB (1999) Damping parameter in Marquardt's method, Technical report IMM-REP-1999-05. IMM, Department of Mathematical Modelling, Technical University of Denmark, Lyngby

Papanikolaou N, Mackie TR, Meger-Wells C, Gehring M, Reckwerdt P (1993) Investigation of the convolution method for polyenergetic spectra. Med Phys 20(5):1327–1336

Partridge M, Ebert M, Hesse BM (2002) IMRT verification by three-dimensional dose reconstruction from portal beam measurements. Med Phys 29(8):1847–1858

Pasma KL, Kroonwijk M, de Boer JC, Visser AG, Heijmen BJ (1998) Accurate portal dose measurement with a fluoroscopic electronic portal imaging device (EPID) for open and wedged beams and dynamic multileaf collimation. Phys Med Biol 43(8):2047–2060

Press WH, Flannery BP, Teukolsky SA, Vetterling WT (1986) Numerical recipes. Cambridge University, Cambridge

Renner WD, Sarfaraz M, Earl MA, Yu CX (2003) A dose delivery verification method for conventional and intensity-modulated radiation therapy using measured field fluence distributions. Med Phys 30(11):2996–3005

Seco J, Evans PM (2006) Assessing the effect of electron density in photon dose calculations. Med Phys 33(2):540–552

Sharpe MB, Battista JJ (1993) Dose calculations using convolution and super-position principles: the orientation of dose spread kernels in divergent x-ray beams. Med Phys 20(6):1685–1694

Sheikh-Bagheri D, Rogers DW (2002) Monte Carlo calculation of nine mega-voltage photon beam spectra using the BEAM code. Med Phys 29(3):391–402

Steciw S, Warkentin B, Rathee S, Fallone BG (2005) Three-dimensional IMRT verification with a flat-panel EPID. Med Phys 32(2):600–612

van Elmpt WJ, Nijsten SM, Schiffeleers RF, Dekker AL, Mijnheer BJ, Lambin P, Minken A (2006) A Monte Carlo based three-dimensional dose reconstruction method derived from portal dose images. Med Phys 33(7):2426–2434

Vassiliev ON, Wareing TA, McGhee J, Failla G, Salehpour MR, Mourtada F (2010) Validation of a new grid-based Boltzmann equation solver for dose calculation in radiotherapy with photon beams. Phys Med Biol 55(3):581–598

Verhaegen F, Seuntiens J (2003) Monte Carlo modelling of external radiotherapy photon beams. Phys Med Biol 48(21):R107–R164

Wendling M, Louwe RJ, McDermott LN, Sonke JJ, van Herk M, Mijnheer BJ (2006) Accurate two-dimensional IMRT verification using a back-projection EPID dosimetry method. Med Phys 33(2):259–273

Xu L, Wan JW (2008) Real-time intensity-based rigid 2D–3D medical image registration using RapidMind multi-core development platform. Conf Proc IEEE EngMed Biol Soc 2008:5382–5385

Yang M, Virshup G, Mohan R, Shaw CC, Zhu XR, Dong L (2008) Improving accuracy of electron density measurement in the presence of metallic implants using orthovoltage computed tomography. Med Phys 35(5):1932–1941

Chapter 13
Visualization of Dose Distributions for Proton

Teiji Nishio and Aya Nishio-Miyatake

Abstract Proton therapy is one of the highly accurate radiation therapies in which the irradiation can be concentrated on a tumor using a scanned or modulated Bragg peak. Therefore, it is very important to evaluate whether prescription dose is delivered to a tumor in order to provide radiation therapy with high dose concentration for patients precisely and safely. Research on imaging of an actual irradiated region in proton therapy has been conducted, which utilizes positron-emitting nuclei generated by target nuclear fragment reactions involving incident protons and nuclei which a human body is composed of in the irradiated region. The proton-irradiated region can be confirmed by detection of pair annihilation gamma rays from the generated positron-emitting nuclei using a positron emission tomography (PET) imaging technique. In the proton treatment room, a beam ON-LINE PET system (BOLP) was constructed for dose-volume delivery-guided proton therapy by visualization of activity distribution in proton irradiation. The daily measured activity images acquired by the BOLPs showed the proton-irradiated region in each patient. Also, it was found that the biological washout effect of positron-emitting nuclei generated in tumor was associated with the proton delivery dose to the tumor.

Keywords Proton therapy • Target nuclear fragmentation reaction • Positron-emitting nuclei • PET imaging technique

---

T. Nishio (✉)
Department of Medical Physics, Graduate School of Medicine, Tokyo Women's Medical University, 8-1, Kawada-cho, Shinjuku-ku, Tokyo 162-8666, Japan
e-mail: nishio.teiji@twmu.ac.jp

A. Nishio-Miyatake
Keen Medical Physics Co. Ltd., 5-32-9 Mutsuura, Kanazawa-ku, Yokohama, Kanagawa 236-0031, Japan

H. Arimura (ed.), *Image-Based Computer-Assisted Radiation Therapy*,
DOI 10.1007/978-981-10-2945-5_13

13.1 Introduction

Proton therapy is one of the highly accurate radiation therapies. When proton beam consisting of protons is irradiated to a thick target, it deposits great energy at the point just before it stops by energy stopping power. This creates a high-dose region called Bragg peak. A spread-out Bragg peak is focused on a tumor in proton therapy, which performs radiation therapy with higher dose concentration. Figure 13.1 shows characteristics of dose distributions in the depth direction in proton therapy and common X-ray therapy. In addition, proton therapy has biological effect on a human body, which is different from photon beam or electron beam. Recently, the number of facilities of proton therapy has been increasing remarkably (PTCOG Data 2016). As an example for a facility of proton therapy, Fig. 13.2 shows National Cancer Center Hospital East Japan (Nishio 1999).

Proton therapy can provide high dose concentration on a target tumor. Without precise irradiation following a treatment plan, a lower rate of treatment control and a higher risk of serious damage than conventional radiotherapy may be caused by proton irradiation to a target region including organs at risk (OAR), as shown in Fig. 13.3.

Although various advances have been made in irradiation technologies to deliver prescription dose to a tumor more accurately for proton and other radiation therapies, it has been impossible to know whether proton irradiation is performed to a

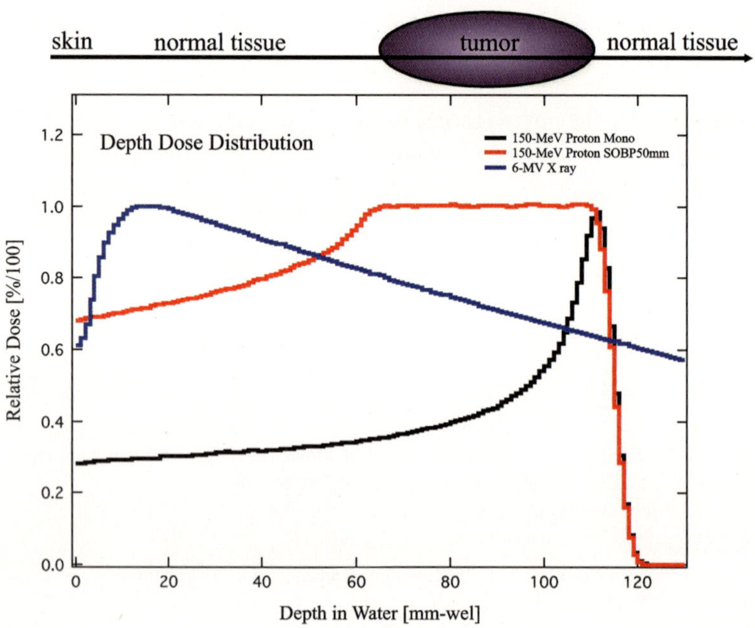

Fig. 13.1 Characteristic of dose distributions in the depth direction in proton therapy and common X-ray therapy

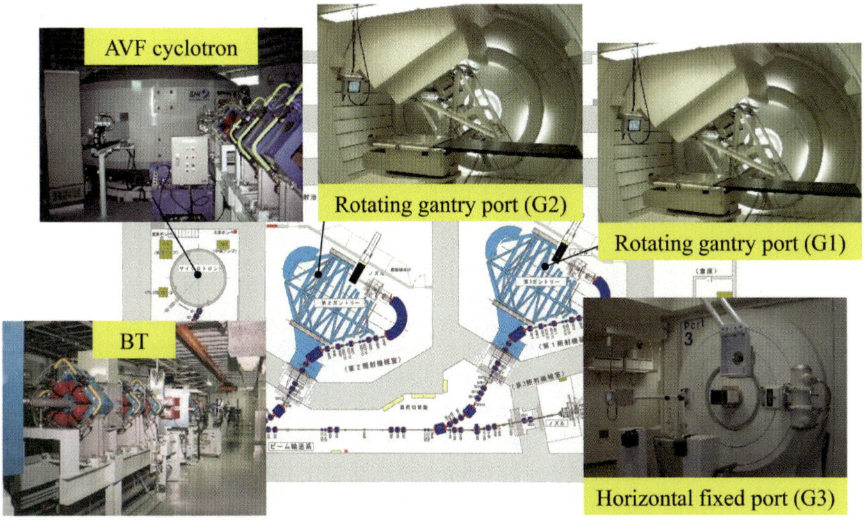

Fig. 13.2 Proton therapy system in National Cancer Center Hospital East Japan

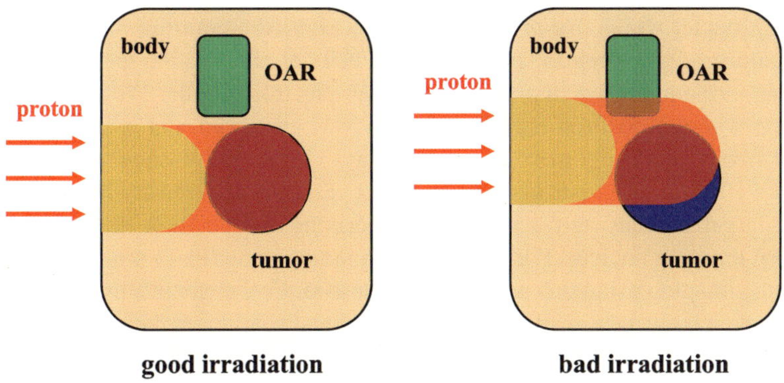

Fig. 13.3 Conceptual diagram expressing differences in dose concentrations depending on accuracy of proton beam irradiation

target tumor following a treatment plan during a patient being irradiated. It is essential to confirm whether prescription dose is delivered to a tumor in order to provide radiation therapy with high dose concentration for patients precisely and safely.

Research on imaging of an actual irradiated region in proton therapy has been conducted, which utilizes positron-emitting nuclei generated by target nuclear fragment reactions between incident protons and nuclei in a human body in the irradiated region.

13.2 Principle of Imaging a Region Irradiated by Proton Beam Using Target Nuclear Fragment Reaction

Proton beam with around 220-MeV kinetic energy is used in proton therapy. There are four nuclear reactions around this energy: elastic and inelastic scattering reactions, Coulomb dissociation reaction, and target nuclear fragment reaction. A reactant nucleus is fragmented into several pieces in Coulomb dissociation reaction and nuclear fragment reaction. Coulomb dissociation reaction occurs when a huge Coulomb force is generated from a reactant nucleus with a large atomic number and another nucleus is at close range. A patient's body is mainly composed of hydrogen nuclei, carbon nuclei, nitrogen nuclei, oxygen nuclei, and calcium nuclei (see Table 13.1) (ICRU Report 46 1992). Therefore, there is a slight possibility of Coulomb dissociation reaction in proton therapy.

Target nuclear fragment reaction is defined as nuclear fragmentation in a limited region where a nucleus collides with another one (Goldhaber 1974). The reaction occurs by incident protons and target nuclei in a patient's body, which is like incident protons ripping nucleons from target nuclei. Many different nuclei which are lighter than target nuclei are generated by the reaction, and its yield is strongly related to energy of incident protons. The generated nuclei include positron-emitting nuclei which are proton-rich nuclei. Positron-emitting nuclei generated by proton irradiation release positrons, and pairs of annihilation gamma rays with 511 keV are emitted when a positron and an electron collide. We can derive the position where a positron-emitting nucleus was generated and its intensity from simultaneous detecting pairs of gamma rays. Figure 13.4 shows a conceptual diagram illustrating target nuclear fragment reaction between an incident proton and a target nucleus and a method for deriving the position of the generated positron-emitting nucleus. Positron emission tomography (PET) is a type of nuclear medicine imaging using this principle and method. Five elements, hydrogen nuclei, carbon nuclei, nitrogen nuclei, oxygen nuclei, and calcium nuclei, are regarded as the main human body's composition, and target nuclear fragment reactions occurred by four of five elements except hydrogen nuclei in an energy range used in proton therapy. Table 13.2 shows target nuclear fragment reactions X(p,A)Y, which we should take into consideration, for imaging of a region irradiated by proton beam and positron-emitting nuclei generated by the reactions. Figure 13.5 shows the partial reaction cross sections of generating positron-emitting nuclei by nuclear fragment reactions about carbon nuclei and oxygen nuclei (NNDC 2016). Data on reaction cross sections of target nuclear fragment reactions for proton beam energy is shown in Fig. 13.5. It is insufficient in an energy range of proton therapy as far as we know from the newest data on the reaction cross sections reported in nuclear physics field which was released by National Nuclear Data Center (NNDC). A recoil shift of nuclei generated by target nuclear fragment reactions can be negligible according to the law of conservation and momentum (law of conservation of four-momentum) in the special theory of relativity, amounts of kinetic energy of incident protons. Imaging an actual proton-irradiated region from

Table 13.1 Examples of composition of human organs

	Element composition [%]						
Body tissue	H	C	N	O	Ca	Others	Mass density [kg/m^3]
Liver (adult)	10.2	13.9	3.0	71.6	0.0	1.3	1060
Adipose tissue (adult)	11.2	51.7	1.3	35.5	0.0	0.3	970
Soft tissue (adult)	10.5	25.6	2.7	60.2	0.0	1.0	1030
Lung (adult)	10.3	10.5	3.1	74.9	0.0	1.2	260
Muscle (adult)	10.2	14.3	3.4	71.0	0.0	1.1	1050
Skeleton sacrum (male)	7.4	30.2	3.7	43.8	9.8	5.1	1290
Skeleton cranium (adult)	5.0	21.2	4.0	43.5	17.6	8.7	1610
Skeleton femur (adult)	7.0	34.5	2.8	36.8	12.9	6.0	1330
Skeleton ribs (adult)	6.4	26.3	3.9	43.6	13.1	6.7	1410

ICRU Report 46 (1992)

information of detected positions and intensity of positron-emitting nuclei generated in a patient's body enables us to verify whether accurate proton irradiation is performed to a target tumor.

Recently, a number of researchers have been studying imaging of a region irradiated by proton beam using target nuclear fragment reactions using PET in order to provide highly accurate proton therapy which takes advantage of high dose concentration. The papers by Bennett et al. indicated the possibility of imaging the region irradiated by high-energy proton beam to matter (Bennett et al. 1975, 1978). Other studies including measurement and simulation of artificial phantoms and real animals for clinical use with images of irradiated regions (Litzenberg et al. 1992, 1999; Miyatake et al. 2011; Miyatake and Nishio 2013; Nishio et al. 2005, 2006; Oelfke et al. 1996; Paans and Schippers 1993; Parodi and Enghardt 2000; Parodi et al. 2002; Parodi et al. 2005; Parodi et al. 2007a, b, Parodi et al. 2007c; Vynckier et al. 1993) and approaches to measured PET images (Hishikawa et al. 2002; Miyatake et al. 2010; Nishio et al. 2001, 2008, 2010) have also reported. Especially, each research team has worked on more actively since commercial PET systems began to spread widely in 2000.

13.3 Beam OFF-LINE and ON-LINE PET Systems

Target nuclear fragment reactions between incident protons and nuclei generate many different positron-emitting nuclei in a region irradiated by proton beam in a patient's body. A positron-emitting nucleus generated in a patient's body decays (β^+ decay) and emits a positron according to the half-life of the nucleus. Thus,

$$ {}^{A}_{Z}X_{N} \rightarrow {}_{Z-1}^{\;\;A}X_{N+1} + e^{+} + \nu^{+}, \tag{13.1}$$

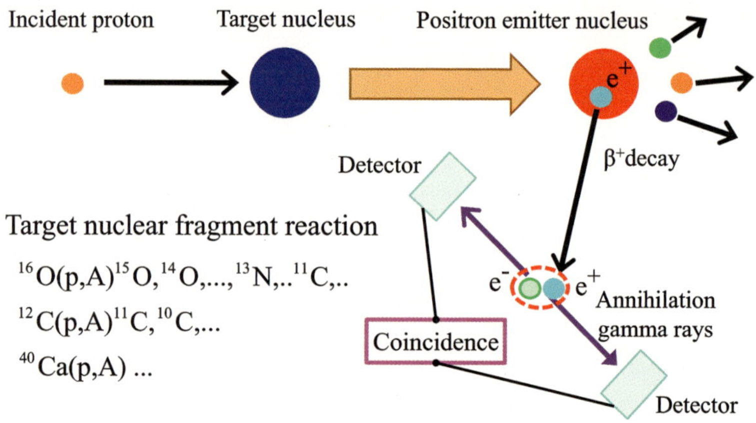

Fig. 13.4 Conceptual diagram expressing target nuclear fragment reaction between an incident proton and a target nucleus and a method for deriving the position of the generated positron-emitting nucleus

Table 13.2 Target nuclear fragment reactions X(p,A)Y which we should take into consideration for imaging of a region irradiated by proton beam and positron-emitting nuclei generated by the reactions

Reaction channel		
X	Y	Half-life [min]
^{12}C	^{11}C	20.39
	^{10}C	0.321
^{16}O	^{15}O	2.037
	^{14}O	1.177
	^{13}N	9.965
	^{11}C	20.39
	^{10}C	0.321
^{14}N	^{13}N	9.965
	^{11}C	20.39
	^{10}C	0.321
^{40}Ca	^{38}K	7.636
	^{30}P	2.498
	^{15}O	2.037
	^{13}N	9.965
	^{11}C	20.39

where ${}^{A}_{Z}X_N$ is the parent isotope, ${}^{A}_{Z-1}X_{N+1}$ is the daughter isotope, e^+ is a positron, and ν^+ is a neutrino. Energy of β^+ decay is expressed by

$$M_X(A,Z)c^2 - M_Y(A,Z-1)c^2 = Q = E_{\beta^+} + m_{e^-}c^2 + m_{e^+}c^2, \qquad (13.2)$$

where $M_X(A,Z)c^2$ is the rest mass energy of the parent nucleus, $M_Y(A,Z-1)c^2$ is the rest mass energy of the daughter nucleus, $m_{e^-}c^2$ is the rest mass energy of an

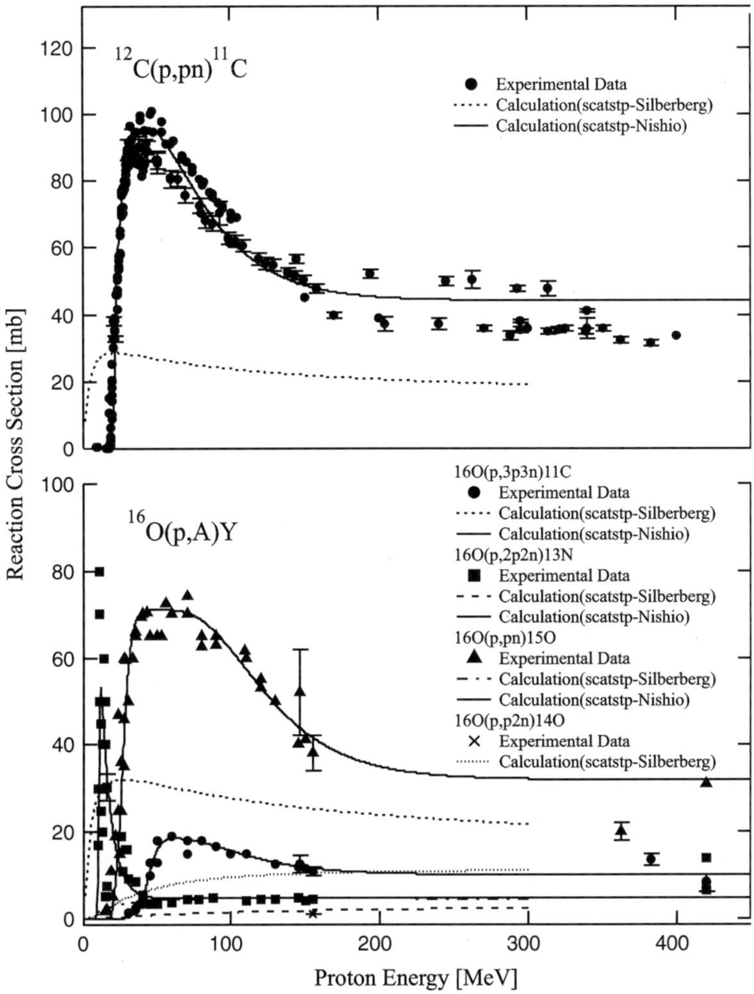

Fig. 13.5 Experimental and calculated partial reaction cross sections of generating positron-emitting nuclei by target nuclear fragment reactions about carbon nuclei and oxygen nuclei (Nishio et al. 2005)

electron, $m_{e^+}c^2$ is the rest mass energy of a positron, and E_{β^+} is the kinetic energy of a positron. Besides, to lead to β^+ decay, the Q value is given by

$$Q \geq m_{e^-}c^2 + m_{e^+}c^2 = 0.511 + 0.511 = 1.022\ [\text{MeV}]. \tag{13.3}$$

The Q value must be 1.022 MeV or more for β^+ decay occurring.

Positrons emitted by β^+ decay lose their energy continuously through interactions with orbital electrons of atoms in a human body. When a positron and an orbital electron collide near the end of the positron track to annihilate, they can produce two gamma rays whose energy is equal to the total of their rest mass energy (1.022 MeV). The energy of the two particles is equivalently divided into the two gamma rays according to the law of conservation of energy and momentum. Each of the gamma rays with 511 keV is released in opposite direction. To be precise, we cannot say that each annihilation gamma ray has an exact energy of 511 keV or that the two annihilation gamma rays travel at exact 180 degrees to each other because the rays obtain energy which the positron has as kinetic energy when annihilation occurs.

A procedure for imaging a region is irradiated by proton beam: (1) target matter or a patient receives proton irradiation in a treatment room, (2) they move to a room where a commercial PET system or PET-CT system has been installed, and (3) PET images of each target are taken. In this procedure, proton treatment system and PET system or PET-CT system have been installed in separate rooms. The proton treatment system following this procedure is called beam OFF-LINE PET system. The most critical issue in this system is that PET images cannot be taken right on the spot after the proton irradiation. The most essential positron-emitting nuclei with large yields for imaging the region irradiated by proton beam are ^{15}O nuclei (half-life, 2 min) generated by a reaction of ^{16}O(p,pn)^{15}O in a human body. We cannot get enough information of ^{15}O nuclei for the imaging because it takes several minutes to start taking PET images after the irradiation in this system. The patient needs to move to the PET room after the proton irradiation, and thus, the patient's conditions in proton irradiation and a PET scan are different. Therefore, the precision of imaging the region deteriorates. The patient has to spend extra time which is a burden to the patient, until finishing the PET scan after proton irradiation. However, this system has the advantages of an easy operation, enough preparation of image-reconstruction algorithms, and functions such as a fusion function between PET images and other medical images (e.g., CT images) or a function of analyzing PET or PET-CT images because commercial PET or PET-CT systems are used.

A system with a PET scanner installed on the beam line in a proton irradiation room is called beam ON-LINE PET system. Installing new PET developed with higher spatial resolution and positional accuracy on the beam line enables us to confirm which region proton beam is delivered in real time during a target tumor in a patient's body being irradiated. Precision of proton irradiation can be observed and kept ensured highly during a treatment period which has the possibility of changing patient's condition such as a reduction in tumor size. Finding out about some changes immediately and coping with them lead to providing patients with high-precision proton therapy. This system also enables us to verify the precision of calculating dose distribution in a patient's body using a proton treatment planning system, which leads to proposing a more optimal treatment plan and judging the most optimal condition of proton beam for the patient.

Beam ON-LINE PET system has some difficulties to obtain a large detection field and to reconstruct three-dimensional images due to a geometrical arrangement of proton beam and PET apparatus. It is necessary to construct a system with a device which can take images in a proton irradiation room such as CBCT (cone-

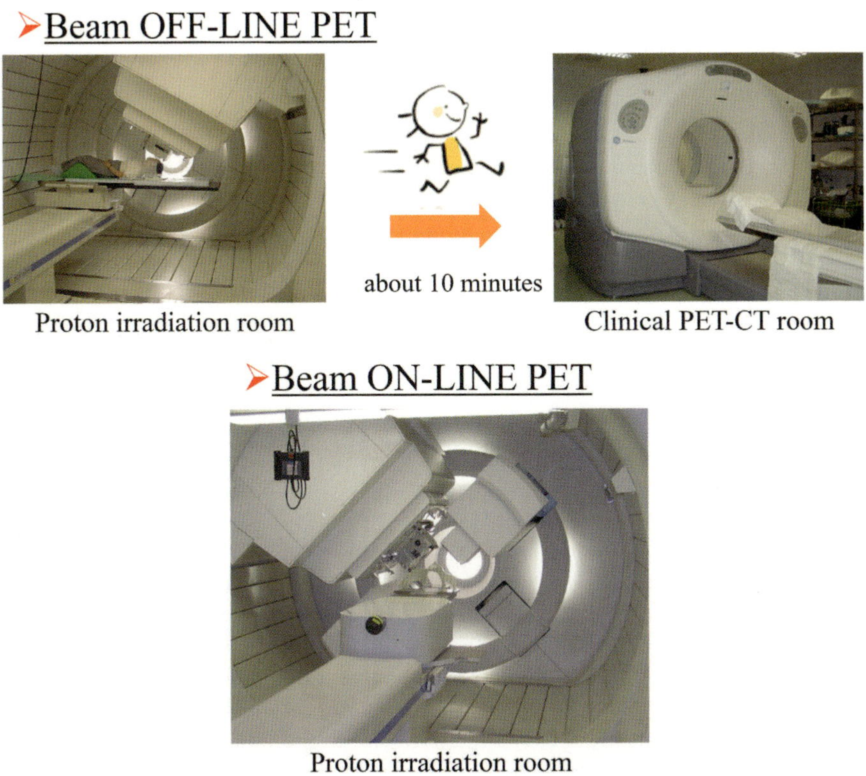

Fig. 13.6 Explanatory diagram of beam OFF-LINE PET system and beam ON-LINE system

beam CT) in order to improve the accuracy of fusion of PET and CT images. However, there is a great advantage of beam ON-LINE system; PET images are immediately taken, keeping the patient condition after proton irradiation. Therefore, it is possible to detect activity of positron-emitting nuclei with faster half-lives including ^{15}O nuclei which is the most essential nuclei for imaging the irradiated region. Furthermore, patients do not need to have extra time for moving to another room to take PET images. This advantage overwhelms above difficulties, and beam ON-LINE PET system would be very useful. Figure 13.6 shows an explanatory diagram of beam OFF-LINE PET system and beam ON-LINE system.

13.4 Studies on Imaging of the Irradiated Region Using Beam OFF-LINE PET System

Imaging of a region irradiated by proton beam using beam OFF-LINE PET system is defined as a procedure: target matter or patients are irradiated by proton beam and move to a room where a commercial PET system or PET-CT system has been installed; after that PET scans of target matter or patients are performed.

Let us show some experiments using a commercial PET system. Targets of polyethylene (CH_2) and water were irradiated by proton beam, and their activities were measured using the PET system. Mono-energy proton beams with about 30 mm FWHM at 138, 179, and 223 MeV were used in this experiment. The targets were irradiated for 10 s with around 10 GyE measured at a point of targets' surface where proton beam arrives. It took about 2 min to start measurement of activity in the targets in the PET scan room after the irradiation. PET scan took 2 min for each irradiation. The width of PET scanning was 144.5 mm in the depth direction per one scan, and an overlap between each scan was 8.5-mm width. The two-dimensional OSEM (ordered-subsets expectation maximization) method (Boellaard et al. 2001) was used to reconstruct PET images from the measured activity data. The spatial resolution of this PET is 4.2–5.8 mm. Figure 13.7 shows the image of measured activity distribution of the positron-emitting nuclei generated in CH_2 target using the PET when the target was irradiated by mono-energy proton beam at 179 MeV.

Target nuclear fragment reactions do not occur between protons from proton beam and other protons from CH_2 target. The positron-emitting nuclei generated in CH_2 target can be narrowed down to only ^{11}C nuclei generated by $^{12}C(p,A)^{11}C$, considering extra time from the end of proton irradiation to the beginning of measurement using PET and results of calculations for yields of various positron-emitting nuclei by target nuclear fragment reactions. Figure 13.8 shows measured activity distributions and measured dose distributions in CH_2 target in the depth direction and in the lateral direction irradiated by mono-energy proton beams at 138, 179, and 223. The range of PET scan and the number of PET scans were changed by the energy of proton beam (see Fig. 13.8 top). Raw data of measured activity was corrected by using half-life of ^{11}C nuclei (20.4 min) as attenuation correction, taking into consideration activity attenuation during PET measurement time. In Fig. 13.8, the intensity of activity in the depth direction which depends on a dose quantity corresponding with stopping power and flux increases gradually up to beam range with an increase of dose and then decreases sharply. In the lateral direction, shapes of activity distributions are similar to shapes of dose distributions. Since a plane at a same depth position in a homogeneous target has almost uniform energy of proton beam, shapes of both distributions depend on flux of proton at the depth position. When a target is irradiated by a proton beam of 2.5 GyE which is generally used in clinical proton therapy, the intensity of activity in the target is estimated at about 3 kB/cc.

The flux of incident protons to a target decreases with nuclear reactions between protons and nuclei in the target as proton beam travels through the target in the

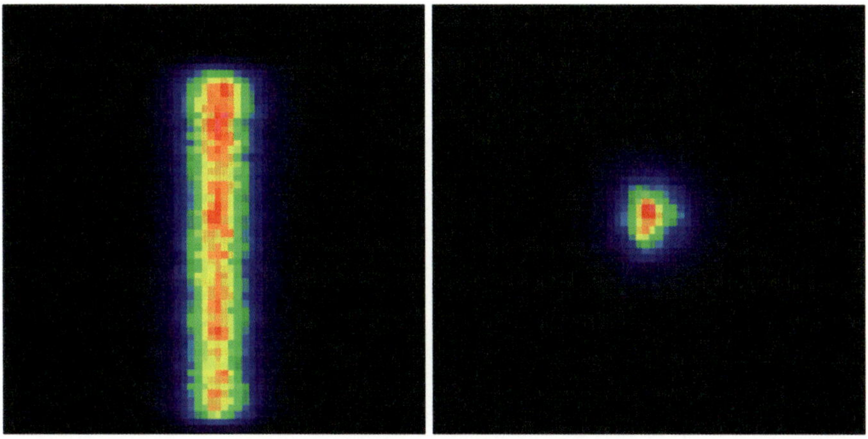

Fig. 13.7 Images of the measured two-dimensional activity distribution in CH_2 target in the depth direction (*left*) and the lateral direction (*right*) (Nishio et al. 2005)

depth direction. The nuclear reaction rate is determined by the total reaction cross section which depends on relative kinetic energy of protons and nuclei in the target. Figure 13.9 shows the experimental results of the total reaction cross section of protons and carbon nuclei. Semi-empirical formulas expressing experimental results approximately for the total reaction cross section have been reported by Sihver et al. (1993) and are as follows. When a target nuclear (mass number, A_t, and atomic number, Z_t) is irradiated by proton beam with kinetic energy $E_p$in the laboratory system, the total reaction cross section on the condition of $E_p \geq 200$ MeV is given by

$$\begin{aligned} \sigma_{\text{reac}}(E_p, A_t, Z_t) &= \sigma_0(A_t) = \pi r_0{}^2\left[1 + A_t{}^{1/3} - b_0\left(1 + A_t{}^{-1/3}\right)\right]^2, \\ b_0 &= 2.247 - 0.915\left(1 + A_t{}^{-1/3}\right), \end{aligned} \tag{13.4}$$

where $r_0 = 1.36$ fm. On the condition of $E_p \geq 200$ MeV and $6 \leq Z_t \leq 8$, it is given by

$$\sigma_{\text{reac}}(E_p, A_t, Z_t) = 0.14\exp(0.0985 E_p) f_{\text{reac}}(E_p, A_t, Z_t)\sigma_0(A_t). \tag{13.5}$$

On the condition of 20 MeV $\leq E_p \leq$ 150 MeV and $6 \leq Z_t \leq 8$, $E_p \leq 150$ MeV and $Z_t < 6$ or $Z_t > 8$, it is given by

$$\sigma_{\text{reac}}(E_p, A_t, Z_t) = f_{\text{reac}}(E_p, A_t, Z_t)\sigma_0(A_t). \tag{13.6}$$

On the condition of 150 MeV $\leq E_p <$ 200 MeV, it is given by

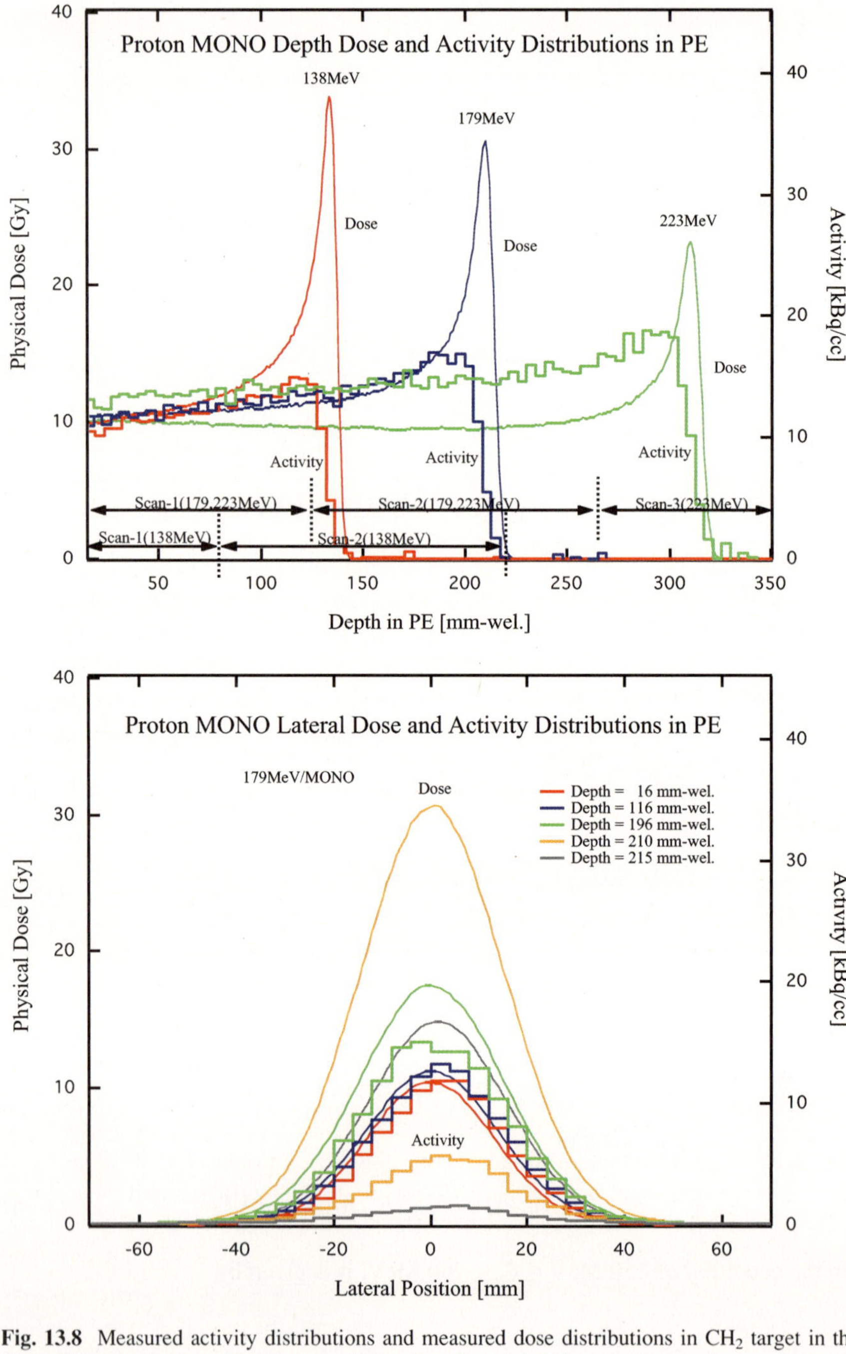

Fig. 13.8 Measured activity distributions and measured dose distributions in CH_2 target in the depth direction (*top*) and in the lateral direction (*bottom*) with mono-energy proton beams at 138, 179, and 223 MeV (Nishio et al. 2005)

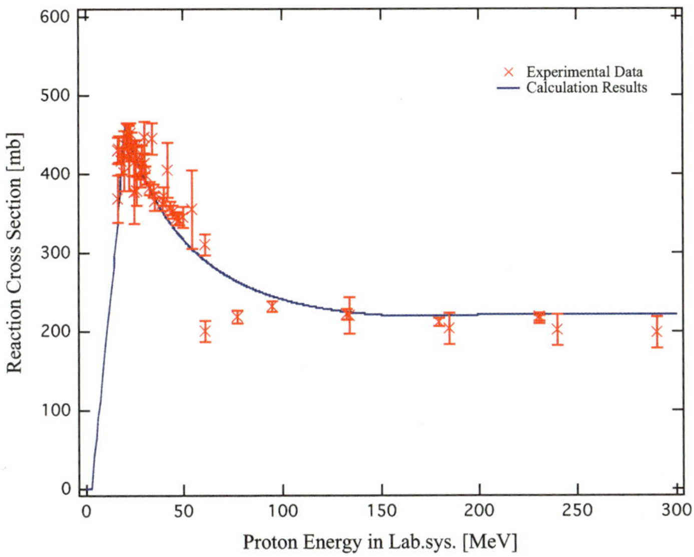

Fig. 13.9 Total reaction cross section of protons and carbon nuclei with kinetic energy of proton beam (Nishio et al. 2005)

$$\sigma_{\text{reac}}\left(E_p, A_t, Z_t\right) = \left[f_{\text{reac}}\left(E_p, A_t, Z_t\right) g_{\text{reac}}\left(E_p, A_t, Z_t\right) + h_{\text{reac}}\left(E_p, A_t, Z_t\right)\right] \sigma_0(A_t). \tag{13.7}$$

These functions f, g, and h depend on kinetic energy of proton beam, and each target nucleus is as follows:

$$\begin{aligned} f_{\text{reac}}\left(E_p, A_t, Z_t\right) &= \left[1.15 + \lambda_1 \exp\left(-E_p/\lambda_2\right)\right] \\ &\quad \times \left[1 - 0.62\exp\left(-E_p/200\right) \sin\left(10.9 E_p{}^{-0.28}\right)\right], \\ g_{\text{reac}}\left(E_p, A_t, Z_t\right) &= 4.00 - 0.02 E_p, \\ h_{\text{reac}}\left(E_p, A_t, Z_t\right) &= 0.02 E_p - 3.00, \end{aligned} \tag{13.8}$$

$$\lambda_1 = \begin{cases} 1.4\ (Z_t \leq 8) \\ 0\ (\text{otherwise}) \end{cases}, \lambda_2 = \begin{cases} 38\ (Z_t = 4) \\ 25\ (Z_t = 5) \\ 10\ (6 \leq Z_t \leq 8) \\ 1\ (\text{otherwise}) \end{cases}. \tag{13.9}$$

Figure 13.9 shows the total reaction cross section of protons and carbon nuclei calculated using Eqs. 13.4, 13.5, 13.6, 13.7, 13.8, and 13.9. The results from calculation seem to be able to draw the results from experiments.

From the total reaction cross section calculated using above equations, the behavior of flux of incident proton beam to CH_2 and water targets in the depth direction is expressed by

$$F(z, A_t, Z_t, n) = F_{\text{in}}(z = 0)q(z)\prod \exp(-\sigma_{\text{reac}}(z, A_t, Z_t)n\Delta), \tag{13.10}$$

where F_{in} is the flux of incident proton beam to the target, z is the charge of incident particle, n is the number of target nuclei per unit density, and Δ is the thickness of the target. E_p can be replaced with z by using the Bethe-Bloch formula of stopping power:

$$-\frac{dE_p}{dz} \approx -\frac{4\pi e^4}{m_e c^2 \beta^2} n Z_t \left\{ \ln\left(\frac{2m_e c^2 \beta^2}{I}\right) - \ln\left(1 - \beta^2\right) - \beta^2 \right\}, \tag{13.11}$$

where I is the mean excitation potential, c is the speed of light, $\beta = v/c$, e is the electron charge, and m_e is the electron mass. q is the factor expressing the effect of range straggling and given by

$$\begin{aligned} q(z) &= \frac{1}{\sqrt{2\pi}\sigma_{\text{Rst}}} \int_z^{\infty} \exp\left(-\frac{(x-R)^2}{2\sigma_{\text{Rst}}{}^2}\right) dx, \\ \sigma_{\text{Rst}}(R) &= \sqrt{0.1569\rho_t \frac{Z_t}{A_t} R \frac{(1-\beta^2/2)}{1-\beta^2} \left(\left(\frac{1}{\rho_t}\frac{dE}{dz}\right)^{-1}_{z\to R}\right)_{\text{mean}}}, \end{aligned} \tag{13.12}$$

where ρ_t is the density of target material.

Figure 13.10 shows the results of calculations using Eq. 13.4 to Eq. 13.12, and the results were normalized to incident flux to the targets, respectively. Data on flux of proton beam in CH_2 and water targets measured from experiments with NIRS-HIMAC/P131 are also shown in Fig. 13.10. The measured values in both targets are a bit lower than the calculated values from the entrance surface of targets to around the range of proton beam, and the measured ones are higher than the calculated ones around the beam range.

The total reaction cross section between incident protons and nuclei in targets includes the partial reaction cross section which shows how large reactions as target nuclei being fragmented by protons are. The partial reaction cross section is one of the most essential parameters to determine the yields of positron-emitting nuclei in target matter or a patient's body after proton irradiation.

Semi-empirical formulas expressing experimental results approximately for the partial reaction cross section have been reported by Sihver et al. (1993). The partial reaction cross section for reactions of ^{12}C(p,A)^{11}C and ^{16}O(p,A)^{11}C,^{13}N,^{14}O,^{15}O is given by

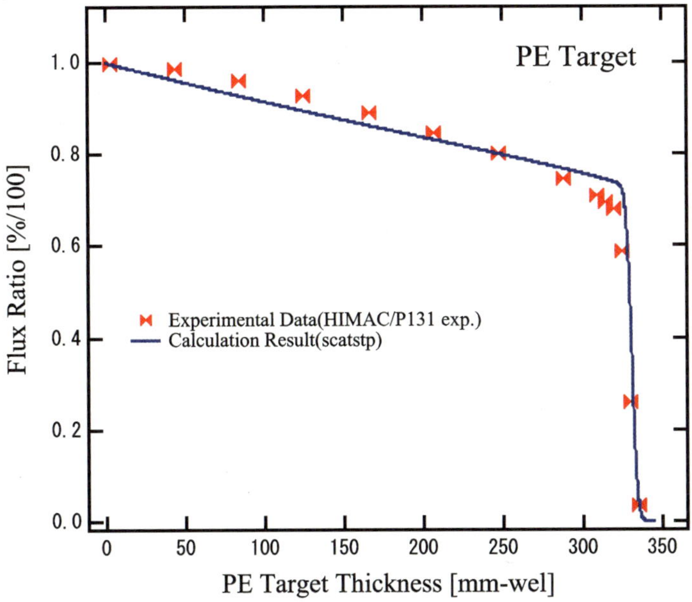

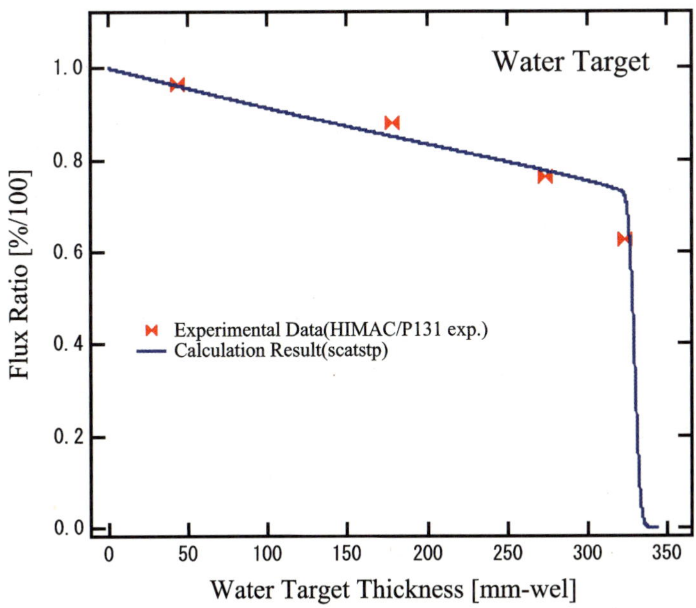

Fig. 13.10 Flux of proton beam in CH_2 and water targets in the depth direction. The marks and lines express the measured and calculated values, respectively (Nishio et al. 2005)

$$\begin{aligned}\sigma_{X\to Y}(E_p) &\\ &= \sigma_R \exp\begin{pmatrix} -2.6{E_p}^{-0.5}(A_t - A_{pr}) - 10.2{E_p}^{-0.26} \\ \times (Z_{pr} - SA_{pr} + 5\times 10^{-4}{A_{pr}}^2)^2 \end{pmatrix}\Omega\eta, \\ \sigma_R &= \frac{232.5({A_t}^{2/3} - 1)[1 - 0.3\ln(A_t/20)]{E_p}^{-0.63}}{1 - \exp(-2.6A_t{E_p}^{-0.5})}, \\ S &= 0.502 - 0.26\left(\tfrac{A_t}{Z_t} - 2\right)^{1.4},\end{aligned} \tag{13.13}$$

where A_{pr} and Z_{pr} are mass number and atomic number of nuclei generated by each reaction and Ω and η are coefficients depending on the generated nuclei and have constant values (see Table 13.3). Figure 13.5 shows the partial reaction cross sections of ^{12}C(p,A)^{11}C and ^{16}O(p,A)^{11}C, ^{13}N, ^{14}O, ^{15}O calculated using values in Figs. 13.9 and 13.10 and Eq. 13.13. There are large differences in the partial reaction cross sections between experimental results and calculation ones under 250-MeV proton beam. Incidentally, the range of proton beam is generally from about 100 MeV to 250 MeV in clinical proton therapy. To reproduce experimental values more accurately, a simple equation was derived by Nishio et al. (2005):

$$\sigma_{X\to Y}(E_p) = \frac{a}{1 + \exp\left(\frac{b - E_p}{c}\right)}\left\{1 - d\left(1 - e\exp\left(-\frac{E_p - f}{g}\right)\right)^h\right\}, \tag{13.14}$$

where the coefficients of parameters are shown in Table 13.4, which depends on nuclei generated by reactions. The results of the partial reaction cross sections were calculated using Eqs. 13.13 and 13.14 with the calculation program of scatstp.

Since a cyclotron operates continuous wave (CW), the intensity of proton beam provided by a cyclotron is regarded as constant during irradiation to a target, and yields of positron-emitting nuclei are constant during the irradiation. When the half-life of positron-emitting nucleus is $T_{1/2}$ and the time of beam irradiation t_i, the total number of generated positron-emitting nuclei within t_i is given by

$$N_R(t_i, F, \sigma_{X\to Y}) = F(z, A_t, Z_t, n)\left[1 - \exp\left(-\sigma_{X\to Y}(E_p)n\Delta\right)\right]. \tag{13.15}$$

Considering a decrease in the number of positron-emitting nuclei by their half-lives, the number of residual positron-emitting nuclei in the target right after irradiation N_{act} is given by

$$N_{\rm act}(t_i, T_{1/2}, F, \sigma_{X\to Y}) = N_R(t_i, F, \sigma_{X\to Y})\left[1 + 2^{-t_i/T_{1/2}} - \frac{T_{1/2}}{t_i \ln 2}\left(1 - 2^{-t_i/T_{1/2}}\right)\right]. \tag{13.16}$$

When the time from the end of proton irradiation to the beginning of measurement using PET is t_s, the time from the end of proton irradiation to the end of measurement using PET t_e, the detection efficiency for a single 511-keV gamma ray

Table 13.3 Coefficients of Ω and η depending on the generated nuclei in Eq. 13.13 (Nishio et al. 2005)

Product	^{11}C	^{13}N	^{14}O	^{15}O
Ω	1.00	0.40	1.00	1.20
η	1.15	0.90	1.15	1.15

Table 13.4 Coefficients of parameters depending on the generated nuclei in Eq. 13.14

Reaction Channel		Parameter							
X	Y	a	b	c	d	e	f	g	h
^{12}C	^{11}C	96.0	21.4	0.9	0.5	1.2	39.0	34.5	2.0
^{16}O	^{15}O	71.0	26.0	2.8	0.6	1.1	41.0	36.0	6.0
^{16}O	^{13}N	66.0	10.4	0.4	0.9	0.8	11.6	6.8	1.0
^{16}O	^{11}C	18.8	43.6	3.6	0.5	1.0	49.0	35.0	4.0

Nishio et al. (2005)

ε, and the solid angle of the total detectors Ω_{sa}, the number of activity counts detected using PET N_{PET} is given

$$N_{\mathrm{PET}}\left(t_i, T_{1/2}, t_s, t_e, F, \sigma_{X\to Y}\right) = N_{\mathrm{act}}\left(t_i, T_{1/2}, F, \sigma_{X\to Y}\right) 2^{-t_s/T_{1/2}}\left[1 - 2^{-(t_e-t_s)/T_{1/2}}\right]\varepsilon^2 \frac{\Omega_{sa}}{4\pi}. \tag{13.17}$$

Figure 13.11 shows activity distributions of CH_2 and water targets in the depth direction which include both results of measurement using PET and calculation using Eqs. 13.14 and 13.17 with mono-energy proton beam at 179 MeV. It also shows changes in the distributions with time after proton irradiation. All the activity distributions shown in Fig. 13.11 were normalized at a depth of 16 mm WEL from the beam entrance of the targets in the activity of 3 min after proton irradiation. The activity distributions of CH_2 target in the case of right after irradiation (only calculated distribution) 3 and 23 min after irradiation are shown and the activity distributions of water target in the case of right after irradiation (only calculated distribution), 3, 5, 7, and 9 min after irradiation. Since the activity of 3 or more minutes after irradiation was almost composed by only ^{11}C nuclei in CH_2 target, the activity of 23 minutes after irradiation was half of that of 3 min after irradiation with both distributions having similar shapes. On the other hand, since the activity of water target was composed of four kinds of nuclei, ^{11}C, ^{13}N, ^{14}O, and ^{15}O, the shapes of activity distributions changed with time. There were some differences in shapes between the measured activity distributions and the calculated ones. These differences would be mainly caused by accuracies of experiments and calculations for the partial reaction cross section which is a major factor in calculating distributions and by accuracy of calculation of flux in the targets. The shapes of measured distributions in distal regions might depend on both accuracy of the PET and the algorithm of image reconstruction. The activity range is defined as the 50 % depth point of distal falloff in the activity distribution which is normalized

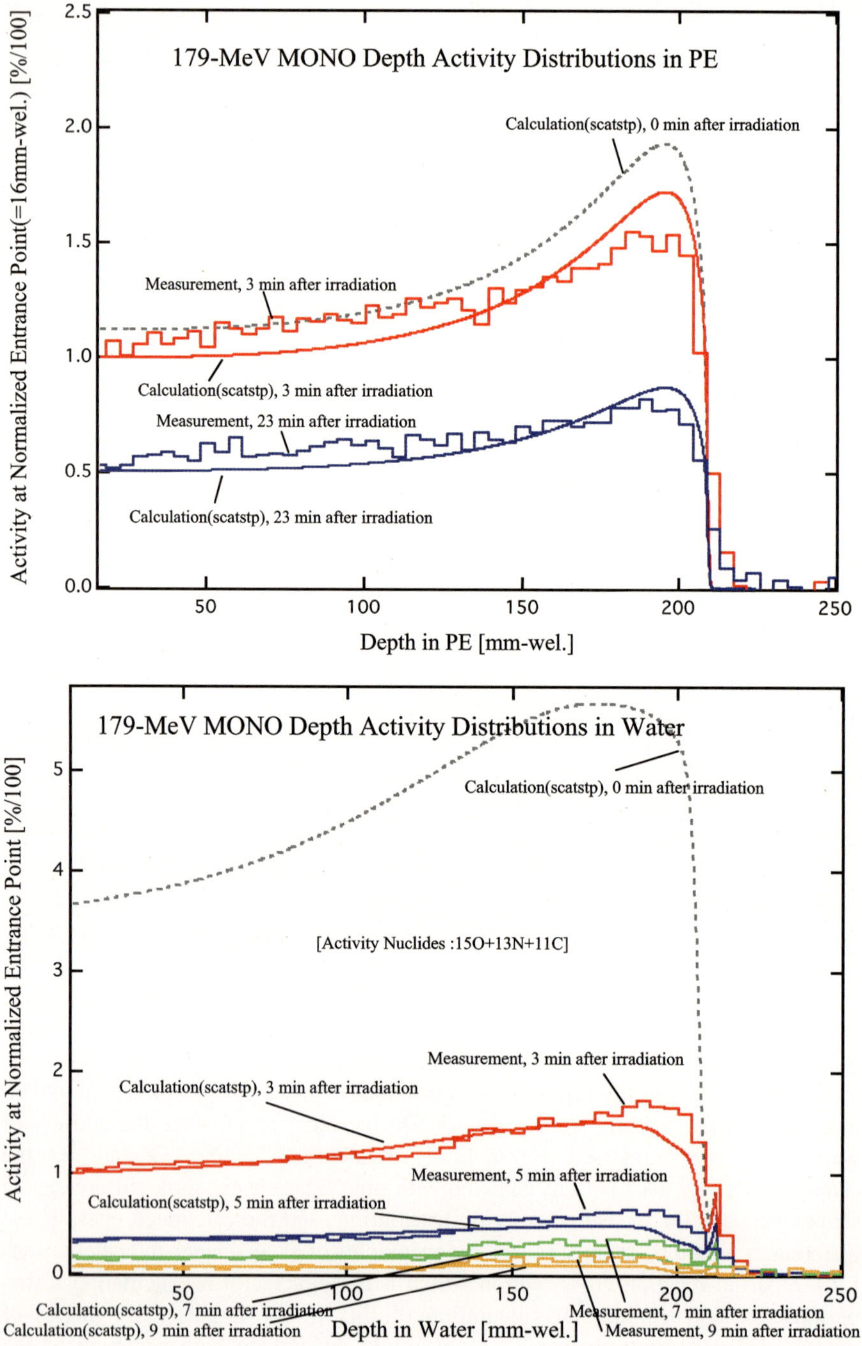

Fig. 13.11 Calculated and measured activity distributions of CH_2 target at 3 and 23 min after irradiation (*top*) and those of water target at 3, 5, 7 and 9 min after irradiation (*bottom*) with monoenergy proton beam of 179 MeV (Nishio et al. 2005)

at peak. The ranges of the CH_2 and water targets were shorter than the physical ranges by about 4 mm and about 2 mm, respectively, because of the threshold energies of the target nuclear fragment reaction. Differences in FWHM of the measured dose and activity distributions in the CH_2 and water targets in the lateral direction were in an accuracy within 1 mm.

13.5 Studies on Imaging of the Irradiated Region Using Beam ON-LINE PET System

The great advantage of proton therapy is high dose concentration on the target tumor, so that it is highly significant to grasp changes in tumor accurately during a period of proton treatment. If there are some changes in a patient's condition such as a reduction in target tumor's size during a comparatively long period of proton treatment, and we don't notice these changes, the patient would be provided the dose distribution which is greatly different from the planned one.

Figure 13.12 shows the dose distributions with a field irradiation in the anterior-posterior direction for the paranasal sinuses tumor; the calculated distribution at the beginning of the treatment is shown in the left side and the calculated distribution in the case of a partial reduction in tumor size in the right side. The planed proton beam is highly concentrated on the tumor without any irradiation to the brain stem as an adjacent organ at risk; however, the tumor is irradiated with lower beam concentration, and the amount of dose on the brain stem increases sharply when the tumor shrinks during the treatment period.

Installing new PET with higher spatial resolution and positional accuracy on the beam line enables us to confirm which region proton beam is delivered in real time during a target tumor in a patient's body being irradiated. The prototype of beam ON-LINE PET system (PT-BOLPs) equipped with a planar-type detector heads with high positional accuracy was built and mounted with its field of view covering the isocenter in the treatment room (see Fig. 13.13). The PT-BOLPs system as well as a commercial PET system can localize positron-emitting nuclei and detect their activity by measuring pairs of annihilation gamma rays coincidently from positron-emitting nuclei generated in a patient's body. The system of detector heads in the PT-BOLPs was a planar positron imaging system (Hamamatsu Photonics K. K., Hamamatsu, Japan) (Uchida et al. 2004) with BGO scintillators. Each detector head consisted of 24 units per photomultiplier tube, and each unit arranged 10 × 10 arrays of BGO crystals whose individual size was 2 mm × 2 mm × 20 mm. The field of view (FOV) which means the useful field size for the detection area was 120.8 mm × 186.8 mm. In the PT-BOLPs system, the detector heads were placed where the center of the detection area matched the isocenter in the treatment room. The distance between the upper and the lower detector heads was 500 mm. This system with high positional accuracy (1.6–2.1 mm FWHM) is able to measure data without dead time if its collection rate of coincident detection of pairs of 511-keV

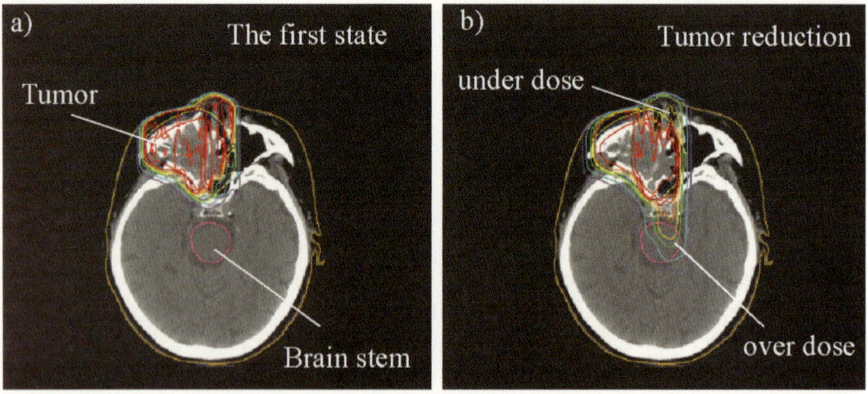

Fig. 13.12 Proton dose distributions with one field irradiation in the anterior-posterior direction for the paranasal sinuses tumor calculated using the proton treatment planning system, (**a**) at the beginning of the treatment, and (**b**) in the case of a partial reduction in tumor size

gamma rays is up to a few thousand counts per second (kcps). PET images are taken without deterioration in image resolution under the collection rates of 20 kcps (Uchida et al. 2004).

When the time from the end of proton irradiation to the beginning of measurement using the PT-BOLPs is t_s, the time from the end of proton irradiation to the end of measurement using the PT-BOLPs t_e, the detection efficiency for a single 511-keV gamma ray ε, and the solid angle of the total detectors Ω_{sa}, the number of activity counts measured using the PT-BOLPs is given by

$$\begin{aligned} & N_{\mathrm{BOLPs}}\left(t_i, T_{1/2}, t_s, t_e, F, \sigma_{X\to Y}\right) \\ & = N_{\mathrm{act}}\left(t_i, T_{1/2}, F, \sigma_{X\to Y}\right) 2^{-t_s/T_{1/2}}\left[1-2^{-(t_e-t_s)/T_{1/2}}\right]\varepsilon^2\frac{\Omega_{sa}}{4\pi} \\ & = F\left(t_i, E_p\right)\left[1-\exp\left(-\sigma_{X\to Y}\left(A_t, Z_t, E_p\right)n\Delta\right)\right]\left[1+2^{-t_i/T_{1/2}}-\frac{T_{1/2}}{t_i \ln 2}\left(1-2^{-t_i/T_{1/2}}\right)\right] \\ & \times 2^{-t_s/T_{1/2}}\left[1-2^{-(t_e-t_s)/T_{1/2}}\right]\varepsilon^2\frac{\Omega_{sa}}{4\pi}. \end{aligned} \tag{13.18}$$

The total detection efficiency of the PT-BOLPs with a distance between the detector heads of 500 mm C_{eff} is as follows:

$$C_{\mathrm{eff}} = \varepsilon^2\frac{\Omega_{sa}}{4\cdot\pi} \approx 0.86^2 \times 0.06 \approx 0.04\ [\%/100]. \tag{13.19}$$

Let us show an experiment using the PT-BOLPs for an animal. Measurement using the PT-BOLPs for a frozen rabbit with about 60 cm long was performed during proton irradiation. Before the measurement, the same procedure for a patient was followed: CT imaging, treatment planning, and proton irradiation. A virtual cylindrical-shaped tumor which had a step around the center and a volume of 8.4 ml

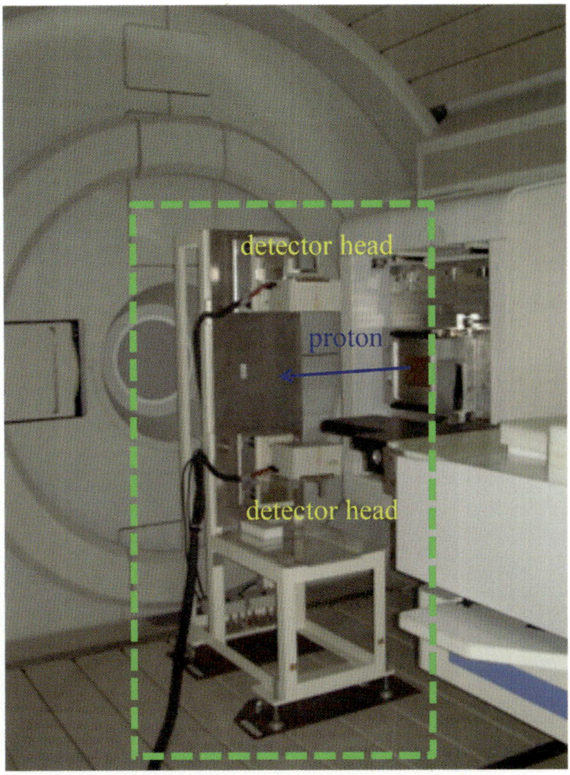

Fig. 13.13 Setup of the PT-BOLPs in the treatment room

was set in the liver of the rabbit on CT images. The virtual tumor was regarded as a target for proton irradiation, and all of the gross tumor volumes (GTV), the clinical target volumes (CTV), and the planning target volumes (PTV) were set to be equal. The proton irradiation of a 4.0-Gy dose to the reference point in PTV with one field irradiation in the posterior-anterior direction (gantry angle, 90° degree) was planned and performed. The maximum range of the irradiated proton beam was 82.4 mmWEL from the surface of the rabbit to the deeper rim of PTV in the beam traveling direction, and the energy was 103 MeV at the point. The size of the irradiation field was 29 mm × 54 mm using the spread-out Bragg peak (SOBP) of 30 mm, and the maximum thickness of PTV was 21 mmWEL in the beam traveling direction. The patient compensator and collimator were prepared following the rabbit's irradiation plan. Figure 13.14 shows the two-dimensional and three-dimensional dose distributions calculated using the proton treatment planning system in the axial, sagittal, and coronal planes for the plan. Figure 13.15 shows the condition of the proton irradiation to the rabbit and the measurement using the PT-BOLPs. Both the center of the detection area of the PT-BOLPs and the reference point of the virtual tumor in the rabbit matched the isocenter. The measurement for the rabbit using the PT-BOLPs was performed for 33 min (beam on, 1 min; beam off, 32 minutes) from the start of the proton irradiation.

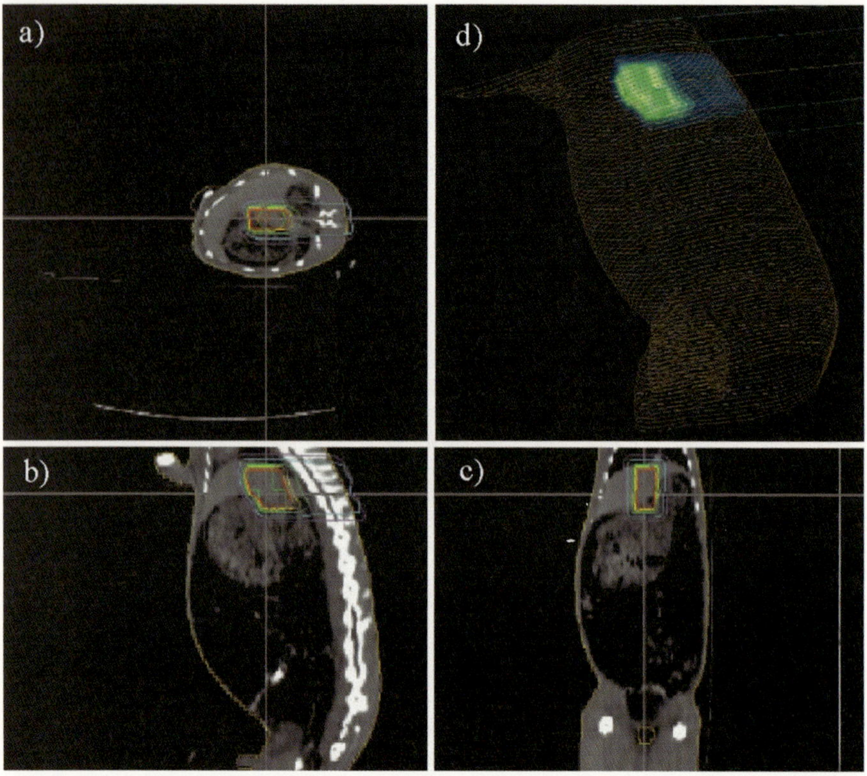

Fig. 13.14 Dose distributions calculated using the proton treatment planning system for the rabbit. Two-dimensional distributions in the axial (**a**), sagittal (**b**), and coronal (**c**) planes and three-dimensional distribution (**d**) are shown (Nishio et al. 2006)

Fig. 13.15 Condition of the proton irradiation to the rabbit and the measurement using the PT-BOLPs (Nishio et al. 2006)

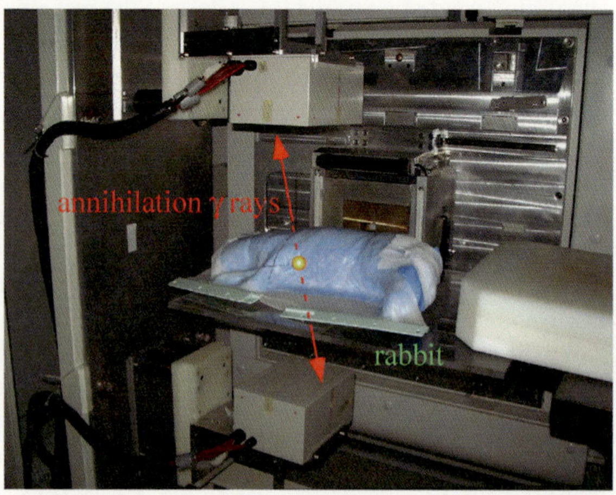

Figure 13.16 shows the calculated dose distributions to the rabbit and the measured PET images using the PT-BOLPs, and the activities are measured for 1 min, 2 min, 4 min, 10 min, and 30 min after the proton irradiation. The activity distributions measured using the PT-BOLPs were related to the dose distributions calculated using the proton treatment planning system in their shapes. The measured PET images were clearer with the detection time increasing. Figure 13.17 shows the detection counts per second of the activity in the rabbit after the irradiation. According to the results of the detection counts (see Fig. 13.17), more than 95 % of total detection of the activity was detected by 10-min measurement after the proton irradiation using the PT-BOLPs. PET images measured for over 10 min would not be much clearer than PET images for 10 min. The data measured using the PT-BOLPs included a large amount of background data such as lots of secondary X-rays, gamma rays, and neutrons generated by proton beam bombarding the device for making the appropriate irradiation fields during the proton irradiation.

Considering that a human body is mainly composed of hydrogen nuclei ^{1}H, carbon nuclei ^{12}C, nitrogen nuclei ^{14}N, and oxygen nuclei ^{16}O, it is predicted that positron-emitting nuclei generated by target nuclear fragment reaction in the proton irradiation to a human body are mainly occupied by ^{15}O nuclei (half-life, $T_{1/2}(^{15}\mathrm{O}) = 122.2$ s), and other nuclei are included: ^{14}O (half-life, $T_{1/2}(^{14}\mathrm{O}) = 70.6$ s), ^{13}N (half-life, $T_{1/2}(^{13}\mathrm{N}) = 9.971\mathrm{min}$), and ^{11}C (half-life, $T_{1/2}(^{11}\mathrm{C}) = 20.4\mathrm{min}$). ^{38}K (half-life, $T_{1/2}(^{38}\mathrm{K}) = 7.6\mathrm{min}$) are also generated from calcium nuclei ^{40}Ca which are one of the main elements of a human bone. However, by dividing the elements of the positron-emitting nuclei generated in a human body into two groups of short half-lives and long ones, the detection rate was approximated by

$$CR(t) = \sum_{i={}^{15}\mathrm{O},\,{}^{14}\mathrm{O},\,{}^{13}\mathrm{N},\,{}^{11}\mathrm{C},\ldots} [CR(t)]_i = \sum_{j={}^{15}\mathrm{O},\,{}^{14}\mathrm{O},\ldots} [CR(t)]_j + \sum_{k={}^{13}\mathrm{N},\,{}^{11}\mathrm{C},\ldots} [CR(t)]_k$$

$$\rightarrow 1977.9 \times \left(\frac{1}{2}\right)^{\frac{t}{110.5}} + 219.7 \times \left(\frac{1}{2}\right)^{\frac{t}{847.6}}, \tag{13.20}$$

where t is the measurement time after the beam stop.

Usefulness of the BOLPs in clinical proton therapy was greatly supported by constructing the PT-BOLPs and the results of studies on it. The next BOLPs: a PET system with high positional accuracy was set in the rotating gantry directly and was developed as a beam ON-LINE PET system mounted on rotating gantry port (BOLPs-RGp) (see Fig. 13.18). A planar-type positron imaging system (Hamamatsu Photonics K. K., Hamamatsu, Japan) with a high positional accuracy (about 2 mm FWHM) and detector heads with BGO scintillators was used for the BOLPs-RGp, which was developed to make the dead region between the detector heads more narrow than the previous system. Each detector head consisted of 36 units per a photomultiplier tube by making each unit gap narrow from the previous 11.0 mm

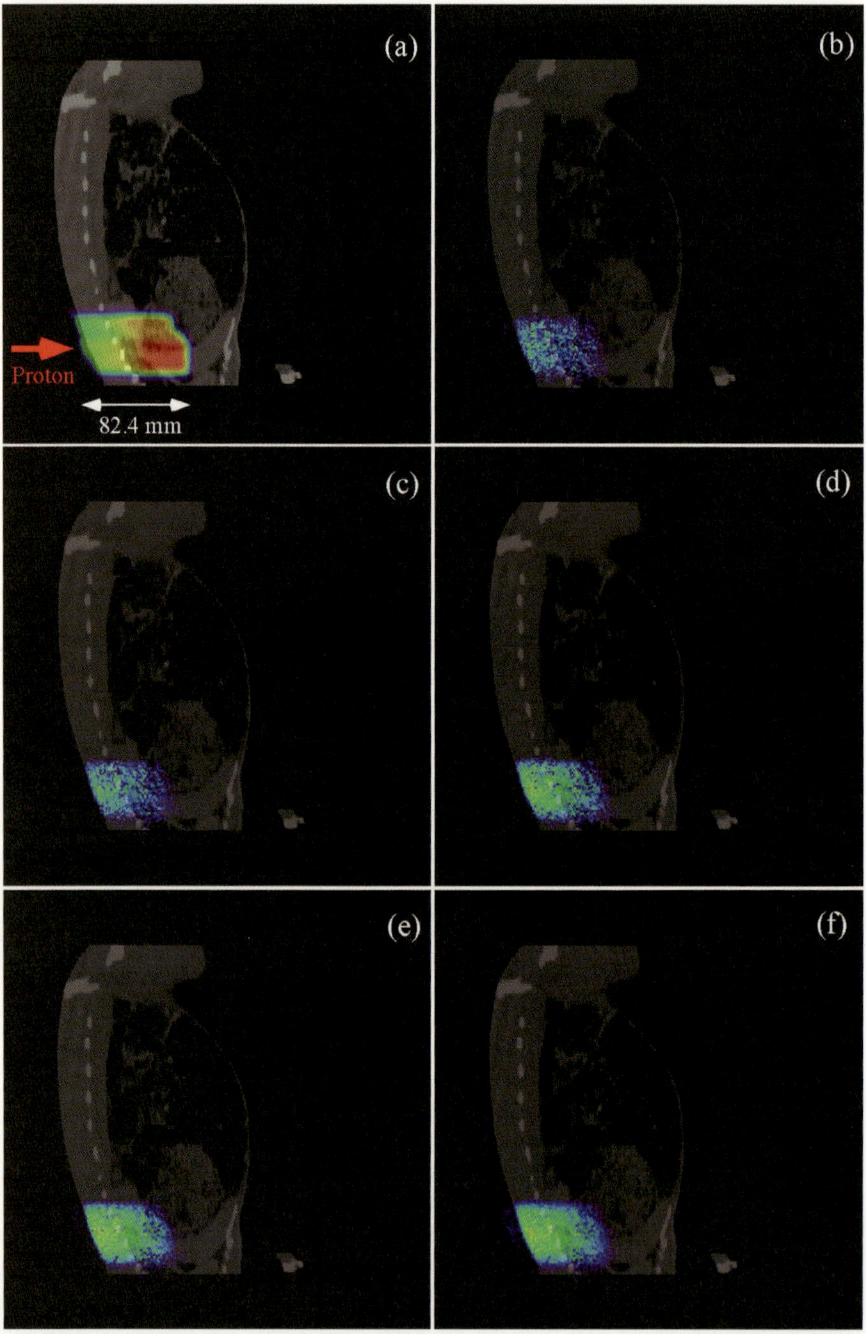

Fig. 13.16 Calculated dose distribution (**a**) and measured PET images using the PT-BOLPs for 1 min (**b**), 2 min (**c**), 4 min (**d**), 10 min (**e**), and 30 min (**f**) after the proton irradiation to the rabbit (Nishio et al. 2006)

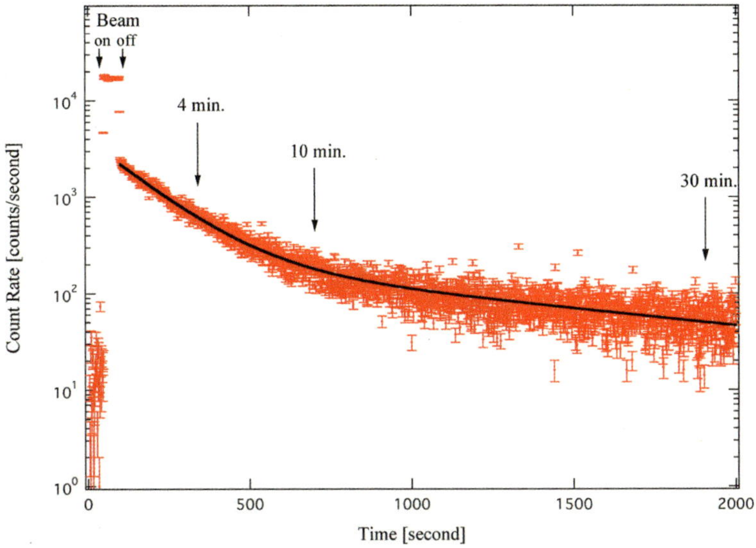

Fig. 13.17 Detection counts per second of the activity using the PT-BOLPs in the rabbit after the irradiation (Nishio et al. 2006)

to 3.3 mm, and each unit arranged 10 × 10 arrays of BGO crystals whose individual size was 2 mm × 2 mm × 20 mm, and the total number of BGO crystals was 7200 (see Fig. 13.19). The FOV widened to 164.8 mm × 167.0 mm from 120.8 mm × 186.8 mm, which is almost enough size to use the BOLPs-RGp for every case in proton therapy. The detector heads were set across from each other on the rotating gantry, and the center of detection area of the BOLPs-RGp was matched to the isocenter in the treatment room. The both opposing detectors rotate together if the gantry rotates, and the FOV is always along the axis of the proton beam direction and observes in beam range direction. The distance between the detector heads can vary from 30 cm to 100 cm continuously. The BOLPs-RGp is able to measure data without dead time if its collection rate for the coincident detection of pairs of 511-keV gamma rays is up to about 4 kcps/cm^2. The basic accuracy of measurements of activity distributions using the BOLPs-RGp was proved by studies on the PT-BOLPs. Activity distributions measured using the BOLPs-RGp were reconstructed by a back projection method with FOV including the axes of the beam direction and the vertical beam direction. The positional accuracy of activity with the gantry rotating is about 1 mm (1 sigma) by an experiment using ^{22}Na point source. A device to observe and analyze activity distributions measured using the BOLPs-RGp was also developed. The measured images are observed as planar images including the axes of the beam direction and the rotating angle of the gantry system using the device (see Fig. 13.20).

Let us show some clinical cases using the BOLPs-RGp for patients. Measurements for each treatment site of the head and neck, prostate, liver, lungs, and brain were performed using the BOLPs-RGp after proton irradiation. Activity of pairs of

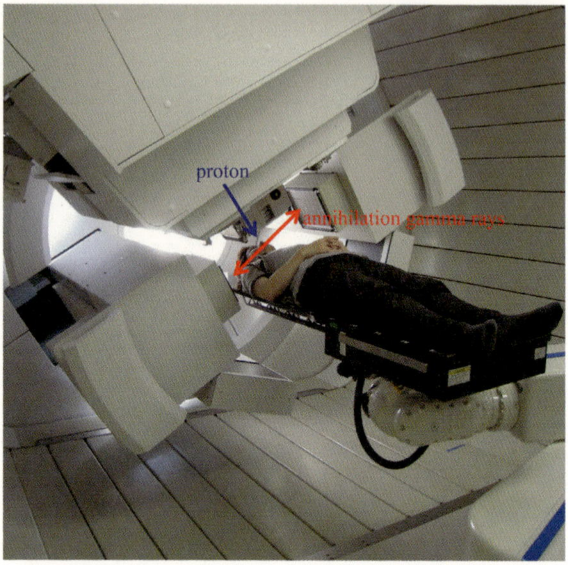

Fig. 13.18 Setup of the BOLPs-RGp in the proton treatment room

annihilation gamma rays was measured using the BOLPs-RGp, and the measurements began when each proton irradiation started, and they ended when 200 s elapsed from the end of each irradiation. Distances between the detector heads were set as close as possible to each of the patients. Activity data measured using the BOLPs-RGp during proton irradiation was almost background data including X-rays, gamma rays, and neutrons as the measurement data using the PT-BOLPs showed that previously. Therefore, the measured activity distributions were reconstructed without the data measured during irradiation. Two coefficients were considered in the reconstruction process using a back projection method. One is the attenuation coefficient, and the other is the collection coefficient of detection activity intensity. The former coefficient of 511-keV gamma rays in each patient's body was calculated using each patient's data on water equivalent length from each patient's CT image which was scanned for planning each treatment. The latter coefficient which depended on the point on the planar detectors was obtained from an experiment. Figure 13.21 shows examples of the calculated dose distributions and activity distributions measured using the BOLPs-RGp of each of the target sites for proton treatments. All the distributions shown in Fig. 13.21 are normalized at the isocenter in the treatment room. The mean detection rates of the activity measured using the BOLPs-RGp for 200 s after the irradiation were 1.58 kcps (head and neck), 1.39 kcps (liver), 0.53 kcps (lungs), 1.08 kcps (prostate), and 1.85 kcps (brain). In all the cases of liver and lungs, respiratory-gated proton beam therapy was performed, and the length of proton irradiation time was longer. Therefore, the measured mean detection rates for these treatment sites were lower than those for other sites by a decrease in activity intensity during proton irradiation. It can be said that all proton irradiation in this study seemed to be performed

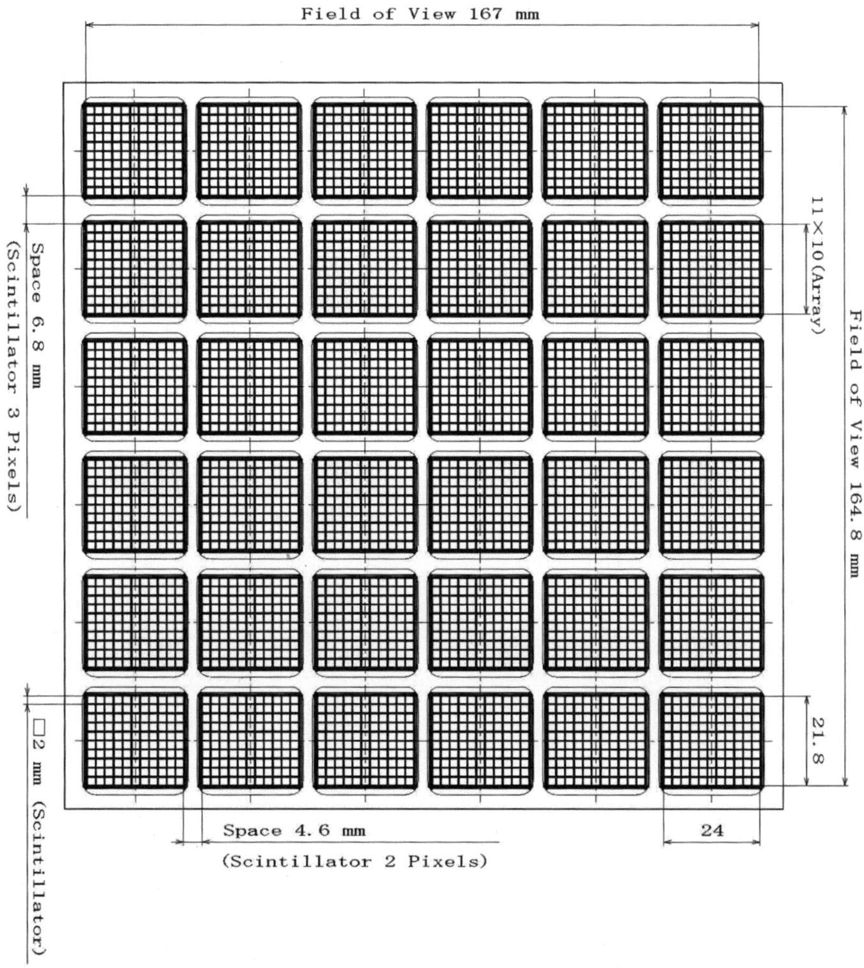

Fig. 13.19 Design for the detector head developed for the BOLPs-RGp

following the planed treatments by comparing calculated dose distributions with measured activity distributions visually.

Proton therapy utilizes Bragg peak which is one of the characteristics of proton dose distribution in the depth direction. That is, when proton beam stops before organs at risk (OAR) under our control, high dose irradiation is delivered to a target tumor located before the OAR in the beam direction. If there are some changes such as a reduction in target tumor size during a period of proton treatment, an unplanned region would be given the high dose irradiation which was supposed to give to the target. Observing changes in shapes of activity distributions which are obtained at daily proton treatment using the BOLPs enables us to verify whether daily proton irradiation is performed precisely. In a period of proton treatment, activity

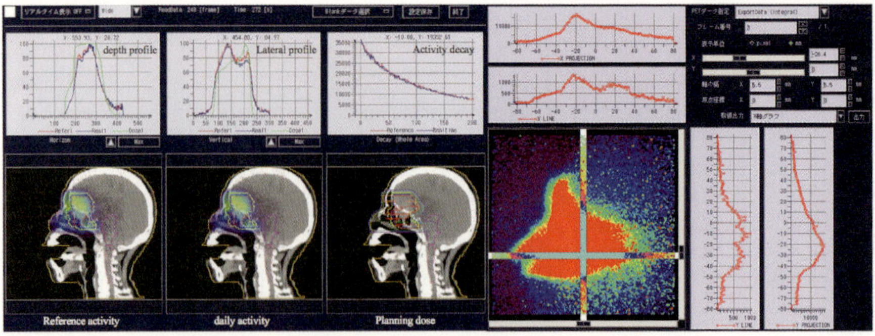

Fig. 13.20 Example screen on the device developed for observing and analyzing activity distributions measured using the BOLPs-RGp

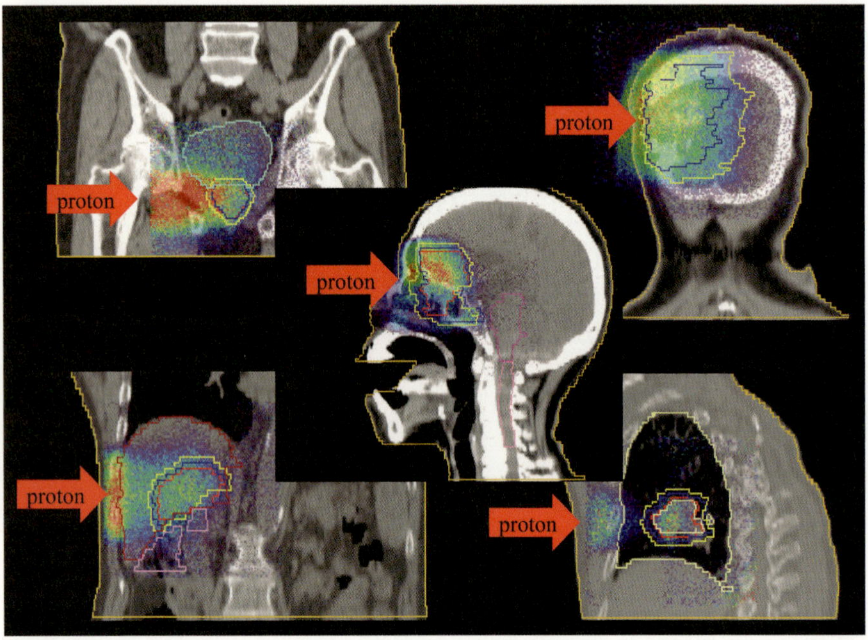

Fig. 13.21 Examples of the calculated dose distributions (color lines) and the activity distributions (color wash) measured using the BOLPs-RGp for each of the target sites. *Red* and *blue* express high and low activity in color wash, respectively

distribution measured at the first treatment day is used as a reference image, and differences between the reference and daily measured activity distributions are observed (see Fig. 13.22). Comparing shapes of these distributions makes it possible to confirm the irradiated regions in a tumor and OAR around the tumor every day and to guarantee the irradiation accuracy during a period of treatment. In the case of the head and neck especially paranasal sinus tumor, it is important to

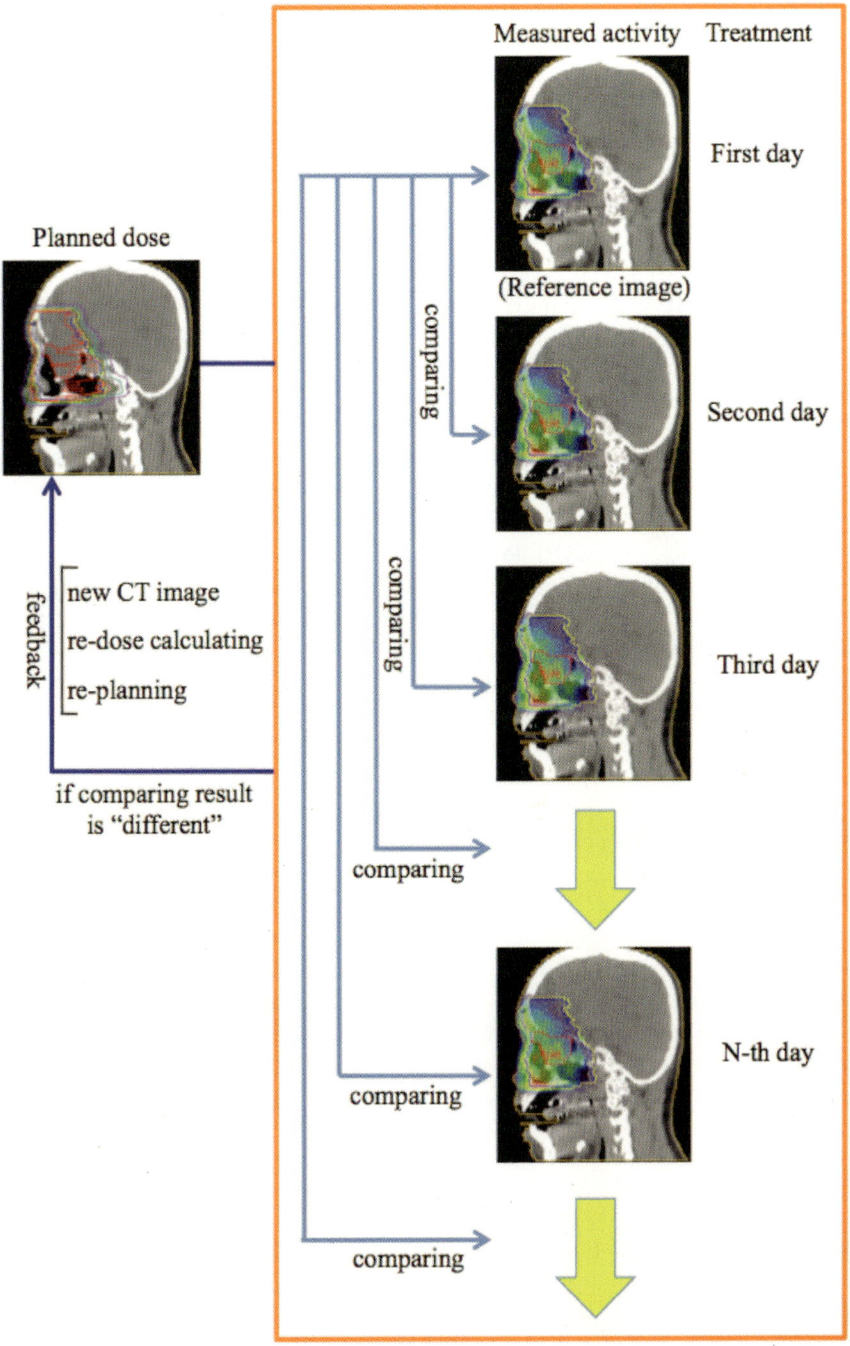

Fig. 13.22 Conceptual diagram of the use of the BOLPs-RGp in clinical proton therapy (Nishio et al. 2010)

perform proton irradiation with high accuracy because OAR such as the brain stem and optic nerves are adjacent to the tumor. In the case of paranasal sinus tumor, a treatment region including matter with different densities such as bone, air, and tumor causes deterioration in accuracy of dose calculation. Therefore, deterioration in dose concentration on the tumor or irradiation to OAR resulting from changes in tumor condition would lead to lowering the rate of treatment control and increasing the risk of serious damage.

Figure 13.23 shows the calculated dose distributions, the daily activity distributions measured using the BOLPs-RGp, and the daily projection profiles of the measured activity in the depth direction in the case of a patient with paranasal sinus tumor. Total prescription dose of 65-GyE was planned. Some changes in the measured activity distributions due to a reduction in tumor size were observed during the treatment days. Daily activity ranges which were obtained from daily measured activity distributions were longer by around 15 mm than the reference activity range which was obtained at the first treatment day, namely, the activity ranges seemed to be extended toward the brain stem. Another CT scan was performed and a new treatment plan was recalculated after prescribing 35-GyE (2.5 GyE $\times$ 14 fx. $=$ 35GyE) dose in this treatment case. We found out that the reduction in the tumor volume from 184 to 125 cc, the change in the maximum beam range by about 20 mmWEL, and the unplanned irradiation to the brain stem. The same procedure was conducted in other three cases of 46 cases of paranasal sinus tumor. Observing changes in measured activity distributions revealed unplanned irradiation to the brain stem caused by reductions in tumor volume and replanned new treatment plans. It indicates that proper proton treatments could be provided to the patients using the BOLP-RGp in clinical proton therapy.

The calculated dose distribution and the activity distribution which was measured for 200 s after the proton irradiation with 3.8-GyE prescription dose at the first treatment day in the case of the patient with liver tumor are shown in the upper Fig. 13.24. In this figure, the high activity region which was related to a necrotic region resulting from a pathological examination before starting proton treatment was observed in the tumor. Two regions of interest (ROI) are set; ROI area A is the necrotic region in the tumor, and ROI area B is the tumor region covering the necrotic region in the liver. The results of the number of detection counts per 20 s of activity in area A and B-A are shown in the lower Fig. 13.24. Area B-A is equivalent to the tumor region except the necrotic region. The results of decay curves in area A and B-A (see the lower right graph in Fig. 13.24) were fitted adequately using a double exponential equation. Shorter half-lives were 31 $\pm$ 8 s and 21 $\pm$ 4 s, and longer ones were 146 $\pm$ 20 s and 134 $\pm$ 11 s in area A and B-A, respectively. Both shorter and longer half-lives in the necrotic region (area A) were longer than those in the tumor region except the necrotic region (area B-A).

Figure 13.25 shows the activity distributions measured for 200 s using the BOLPs-RGp after each proton irradiation for the same patient. The high activity in the necrotic region decreased to the similar activity in the non-necrotic region around the necrosis with an increase of prescription dose. In the region of area A

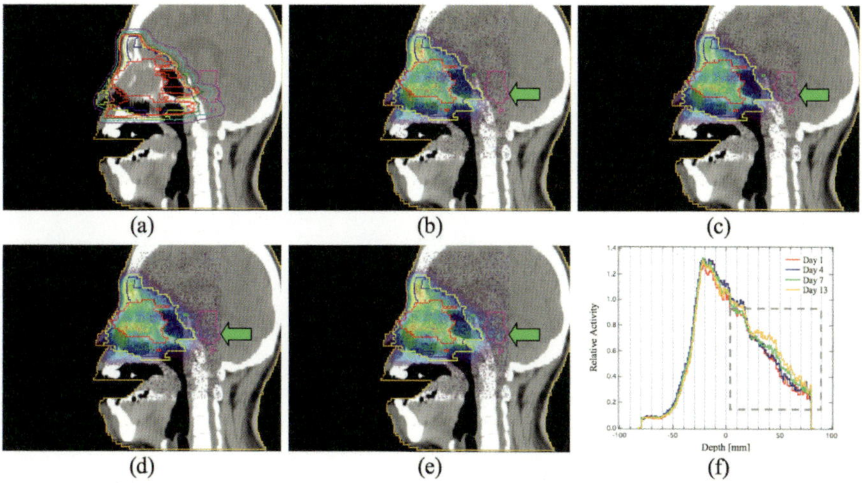

Fig. 13.23 In the case of the patient with paranasal sinus tumor, (**a**) the calculated dose distribution, the measured activity distributions using the BOLPs-RGp: (**b**) the first day, (**c**) the fourth day, (**d**) the 7th day, (**e**) the 13th day, and (**f**) the projection profiles in the depth direction (Nishio et al. 2010)

and B shown in the lower Fig. 13.24, the ratio F of the number of detection counts of activity at each prescription dose to that at the first treatment day is given by

$$F(D) = \frac{\int_0^{S_A} \left({dN(D)}/{dS} \right) dS \Big/ \int_0^{S_A} dS}{\int_{S_A}^{S_B} \left({dN(D)}/{dS} \right) dS \Big/ \int_{S_A}^{S_B} dS}, \tag{13.21}$$

where D is the delivery dose, N is the detection number, S_A is the square of area A, and S_B is the square of area B. The result of calculations using Eq. 13.21 was shown in Fig. 13.25. The activity in the necrotic region noticeably decreased with an increase of prescription dose. This result indicates that each prescription dose can be determined for each one of patients, in consideration of individual sensibility to doses, which is absolutely essential for the next step in proton therapy. Dose-volume delivery-guided proton therapy (DGPT) which is a proton therapy with observation of individual sensibility to doses during a treatment period will be established as the most advanced and unique proton therapy.

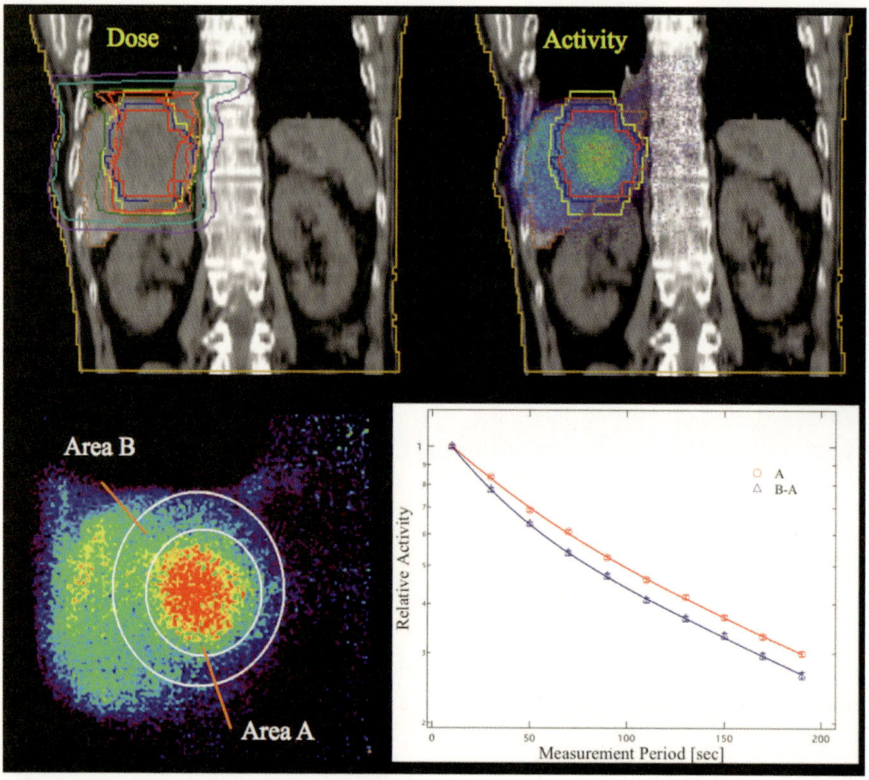

Fig. 13.24 Calculated dose distribution, the measured activity distribution, and the results of the number of detection counts per 20 s of activity in area A and B-A using the BOLPs-RGp in the case of the liver tumor including the necrotic region (Nishio et al. 2010)

13.6 Summary

The BOLPs were developed for imaging of regions irradiated by proton beam using target nuclear fragment reactions, and the imaging was realized. The results of these studies on the BOLPs indicate that the clinical use of the BOLPs-RGp leads to dose concentration on target tumors, a reduction in doses which are delivered to organs at risk, and the potential to verify dose sensibility of each patient during a period of proton treatment. We are able to take advantage of various techniques, technologies, and results of imaging activity from positron-emitting nuclei generated in a patient's body by radiation irradiation for the fields of not only proton therapy but also popular high-energy X-ray therapy and other particle therapies (Nishio et al. 2007). The results of these studies for providing proton therapy with more accuracy and safety would expand in many fields of cancer treatment.

There are a lot of matters to solve in order to establish techniques and technology for imaging of proton-irradiated regions. Lots of values of cross section of target

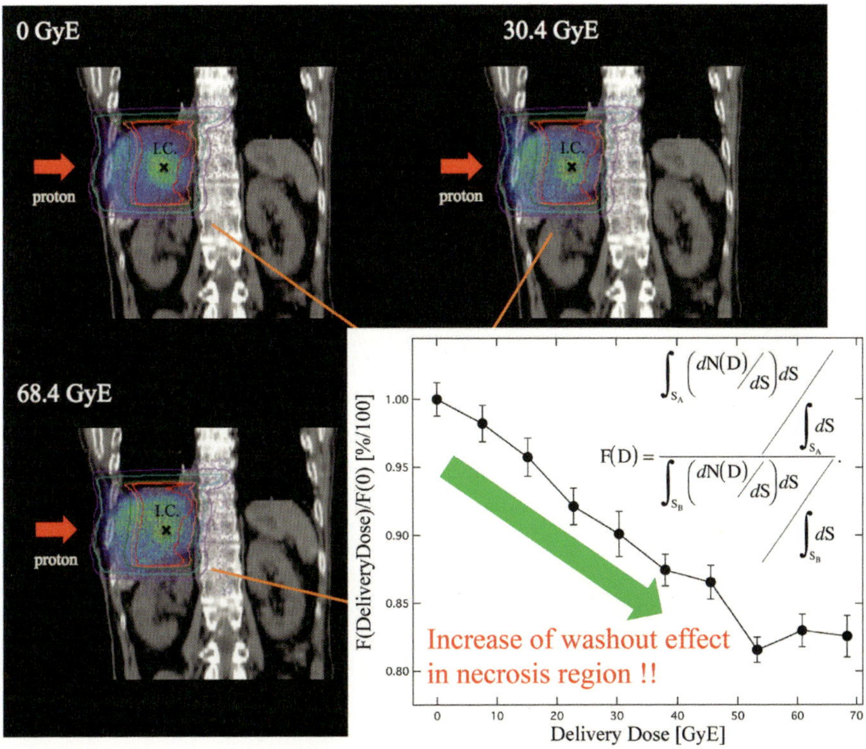

Fig. 13.25 Activity distributions measured for 200 s using the BOPS-RGp after each proton irradiation in the case of the liver tumor including the necrotic region and the ratio of the measured counts of activity using Eq. 13.21 (Nishio et al. 2010)

nuclear fragment reactions have been left with uncertainty. It is necessary to obtain the cross section data systematically (Matsushita et al. 2016), and views and knowledge from basic physics including nuclear physics must be the key to obtain that. It is also necessary to establish methods of assigning information of CT images to elemental composition of organs accurately and to develop techniques of simulating activity distribution (Miyatake et al. 2011; Miyatake and Nishio 2013). To solve those necessities, collaboration with other fields such as basis physics is needed over the boundaries of fields. One of the most significant studies for the radiation therapy future is the realization of tailor-made particle therapy for each patent with observation of individual response to doses from tumors. A further study is being done using the results of these studies. Tumor response observation system of observing dose response has both PET system and Compton camera system, which can detect prompt and annihilation gamma rays emitted from irradiated regions during and after irradiation with high positional accuracy and high efficiency (see Fig. 13.26) (JST SENTAN). The important thing is to carry out research and development in order to improve the standard of cancer treatment and

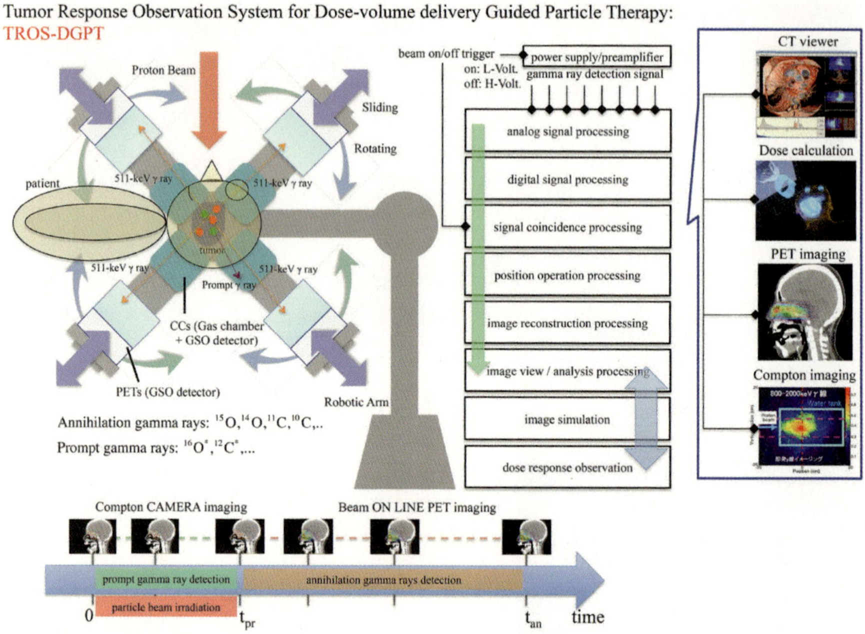

Fig. 13.26 Conceptual diagram of tumor response observation system for dose-volume delivery-guided particle therapy, TROS-DGPT

provide high accurate cancer treatment to more patients by establishing cooperative relationship over various fields.

References

Bennett GW, Goldberg AC, Levine GS, Guthy J, Balsamo J, Archambeau JO (1975) Beam localization via O-15 activation in proton-radiation therapy. Nucl Inst Methods 125:333–338

Bennett GW, Archambeau JO, Archambeau BE, Meltzer JI, Wingate CL (1978) Visualization and transport of positron emission from proton activation in vivo. Science 200:1151–1153

Boellaard R, Lingen AV, Lammertsma AA (2001) Experimental and clinical evaluation of iterative reconstruction (OSEM) in dynamic PET: quantitative characteristics and effects on kinetic modeling. J Nucl Med 42:808–817

Goldhaber AS (1974) Statistical models of fragmentation processes. Phys Lett B53(4):306–308

Hishikawa Y, Kagawa K, Murakami M, Sakai H, Akagi T, Abe M (2002) Usefulness of positron-emission tomographic images after proton therapy. Int J Radiat Oncol Biol Phys 53:1388–1391

ICRU Report 46 (1992) Photon, electron, proton and neutron interaction date for body tissues. JST SENTAN Grant Number 13A1101

Litzenberg DW, Bajema JF, Becchetti FD, Brown JA, Roberts DA, Caraher J, Hutchins G, Ronningen R, Smith R, Abbot M (1992) On-line monitoring and PET imaging of proton radiotherapy beams. IEEE MIC, Orlando, FL, 25–31 October 1992, pp 954–956

Litzenberg DW, Roberts DA, Lee MY, Pham K, Vander Molen AM, Ronningen R, Becchetti FD (1999) On-line monitoring of radiotherapy beams: experimental results with proton beams. Med Phys 26:992–1006

Matsushita K, Nishio T, Tanaka S, Tsuneda M, Sugiura A, Ieki K (2016) Measurement of proton-induced target fragmentation cross-section in carbon. Nucl Phys A 946:104–116

Miyatake A, Nishio T, Ogino T, Saijo N, Esumi H, Uesaka M (2010) Measurement and verification of positron emitter nuclei generated at each treatment site by target nuclear fragment reactions in proton therapy. Med Phys 37(8):4445–4455

Miyatake A, Nishio T, Ogino T (2011) Development of activity pencil beam algorithm using measured distribution data of positron emitter nuclei generated by proton irradiation of targets containing ^{12}C, ^{16}O and ^{40}Ca nuclei in preparation of clinical application. Med Phys 38 (10):5818–5829

Miyatake A, Nishio T (2013) Application of activity pencil beam algorithm using measured distribution data of positron emitter nuclei for therapeutic SOBP proton beam. Med Phys 40 (9):091709-1-9

Nishio T (1999) Proton therapy facility at National Cancer Center, Kashiwa, Japan. J Energy Soc 41(11):1134–1138

Nishio T, Ogino T, Shimbo M, Katsuta S, Murakami T, Sato T, Kojima Y, Murakami K, Ikeda H (2001) Distributions of β+ decayed nucleus produced from the target fragment reaction in (CH2) n and patient liver targets by using a proton beam for therapy. Abstracts of the XXXIV PTCOG MEETING in Boston, pp 15–16

Nishio T, Sato T, Kitamura H, Murakami K, Ogino T (2005) Distributions of β+ decayed nuclei generated in the CH2 and H2O targets by the target nuclear fragment reaction using therapeutic MONO and SOBP proton beam. Med Phys 32:1070–1082

Nishio T, Ogino T, Nomura K, Uchida H (2006) Dose–volume delivery guided proton therapy using beam on-line PET system. Med Phys 33:4190–4197

Nishio T, Inaniwa T, Inoue K, Miyatake A, Nakagawa K, Yoda K, Ogino T (2007) Experimental verification of the utility of positron emitter nuclei generated by photonuclear reactions for the X-ray beam monitoring in a phantom. Radiat Med 25(10):516–522

Nishio T, Miyatake A, Inoue K, Katsuta S, Gomi-Miyagishi T, Kohno R, Kameoka S, Nakagawa K, Ogino T (2008) Experimental verification of proton beam monitoring in a human body by use of activity image of positron-emitting nuclei generated by nuclear fragmentation reaction. Radiol Phys Technol 1(1):44–54

Nishio T, Miyatake A, Ogino T, Nakagawa K, Saijo N, Esumi H (2010) The development and clinical use of a Beam ON-LINE PET system mounted on a rotating gantry port in proton therapy. Int J Radiat Oncol Biol Phys 76(1):277–286

NNDC (2016) http://www.nndc.bnl.gov/

Oelfke U, Lam GK, Atkins MS (1996) Proton dose monitoring with PET: quantitative studies in Lucite. Phys Med Biol 41:177–196

Paans AMJ, Schippers JM (1993) Proton therapy in combination with PET as monitor: a feasibility study. IEEE Trans Nucl Sci 40:1041–1044

Parodi K, Enghardt W (2000) Potential application of PET in quality assurance of proton therapy. Phys Med Biol 45:N151–N156

Parodi K, Enghardt W, Haberer T (2002) In-beam PET measurements of β+ radioactivity induced by proton beams. Phys Med Biol 47:21–36

Parodi K, Pönisch F, Enghardt W (2005) Experimental study on the feasibility of in-beam PET for accurate monitoring of proton therapy. IEEE Trans Nucl Sci 52:778–786

Parodi K, Paganetti H, Shih HA, Michaud S, Loeffler JS, Delaney TF, Liebsch NJ, Munzenrider JE, Fischman AJ, Knopf A, Bortfeld T (2007c) Patient study of in vivo verification of beam delivery and range, using positron emission tomography and computed tomography imaging after proton therapy. Int J Radiat Oncol Biol Phys 68:920–934

Parodi K, Ferrari A, Sommerer F, Paganetti H (2007a) Clinical CT-based calculations of dose and positron emitter distributions in proton therapy using the FLUKA Monte Carlo code. Phys Med Biol 52:3369–3387

Parodi K, Paganetti H, Cascio E, Flanz JB, Bonab AA, Alpert NM, Lohmann K, Bortfeld T (2007b) PET/CT imaging for treatment verification after proton therapy-a study with plastic phantoms and metallic implants. Med Phys 34:419–435

PTCOG Data (2016): http://www.ptcog.ch/index.php/facilities-in-operation

Sihver L, Tsao CH, Silberberg R, Kanai T, Barghouty AF (1993) Total reaction and partial cross section calculations in proton-nucleus and nucleus-nucleus reactions. Phys Rev C47:1225–1236

Uchida H, Okamoto T, Ohmura T, Shimizu K, Satoh N, Koike T, Yamashita T (2004) A compact planar positron imaging system. Nucl Inst Methods A516:564–574

Vynckier S, Derreumaux S, Richard F, Bol A, Michel C, Wambersie A (1993) Is it possible to verify directly a proton-treatment plan using positron emission tomography? Radiother Oncol 26:275–277

Part V
Computerized Prediction of Treatment Outcomes

Chapter 14
Computerized Prediction of Treatment Outcomes and Radiomics Analysis

Issam El Naqa

Abstract Imaging has been traditionally used in radiotherapy for the purposes of tumor delineation and treatment planning. Recent evidence suggests that such imaging information could be also used as biomarkers for predicting response and personalized treatment as part of an emerging field called "radiomics." In this chapter, we discuss the application of imaging-based approaches to predict radiotherapy outcomes from single and hybrid imaging modalities. We describe the different steps involved in radiomics analysis and present examples from our own experiences. We highlight the current challenges and future potentials for image-based decision support in radiotherapy.

Keywords Radiotherapy • Outcomes prediction • Radiomics

14.1 Introduction

kV X-ray computed tomography (kV-CT) has been historically considered the standard modality for treatment planning in 3D conformal (3DCRT) or intensity-modulated radiotherapy (IMRT) because of its ability to provide electron density information for heterogeneous dose calculations (Khan 2007; Webb 2001). However, additional information from other imaging modalities could be also used to improve treatment monitoring and prognosis in different cancer sites (El Naqa et al. 2009; Kumar et al. 2012; Lambin et al. 2012). Physiological information (tumor metabolism, proliferation, necrosis, hypoxic regions, etc.) can be collected directly from nuclear imaging modalities such as single-photon emission computed tomography (SPECT) and positron emission tomography (PET) or indirectly from magnetic resonance imaging (MRI) (Condeelis and Weissleder 2010; Willmann et al. 2008). The complementary nature of these different imaging modalities has led to efforts toward combining information to achieve better treatment outcomes. For instance, PET/CT has been utilized for staging, planning, and assessment of

I. El Naqa, PhD, DABR (✉)
Department of Radiation Oncology, Physics Division, University of Michigan, Ann Arbor, MI 48103, USA
e-mail: ielnaqa@med.umich.edu

H. Arimura (ed.), *Image-Based Computer-Assisted Radiation Therapy*,
DOI 10.1007/978-981-10-2945-5_14

response to radiation therapy in lung (Verhagen et al. 2004; Bradley et al. 2004a, b; Bradley 2004; Erdi et al. 2000; Mac Manus and Hicks 2003; Mac Manus et al. 2003; MacManus et al. 2003; Pandit et al. 2003; Toloza et al. 2003), gynecological (Mutic et al. 2003; Miller and Grigsby 2002), and colorectal cancers (Ciernik 2004). Similarly, MRI has been applied in tumor delineation and assessing toxicities in head and neck cancer (Newbold et al. 2006; Piet et al. 2008). Most recently, PET/MR has started to make its appearance in the field (Zaidi et al. 2007; Thorwarth et al. 2013). There are accumulating evidences that pretreatment or posttreatment information from anatomical or particularly functional imaging could be used to monitor and predict treatment outcomes in radiotherapy. For instance, changes in tumor volume captured on CT images may be predictive of local control in lung cancer (Seibert et al. 2007; Ramsey et al. 2006). Interestingly, a study showed that rectum status (full/empty) or the presence of bowel gas at the time of treatment simulations predicts for treatment failure (Stasi et al. 2006) and the risk of rectal bleeding(de Crevoisier et al. 2005), probably due to a shift of the dose field compared to anatomy upon delivery. However, functional/molecular imaging and in particular fluorodeoxyglucose (FDG)-PET, a glucose metabolism analog, has shown promise as a potential prognostic factor for predicting radiotherapy efficacy or potential side effects. The primary focus in the literature to this point has been directed toward simple metrics describing the FDG image, especially maximum standardized uptake values (SUV_{max}). A few attempts have been made to extend this analysis to include image features. A visual assessment method was used in Kalff et al. to evaluate heterogeneity in FDG images for patients with locally advanced rectal carcinoma (Kalff et al. 2006). Hicks et al. applied a simple pattern recognition technique to FDG images for lung cancer and found that normal tissue inflammatory changes were linked to tumor responsiveness (Hicks et al. 2004). A shape metric based on the deviation from an idealized ellipsoid structure (i.e., eccentricity) was found to have strong association with survival in patients with soft tissue sarcoma (STS) (O'Sullivan et al. 2003, 2005). Beside FDG-PET, other PET tracers have been shown to be useful in interrogating tumor properties such as: hypoxia by fluoromisonidazole (FMISO) or copper (II)-diacetyl-bis (N4-methylthiosemicarbazone (Cu-ATSM) and deoxyribonucleic acid (DNA) synthesis and cell proliferation by fluorothymidine (FLT) (Shields 2006). On the other hand, dynamic contrast-enhanced MRI (DCE-MRI), a perfusion surrogate, was used to assess treatment response of soft tissue sarcoma (Shapeero et al. 2002; van Rijswijk et al. 2003; Vanel et al. 2004), and apparent diffusion coefficient (ADC) values from diffusion-weighted MRI (DW-MRI), a measure of water molecule diffusion (Brownian motion) in tissue, were significantly correlated with sarcoma response to radiotherapy (Einarsdottir et al. 2004). Recently, hybrid imaging modalities PET/CT and PET/MR have been applied. Benz et al. showed that combined assessment of metabolic and volumetric changes predicts tumor response in patients with sarcoma (Benz et al., Benz M et al. 2008). Similarly, Yang et al. showed that the combined evaluation of contrast-enhanced CT and FDG-PET/CT predicts the clinical outcomes in patients with aggressive non-Hodgkin's lymphoma (Yang et al. 2009). Denecke et al. compared CT, MRI, and FDG-PET in the prediction of outcomes to neoadjuvant radiochemotherapy in patients with locally advanced primary rectal cancer, demonstrating sensitivities of 100 % for FDG-PET, 54 % for CT, and 71 % for MRI and specificities of 60 % for FDG-PET, 80 % for CT, and 67 % for MRI (Denecke et al. 2005).

In this chapter, we discuss the development of image-based models to predict radiotherapy outcomes from single and hybrid imaging modalities.

14.2 Imaging as a Biomarker of Radiotherapy Response (Radiomics)

The extraction of quantitative information from imaging modalities and relating information to biological and clinical endpoints is a new emerging field referred to as "radiomics" (Lambin et al. 2012; Kumar et al. 2012).

Radiomics could be thought of as consisting of two main steps: (1) extraction of relevant static and dynamic imaging features and (2) incorporating these features into mathematical model to predict outcomes as discussed in the following subsections.

14.2.1 Image Feature Extraction

The features extracted from images could be divided into static (time invariant) and dynamic (time variant) features according to the acquisition protocol at the time of scanning and into pre- or intra-treatment features according to the scanning time point (El Naqa 2014).

14.2.1.1 Static Image Features

(a) *Standardized uptake value (SUV) or Hounsfield unit (HU) descriptors*: SUV is a standard image quantification method particularly used in PET analysis (Strauss and Conti 1991); likewise, HU is used in CT. In this case, raw intensity values are converted into SUVs/HUs, and statistical descriptors such as maximum, minimum, mean, standard deviation (SD), and coefficient of variation (CV) are extracted.
(b) Total *lesion glycolysis (TLG)*: This is also used in FDG-PET and is defined as the product of volume and mean SUV (Benz et al., Benz M et al. 2008; Erdi et al. 2000; Larson et al. 1999).
(c) *Intensity volume histogram (IVH)*: This is analogous to the dose-volume histogram (DVH) widely used in radiotherapy treatment planning in reducing complicated 3D data into a single easier to interpret curve. Each point on the

IVH defines the absolute or relative volume of the structure that exceeds a variable intensity threshold as a percentage of the maximum intensity (El Naqa et al. 2009). This method would allow for extracting several metrics from images for outcome analysis such as I_x (minimum intensity to x % highest intensity volume), V_x (percentage volume having at least x % intensity value), and descriptive statistics (mean, minimum, maximum, standard deviation, etc.). We have reported the use of the IVH for predicting local control in lung cancer (Vaidya et al. 2012), where a combined metric from PET and CT image-based model provided a superior prediction power compared to commonly used dosimteric-based models of local treatment response. More details are provided in the example of Sect. 14.3.1.

(d) *Morphological features*: These are generally geometrical shape attributes such as eccentricity (a measure of non-circularity), which is useful for describing tumor growth directionality, and Euler number (the number of connected objects in a region minus the solidity (this is a measurement of convexity), which may be a characteristics of benign lesions (Jain 1989; O'Sullivan et al. 2005). An interesting demonstration of this principle is that a shaped-based metric based on the deviation from an idealized ellipsoid structure (i.e., eccentricity) was found to have strong association with survival in patients with sarcoma (O'Sullivan et al. 2003, 2005).

(e) *Texture features*: Texture in imaging refers to the relative distribution of intensity values within a given neighborhood. It integrates intensity with spatial information resulting in higher-order histograms when compared to common first-order intensity histograms. It should be emphasized that texture metrics are independent of tumor position, orientation, size, and brightness and take into account the local intensity spatial distribution (Castleman 1996; Haralick et al. 1973). This is a crucial advantage over direct (first-order) histogram metrics (e.g., mean and standard deviation), which only measures intensity variability independent of the spatial distribution in the tumor microenvironment. Texture methods are broadly divided into three categories: statistical methods (e.g., high-order statistics, co-occurrence matrices, moment invariants), model-based methods (e.g., Markov random fields, Gabor filter, wavelet transform), and structural methods (e.g., topological descriptors, fractals) (Zhang and Tan 2002; Castellano et al. 2004). Among these methods, statistical approaches based on the co-occurrence matrix and its variants such as the gray-level co-occurrence matrix (GLCM), neighborhood gray-tone difference matrix (NGTDM), run-length matrix (RLM), and gray-level size zone matrix (GLSZM) have been widely applied for characterizing tumor heterogeneity in images (Chicklore et al. 2013). Four commonly used features from the GLCM include energy, entropy, contrast, and homogeneity (Haralick et al. 1973). The NGTDM is thought to provide more humanlike perception of texture such as coarseness, contrast, busyness, and complexity. RLM and GLSZM emphasize regional effects. More details are provided in the example of 14.3.2.

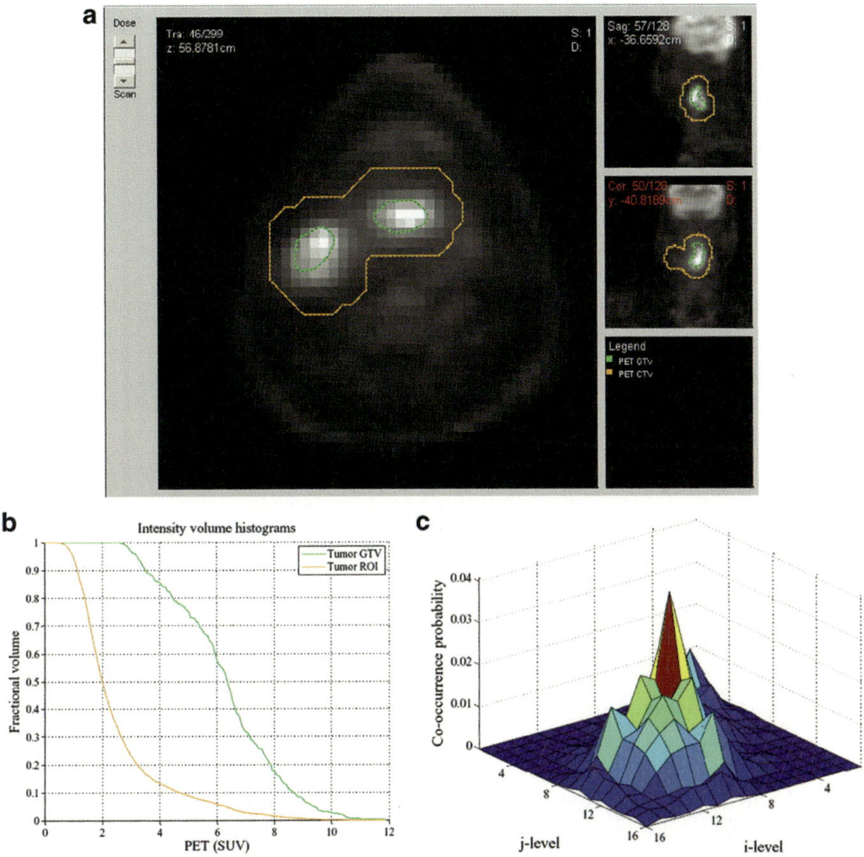

Fig. 14.1 (**a**) A pretreatment PET scan of a head and neck cancer case of patient who died from disease after radiotherapy treatment. The head and neck tumor region of interest (*brown*) and the gross tumor volume (GTV) (*green*) were outlined by the physician. (**b**) an IVH plot, where Ix and Vx parameters are derived. (**c**) A texture map plot of the GTV heterogeneity through intensity spatial mapping

An example of different feature extraction from PET in the case of head and neck cancer is shown in Fig. 14.1.

14.2.1.2 Dynamic Image Features

The dynamic features are extracted from time-varying acquisitions such as dynamic PET or MR. These features are based on kinetic analysis using tissue compartment models and parameters related to transport and binding rates (Watabe et al. 2006; Tofts 1997). Recently, using kinetic approaches, Thorwarth et al. published provocative data on the scatter of voxel-based measures of local perfusion and hypoxia in the head and neck (Thorwarth et al. 2006, 2007). Tumors showing widespread in

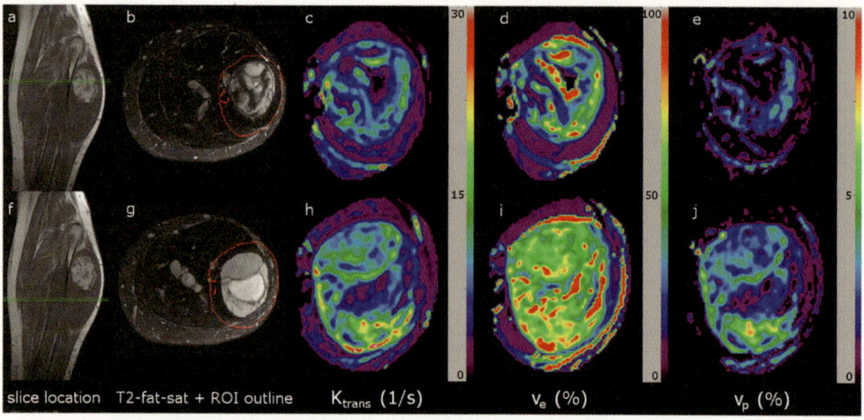

Fig. 14.2 Dynamic features extracted from DCE-MRI in case of soft tissue sarcoma in the *lower leg*. Data are presented for two slices (*top* and *bottom row*, respectively), showing (*a, f*) slice position on a coronal T1-weighted image, (*b, g*) a fat-saturated high-resolution T2-weighted image of the slice with region-of-interest outlined, (*c, h*) the trans-endothelial transfer constant K_{trans} (in 1/s), (*d, i*) the extravascular, extracellular space volume fraction *ve* (%), and (*e, j*) the blood volume fraction (*bv*) (%)

both characteristics showed less reoxygenation during RT and had worse local control. An example from DCE-MRI is shown in Fig. 14.2, in which a three-compartment model is used and extracted parameters include the transfer constant (K_{trans}), the extravascular-extracellular volume fraction (*ve*), and the blood volume (*bv*) (Sourbron and Buckley, Sourbron and Buckley 2011). A rather interesting approach to improve the robustness of such features is the use of advanced 4D iterative techniques (Reader et al. 2006). Further improvement could be achieved by utilizing multi-resolution transformations (e.g., wavelet transform) to stabilize kinetic parameter estimates spatially (Turkheimer et al. 2006).

14.2.2 Outcome Modeling

Outcomes in radiation oncology are generally characterized by two metrics: tumor control probability (TCP) and the surrounding normal tissue complication probability (NTCP) (Steel 2002; Webb 2001). The dose-response explorer system (DREES) is a dedicated software tool for modeling of radiotherapy outcome (El Naqa et al. 2006c). A detailed review of outcome modeling in radiotherapy is presented in our previous work (El Naqa 2013). In the context of image-based treatment outcome modeling, the observed outcome (e.g., TCP or NTCP) is considered to be adequately captured by extracted image features (El Naqa et al. 2009; El-Naqa et al. 2004), where complementary imaging information are built into a data-driven model such as classical logistic regression approaches or more advanced machine learning techniques.

14.2.2.1 Outcome Modeling by Logistic Regression

Logistic modeling is a common tool for multi-metric modeling. In our previous work (Deasy and El Naqa 2007; El Naqa et al. 2006a), a logit transformation was used:

$$f(\mathbf{x}_i) = \frac{e^{g(\mathbf{x}_i)}}{1 + e^{g(\mathbf{x}_i)}}, i = 1, \ldots, n, \tag{14.1}$$

where n is the number of cases (patients), and $\mathbf{x}_i$ is a vector of the input variable values (i.e., image features) used to predict $f(\mathbf{x}_i)$ for outcome y_i (i.e., TCP or NTCP) of the i_{th}:

$$g(\mathbf{x}_i) = \beta_o + \sum_{j=1}^{d} \beta_j x_{ij}, i = 1, \ldots, n, j = 1, \ldots, d, \tag{14.2}$$

where d is the number of model variables, and the β's are the set of model coefficients determined by maximizing the probability that the data gave rise to the observations.

14.2.2.2 Outcome Modeling by Machine Learning

Machine learning represents a wide class of artificial intelligence techniques (e.g., neural networks, decision trees, support vector machines), which are able to emulate human intelligence by learning the surrounding environment from the given input data. These methods are increasingly being utilized in radiation oncology because of their ability to detect nonlinear patterns in the data (El Naqa et al. 2015a). This is due to their ability to detect complex patterns in heterogeneous datasets with superior results when compared to state of the art in each of these disciplines. In particular, neural networks were extensively investigated to model post-radiation treatment outcomes for cases of lung injury (Munley et al. 1999; Su et al. 2005) and biochemical failure and rectal bleeding in prostate cancer (Gulliford et al. 2004; Tomatis et al. 2012). A rather more robust approach of machine learning methods is kernel-based methods and its favorite technique of support vector machines (SVMs), which are universal constructive learning procedures based on the statistical learning theory (Vapnik 1998). Learning is defined in this context as estimating dependencies from data (Hastie et al. 2001).

There are two common types of learning: supervised and unsupervised. Supervised learning is used to estimate an unknown (input, output) mapping from known (input, output) samples (e.g., classification or regression). In unsupervised learning, only input samples are given to the learning system (e.g., clustering or dimensionality reduction). In image-based outcome modeling, we focus mainly on supervised learning, wherein the endpoints of the treatments such as TCP or NTCP are provided by experienced oncologists in our case.

For discrimination between patients who are at low risk versus patients who are at high risk of radiation therapy, the main idea of SVM would be to separate these two classes with "hyperplanes" that maximize the margin between them in the nonlinear feature space defined by implicit kernel mapping as shown in Fig. 14.3. The objective here is to minimize the bounds on the generalization error of a model on unseen data before rather than minimizing the mean-square error over the training dataset itself (data fitting). Mathematically, the optimization problem could be formulated as minimizing the following cost function:

$$L(\mathbf{w}, \xi) = \frac{1}{2}\mathbf{w}^T\mathbf{w} + C\sum_{i=1}^{n} \xi_i \tag{14.3}$$

subject to the constraint:

$$\begin{aligned} y_i(\mathbf{w}^T \Phi(\mathbf{x}_i) + b) \geq 1 - \zeta_i \qquad i = 1, 2, ..., n \\ \zeta_i \geq 0 \ \text{ for all } i \end{aligned} \tag{14.4}$$

where $\mathbf{w}$is a weighting vector and $\Phi(\cdot)$is a nonlinear mapping function. The ζ_i represents the tolerance error allowed for each sample to be on the wrong side of the margin (called hinge loss). Note that minimization of the first term in Eq. (14.3) increases the separation (margin) between the two classes, whereas minimization of the second term improves fitting accuracy. The trade-off between complexity (or margin separation) and fitting error is controlled by the regularization parameter C. However, such a nonlinear formulation would suffer from the curse of dimensionality (i.e., the dimensions of the problem become too large to solve) (Haykin 1999; Hastie et al. 2001). Therefore, the dual optimization problem is solved instead of Eq. (14.3), which is convex complexity becomes dependent only on the number of samples and not on the dimensionality of the feature space. The prediction function in this case is characterized by only a subset of the training data, each of which are then known as "support vectors" s_i:

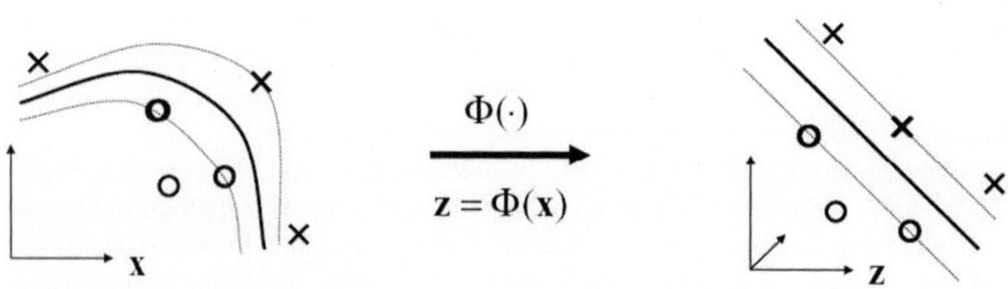

Fig. 14.3 Kernel-based mapping from a lower dimensional space (X) to a higher dimensional space (Z) called the feature space, where non-linearly separable classes become linearly separable

$$f(\mathbf{x}) = \sum_{i=1}^{n_s} \alpha_i y_i K(\mathbf{s}_i, \mathbf{x}) + \alpha_0, \tag{14.5}$$

where n_s is the number of support vectors (i.e., samples at the boundary as in fig. 14.3), α_i are the dual coefficients determined by quadratic programming, and $K(\cdot, \cdot)$ is the kernel function. Typical kernels (mapping functionals) include:

$$\begin{aligned} &\text{Polynomials} &&: K(\mathbf{x}, \mathbf{x}') = (\mathbf{x}^T\mathbf{x}' + c)^q \\ &\text{Radial basis function (RBF)} &&: K(\mathbf{x}, \mathbf{x}') = \exp\left(-\frac{1}{2\sigma^2}\|\mathbf{x} - \mathbf{x}'\|^2\right), \end{aligned} \tag{14.6}$$

where c is a constant, q is the order of the polynomial, and σ is the width of the radial basis functions. Note that the kernel in these cases acts as a similarity function between sample points in the feature space. Moreover, kernels enjoy closure properties, i.e., one can create admissible composite kernels by weighted addition and multiplication of elementary kernels. This flexibility allows for the construction of a neural network by using a combination of sigmoidal kernels. Alternatively, one could choose a logistic regression equivalent kernel by proper choice of the objective function in Eq. (14.3). In Fig. 14.4, we show an example for the application of machine learning to predict local failure in lung cancer (El Naqa et al. 2010).

14.3 Radiomics Examples in Different Cancer Sites

In the following, we will provide two representative cases of image-based outcome modeling and discuss the processes involved in such development. In one case, we will use separate extracted features from PET and CT for predicting tumor control in lung cancer. In the other case, fused extracted features from PET and MR are used to predict distant metastasis to the lung in soft tissue sarcoma.

14.3.1 Predicting TCP in Lung Cancer

In a retrospective study of 30 non-small cell lung cancer (NSCLC) patients, 30 features were extracted from both PET and CT images with and without motion correction as shown in Fig. 14.5.

The features included tumor volume; SUV/HU measurements, such as mean, minimum, maximum, and the standard deviation; IVH metrics; and texture-based features such as energy, contrast, local homogeneity, and entropy. The data corrected for motion artifacts based on a population-averaged probability spread function (PSF) using deconvolution methods derived from four 4D CT datasets

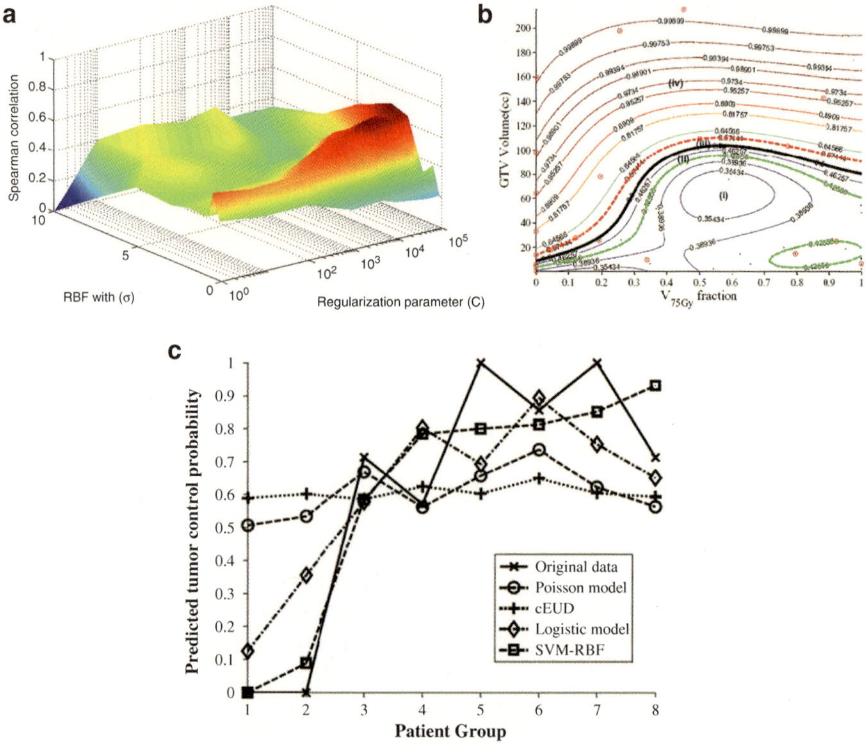

Fig. 14.4 Kernel-based modeling of TCP in lung cancer using gross tumor volume (GTV) and volume receiving 75 Gy (V75) with support vector machine (SVM) and a radial basis function (RBF) kernel. (**a**) Kernel-based modeling of TCP in lung cancer using the GTV volume and V75 with support vector machine (SVM) and a radial basis function (RBF) kernel. (**a**) Scatter plot of patient data (*black dots*) being superimposed with failure cases represented with red circles. Kernel parameter selection on leave-one-out cross-validation (LOO-CV) with peak predictive power attained at $\sigma=2$ and $C=10{,}000$. (**b**) Plot of the kernel-based local failure (1-TCP) nonlinear prediction model with four different risk regions: (1) area of low-risk patients with high confidence prediction level, (2) area of low-risk patients with lower confidence prediction level, (3) area of high-risk patients with lower confidence prediction level, and (4) area of high-risk patients with high confidence prediction level. Note that patients within the "margin" (cases ii and iii) represent intermediate-risk patients, which have border characteristics that could belong to either risk group. (**c**) A TCP comparison plot of different models as a function of patients' being binned into equal groups using the model with highest predictive power (SVM-RBF). The SVM-RBF is compared to Poisson-based TCP, cEUD, and best two-parameter logistic model. It is noted that prediction of low-risk (*high control*) patients is quite similar; however, the SVM-RBF provides a significant superior performance in predicting high-risk (*low control*) patients

(El Naqa et al. 2006b). An example of such features in this case is shown in Fig. 14.6.

Using modeling approaches described in Sect. 14.2.2 and implemented in the DREES software, Fig. 14.7 shows the results for predicting local failure, which

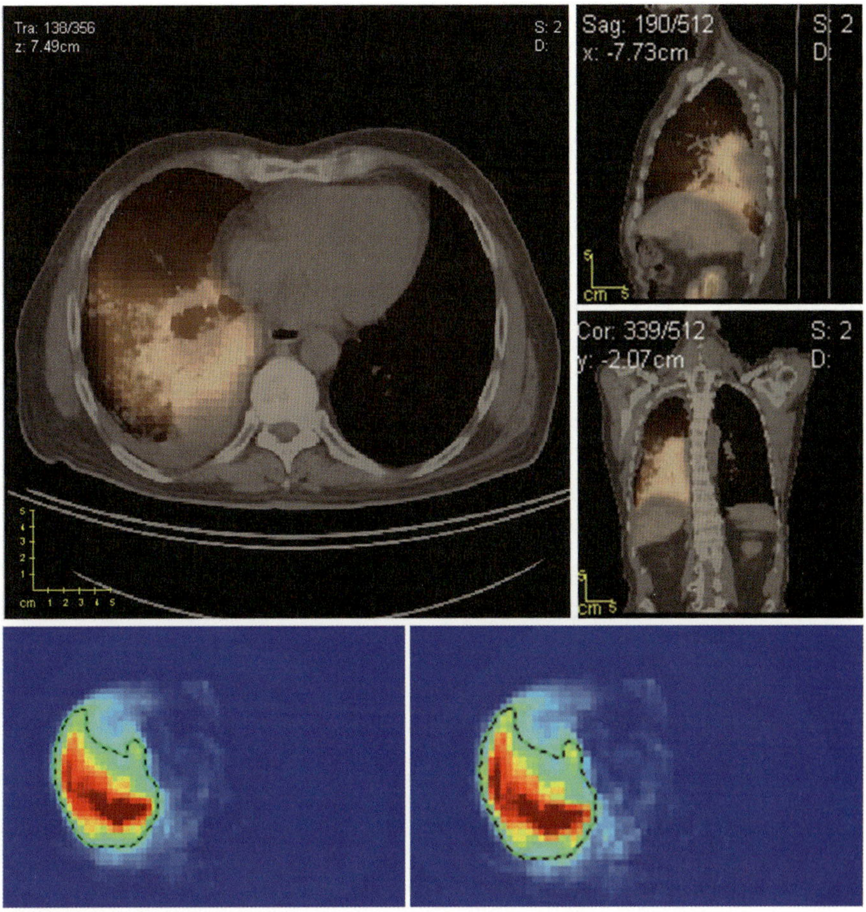

Fig. 14.5 A pretreatment PET/CT scan of a lung cancer patient who failed locally after radiotherapy treatment. *Top row* shows scan samples in different views (transverse, sagittal, coronal). The *bottom row* shows the motion probability spread function (PSF) for not motion-corrected and motion-corrected (*left to right*)

consisted of a model of two parameters from features from both PET and CT based on intensity volume histograms provided the best.

14.3.2 Predicting Distant Metastasis in Soft Tissue Sarcoma

A dataset of 51 patients with histologically proven STS was retrospectively analyzed. All patients had pretreatment FDG-PET and MR scans. MR data comprised of T1-weighted (T1w), T2 fat-saturated (T2FS), and T2 short tau inversion recovery (STIR) sequences as shown in Fig. 14.8.

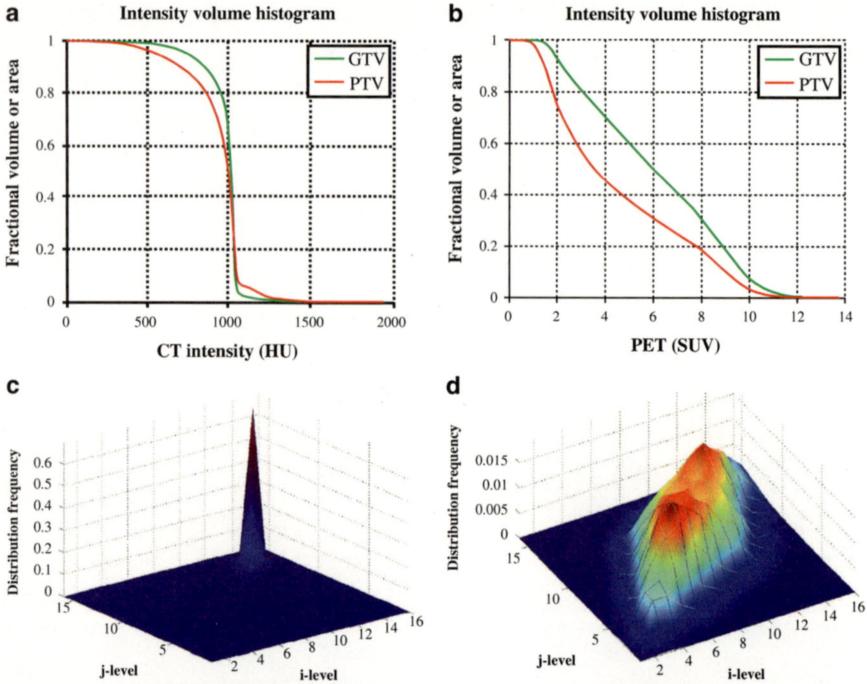

Fig. 14.6 (**a**) Intensity volume histograms (IVH) of (b) CT and (**b**) PET, respectively. (**c**) and (**d**) are the texture maps of the corresponding region of interest for CT (intensity bins equal 100 HU) and PET (intensity bins equal 1 unit of SUV), respectively. Note the variability between CT and PET features: the PET-IVH and co-occurrence matrices show much greater heterogeneity for this patient. Importantly, patients vary widely in the amount of PET and CT gross disease image heterogeneity between patients

A volume fusion process was carried out to combine information from two different volumes (PET and MR) into a single composite volume that is potentially more informative for texture analysis. Fusion of the scans was performed using the discrete wavelet transform (DWT) and a band-pass frequencies enhancement technique (Vallieres et al. 2015). In total, 41 different texture features were extracted out of the tumor regions of five different types of scans: FDG-PET, T1w and T2FS, fused FDG-PET/T1, and fused FDG-PET/T2FS scans. The texture features consisted of 3 features from first-order histograms, 7 features from GLCM, 13 features from GLRLM, 13 features from GLSZM, and 5 features from NGTDM. Optimal features were found using texture optimization based on imbalance-adjusted 0.632+ bootstrap resampling method (Sahiner et al. 2008). The resulting model consisted of four texture features representing variations in size and intensity of the different tumor subregions. It yielded a performance estimate in bootstrapping evaluations, with an area under the receiver-operating characteristic curve (AUC) of 0.984 ± 0.002, a sensitivity of 0.955 ± 0.006, a specificity of 0.926 ± 0.004, and an accuracy of 0.934 ± 0.003 as shown in Fig. 14.9.

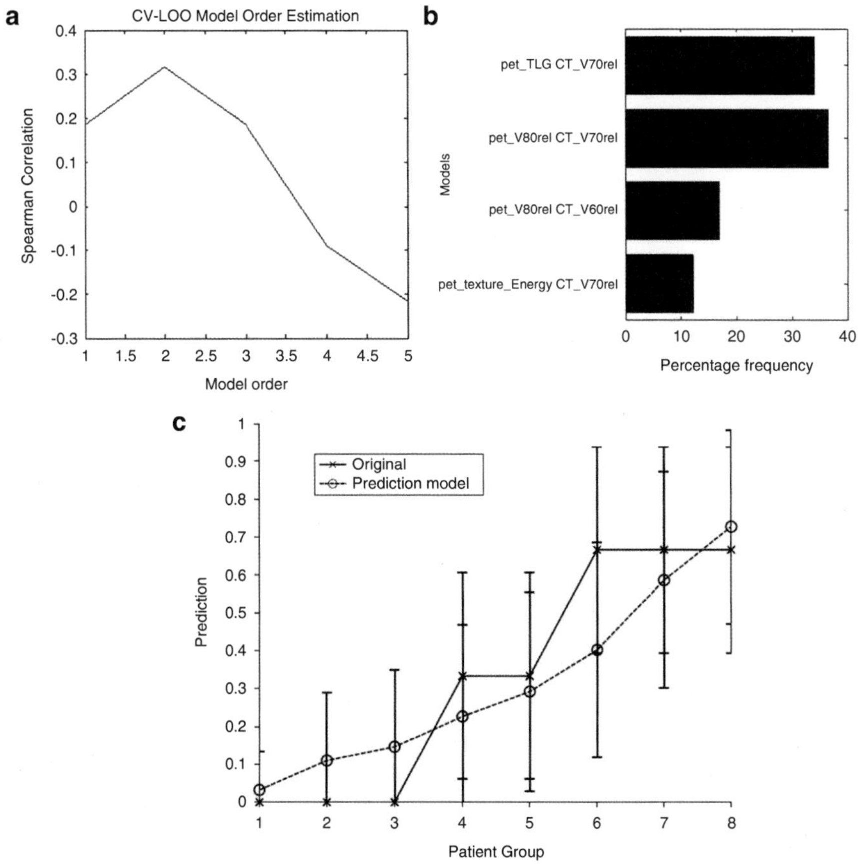

Fig. 14.7 Image-based modeling of local failure from PET/CT features. (**a**) Model order selection using leave-one-out cross-validation. (**b**) Most frequent model selection using bootstrap analysis where the y-axis represents the model selection frequency on resampled bootstrapped samples. (**c**) Plot of local failure probability as a function of patients binned into equal-size groups showing the model prediction of treatment failure risk and the original data (Reproduced with permission from Vaidya et al. 2012)

14.4 Discussion and Conclusions

The use of imaging in outcome modeling of radiotherapy response has witnessed rapid increase in recent years adding more value to already existing use of imaging in cancer treatment in general and radiotherapy in particular. However, there are several issues that are currently limiting its rapid progression. It is well recognized that image acquisition protocols may impact the reproducibility of extracted features from image modalities, which may consequently impact the robustness and stability of these features for treatment prediction. This includes static features such as SUV/HU descriptors and texture features. Interestingly, texture-based features

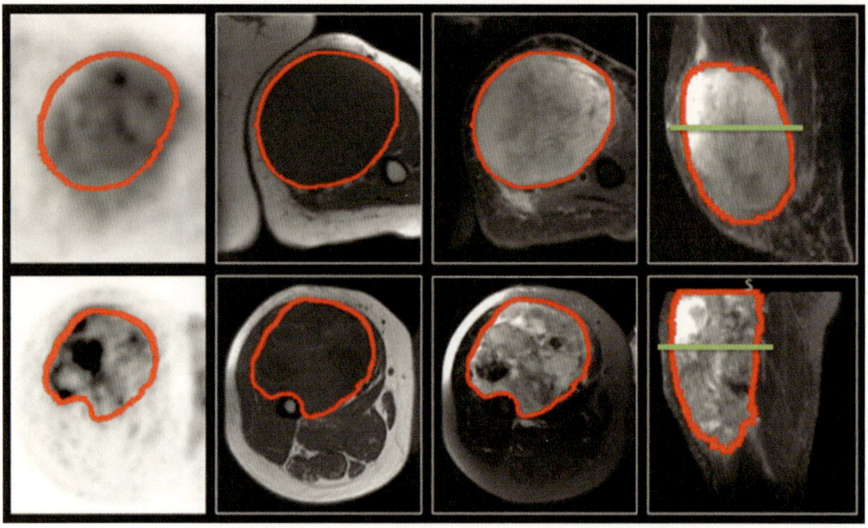

Fig. 14.8 FDG-PET and MR diagnostic images of two patients with soft tissue sarcomas of the extremities. *Top row*: patient that did not develop lung metastases. *Bottom row*: patient that eventually developed lung metastases. From *left* to *right*: FDG-PET, MR T1w, T2FS, and STIR (sagittal). The lines in the images of the fourth column which correspond to the plane shown in the previous images were taken

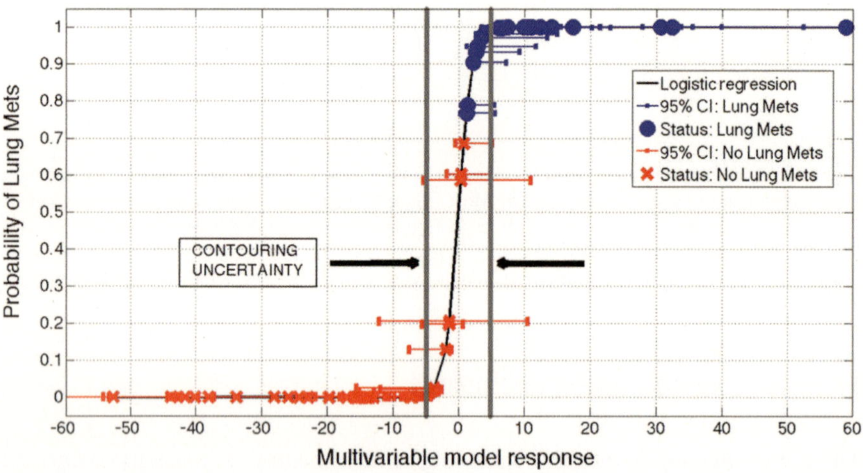

Fig. 14.9 Probability of developing lung metastases as a function of the response of the final multivariable model identified in this work, for all patients of the retrospective cohort (Reproduced from Vallières et al. 2015).

were shown to have a reproducibility similar to or better than that of simple SUV descriptors (Tixier et al. 2012). This demands protocols for standardized acquisition. In addition, factors that may impact the stability of these features also include signal-to-noise ratio (SNR), partial volume effect, motion artifacts, parameter settings, resampling size, and image quantization (El Naqa et al. 2009; Cheng et al. 2013). Nevertheless, advances in hardware and software technologies will further facilitate wider application of advanced image processing techniques to medical imaging to achieve better clinical results. For instance, pre-processing methods such as denoising and deconvolution methods already help in mitigating such artifacts (El Naqa et al. 2005; Zaidi et al. 2012); however, more advanced image restoration methods based on nonlocality and sparsity may be more fruitful (Gunturk and Li 2012). Outcome modeling using logistic regression has become a de facto standard; however, more advanced modeling techniques may provide further predictive power particularly when dealing with more complex and nonlinear relationships among features and between clinical outcomes. We believe that the synergy between image analysis and machine learning (El Naqa et al. 2015b) could provide powerful tools to strengthen and further the utilization of image-based outcome modeling in clinical practice toward improved clinical decision-making and personalized medicine in the future.

Acknowledgments Part of this work was supported by the Canadian Institutes of Health Research (CIHR) under grant MOP-136774 and by the Stuart and Barbara Padnos Research Fund (grant#G017459, University of Michigan Cancer Center). The author would like also to thank Dr. Carolyn Freeman, Mrs. Monica Serban, Mrs. Krishinima Jeyaseelan, Dr. Ives Levesque and Mr. Martin Carrier-Vallières, and Dr. Jan Seuntjens from McGill University for their collaboration on the Sarcoma Project.

References

Benz MR, Allen-Auerbach MS, Eilber F C, Chen HJJ, Dry S, Phelps ME, Czernin J, Weber WA (2008) Combined assessment of metabolic and volumetric changes for assessment of tumor response in patients with soft-tissue sarcomas. J Nucl Med 49:1579–1584

Bradley J (2004) The radiological society of North America. Chicago. Nov 28–Dec 3, vol. Series

Bradley J, Thorstad WL, Mutic S, Miller T R, Dehdashti F, Siegel B A, Bosch W, Bertrand R J (2004a) Impact of FDG-PET on radiation therapy volume delineation in non-small-cell lung cancer. Int J Radiat Oncol Biol Phys 59:78–86

Bradley JD, Perez CA, Dehdashti F, Siegel BA (2004b) Implementing biologic target volumes in radiation treatment planning for non-small cell lung cancer. J Nucl Med 45(Suppl 1):96S–101S

Castellano G, Bonilha L, Li LM, Cendes F (2004) Texture analysis of medical images. Clin Radiol 59:1061–1069

Castleman KR (1996) Digital image processing. Prentice Hall, Englewood Cliffs

Cheng NM, Fang YH, Yen TC (2013) The promise and limits of PET texture analysis. Ann Nucl Med 27:867–869

Chicklore S, Goh V, Siddique M, Roy A, Marsden P, Cook GR (2013) Quantifying tumour heterogeneity in 18F-FDG PET/CT imaging by texture analysis. Eur J Nucl Med Mol Imaging 40:133–140

Ciernik IF (2004) Radiotherapy of rectal cancer. Schweiz Rundsch Med Prax 93:1441–1446
Condeelis J, Weissleder R (2010) In vivo imaging in cancer. Cold Spring Harb Perspect Biol 2: a003848
de Crevoisier R, Tucker SL, Dong L, Mohan R, Cheung R, Cox JD, Kuban DA (2005) Increased risk of biochemical and local failure in patients with distended rectum on the planning CT for prostate cancer radiotherapy. Int J Radiat Oncol Biol Phys 62:965–973
Deasy JO, El Naqa I (2007) In: Mehta M, Bentzen S (eds) Radiation oncology advances. Springer, New York
Denecke T, Rau B, Hoffmann KT, Hildebrandt B, Ruf J, Gutberlet M, Hünerbein M, Felix R, Wust P, Amthauer H (2005) Comparison of CT, MRI and FDG-PET in response prediction of patients with locally advanced rectal cancer after multimodal preoperative therapy: Is there a benefit in using functional imaging? Eur Radiol 15:1658–1666
Einarsdottir H, Karlsson M, Wejde J, Bauer HCF (2004) Diffusion-weighted MRI of soft tissue tumours. Eur Radiol 14:959–963
El Naqa I (2013) In: Starkschall G, Siochi C (eds) Informatics in radiation oncology. CRC Press/Taylor and Francis, Boca Raton, pp 257–275
El Naqa I (2014) The role of quantitative PET in predicting cancer treatment outcomes. Clin Transl Imaging 2:305–320
El-Naqa I, Yang Y, Galatsanos NP, Nishikawa RM, Wernick MN (2004) A similarity learning approach to content-based image retrieval: application to digital mammography. IEEE Trans Med Imaging 23:1233–1244
El Naqa I, Kawrakow I, Fippel M, Siebers JV, Lindsay PE, Wickerhauser MV, Vicic M, Zakarian K, Kauffmann N, Deasy JO (2005) A comparison of Monte Carlo dose calculation denoising techniques. Phys Med Biol 50:909–922
El Naqa I, Bradley JD, Lindsay PE, Blanco AI, Vicic M, Hope AJ, Deasy JO (2006a) Multi-variable modeling of radiotherapy outcomes including dose-volume and clinical factors. Int J Radiat Oncol Biol Phys 64:1275–1286
El Naqa I, Low D, Bradley J, Vicic M, Deasy J (2006b) Deblurring of breathing motion artifacts in thoracic PET images by deconvolution methods. Med Phys 33:3587–3600
El Naqa I, Suneja G, Lindsay PE, Hope AJ, Alaly JR, Vicic M, Bradley JD, Apte A, Deasy JO (2006c) Dose response explorer: an integrated open-source tool for exploring and modelling radiotherapy dose-volume outcome relationships. Phys Med Biol 51:5719–5735
El Naqa I, Grigsby P, Apte A, Kidd E, Donnelly E, Khullar D, Chaudhari S, Yang D, Schmitt M, Laforest R, Thorstad W, Deasy JO (2009) Exploring feature-based approaches in PET images for predicting cancer treatment outcomes. Pattern Recogn 42:1162–1171
El Naqa I, Deasy JO, Mu Y, Huang E, Hope AJ, Lindsay PE, Apte A, Alaly J, Bradley JD (2010) Datamining approaches for modeling tumor control probability. Acta Oncol 49:1363–1373
El Naqa I, Li R, Murphy MJ (eds) (2015a) Machine learning in radiation oncology: theory and application. Springer International Publishing, Cham
El Naqa I, Li R, Murphy MJ (eds) (2015b) Machine learning in radiation oncology: theory and application. Springer International Publishing, Cham
Erdi YE, Macapinlac H, Rosenzweig KE, Humm JL, Larson SM, Erdi AK, Yorke ED (2000) Use of PET to monitor the response of lung cancer to radiation treatment. Eur J Nucl Med 27:861–866
Gulliford SL, Webb S, Rowbottom CG, Corne DW, Dearnaley DP (2004) Use of artificial neural networks to predict biological outcomes for patients receiving radical radiotherapy of the prostate. Radiother Oncol 71:3–12
Gunturk BK, Li X (eds) (2012) Image restoration: fundamentals and advances. CRC Press/Taylor and Francis group, Boca Raton
Haralick R, Shanmugam K, Dinstein I (1973) Texture features for image classification. IEEE Trans Sys Man Cyb SMC 3:610–621
Hastie T, Tibshirani R, Friedman JH (2001) The elements of statistical learning : data mining, inference, and prediction: with 200 full-color illustrations. Springer, New York

Haykin S (1999) Neural networks: a comprehensive foundation. Prentice Hall, New York

Hicks RJ, Mac Manus MP, Matthews JP, Hogg A, Binns D, Rischin D, Ball DL, Peters LJ (2004) Early FDG-PET imaging after radical radiotherapy for non-small-cell lung cancer: Inflammatory changes in normal tissues correlate with tumor response and do not confound therapeutic response evaluation Int J Radiat Oncol Biol Phys 60:412–418

Jain AK (1989) Fundamentals of digital image processing. Prentice Hall, Englewood Cliffs

Kalff V, Duong C, Drummond EG, Matthews JP, Hicks RJ (2006) Findings on 18F-FDG PET scans after neoadjuvant chemoradiation provides prognostic stratification in patients with locally advanced rectal carcinoma subsequently treated by radical surgery. J Nucl Med 47:14–22

Khan FM (2007) Treatment planning in radiation oncology. Lippincott Williams & Wilkins, Philadelphia

Kumar V, Gu Y, Basu S, Berglund A, Eschrich SA, Schabath MB, Forster K, Aerts HJ, Dekker A, Fenstermacher D, Goldgof DB, Hall LO, Lambin P, Balagurunathan Y, Gatenby R A, Gillies R J (2012) Radiomics: the process and the challenges. Magn Reson Imaging 30:1234–1248

Lambin P, Rios-Velazquez E, Leijenaar R, Carvalho S, van Stiphout RG, Granton P, Zegers CM, Gillies R, Boellard R, Dekker A, Aerts H J (2012) Radiomics: extracting more information from medical images using advanced feature analysis. Eur J Cancer 48:441–446

Larson SM, Erdi Y, Akhurst T, Mazumdar M, Macapinlac HA, Finn RD, Casilla C, Fazzari M, Srivastava N, Yeung HW, Humm JL, Guillem J, Downey R, Karpeh M, Cohen AE, Ginsberg R (1999) Tumor treatment response based on visual and quantitative changes in global tumor glycolysis using PET-FDG imaging. The visual response score and the change in total lesion glycolysis. Clin Positron Imaging 2:159–171

Mac Manus MP, Hicks RJ (2003) PET scanning in lung cancer: current status and future directions. Semin Surg Oncol 21:149–155

Mac Manus MP, Hicks RJ, Matthews JP, McKenzie A, Rischin D, Salminen EK, Ball DL (2003) Positron emission tomography is superior to computed tomography scanning for response-assessment after radical radiotherapy or chemoradiotherapy in patients with non-small-cell lung cancer. J Clin Oncol 21:1285–1292

MacManus MR, Hicks R, Fisher R, Rischin D, Michael M, Wirth A, Ball DL (2003) FDG-PET-detected extracranial metastasis in patients with non-small cell lung cancer undergoing staging for surgery or radical radiotherapy – survival correlates with metastatic disease burden. Acta Oncol 42:48–54

Miller TR, Grigsby PW (2002) Measurement of tumor volume by PET to evaluate prognosis in patients with advanced cervical cancer treated by radiation therapy. Int J Radiat Oncol Biol Phys 53:353–359

Munley MT, Lo JY, Sibley GS, Bentel GC, Anscher MS, Marks LB (1999) A neural network to predict symptomatic lung injury. Phys Med Biol 44:2241–2249

Mutic S, Malyapa RS, Grigsby PW, Dehdashti F, Miller TR, Zoberi I, Bosch WR, Esthappan J, Low DA (2003) PET-guided IMRT for cervical carcinoma with positive para-aortic lymph nodes-a dose-escalation treatment planning study. Int J Radiat Oncol Biol Phys 55:28–35

Newbold K, Partridge M, Cook G, Sohaib SA, Charles-Edwards E, Rhys-Evans P, Harrington K, Nutting C (2006) Advanced imaging applied to radiotherapy planning in head and neck cancer: a clinical review. Br J Radiol 79:554–561

O'Sullivan F, Roy S, Eary J (2003) A statistical measure of tissue heterogeneity with application to 3D PET sarcoma data. Biostat 4:433–448

O'Sullivan F, Roy S, O'Sullivan J, Vernon C, Eary J (2005) Incorporation of tumor shape into an assessment of spatial heterogeneity for human sarcomas imaged with FDG-PET. Biostat 6:293–301

Pandit N, Gonen M, Krug L, Larson SM (2003) Prognostic value of [18F]FDG-PET imaging in small cell lung cancer. Eur J Nucl Med Mol Imaging 30:78–84

Piet D, Frederik De K, Vincent V, Sigrid S, Robert H, Sandra N (2008) Diffusion-weighted magnetic resonance imaging to evaluate major salivary gland function before and after radiotherapy. Int J Radiat Oncol Biol Phys 71:1365

Ramsey CR, Langen KM, Kupelian PA, Scaperoth DD, Meeks SL, Mahan SL, Seibert RM (2006) A technique for adaptive image-guided helical tomotherapy for lung cancer. Int J Radiat Oncol Biol Phys 64:1237–1244

Reader AJ, Matthews JC, Sureau FC, Comtat C, Trebossen R, Buvat I (2006) Nuclear science symposium conference record, 2006. IEEE,Oct 29 2006–Nov 1 2006), vol. Series 3) pp 1752–1756

Sahiner B, Chan H-P, Hadjiiski L (2008) Classifier performance prediction for computer-aided diagnosis using a limited dataset. Med Phys 35:1559–1570

Seibert RM, Ramsey CR, Hines JW, Kupelian PA, Langen KM, Meeks SL, Scaperoth DD (2007) A model for predicting lung cancer response to therapy. Int J Radiat Oncol Biol Phys 67:601–609

Shapeero LG, Vanel D, Verstraete KL, Bloem JL (2002) Fast magnetic resonance imaging with contrast for soft tissue sarcoma viability. Clin Orthop Relat Res:212–227

Shields AF (2006) Positron emission tomography measurement of tumor metabolism and growth: its expanding role in oncology. Mol Imaging Biol 8:141–150

Sourbron SP, Buckley DL (2011) On the scope and interpretation of the Tofts models for DCE-MRI. Magn Reson Med 66:735–745

Stasi M, Munoz F, Fiorino C, Pasquino M, Baiotto B, Marini P, Malinverni G, Valdagni R, Gabriele P (2006) Emptying the rectum before treatment delivery limits the variations of rectal dose – volume parameters during 3DCRT of prostate cancer. Radiother Oncol 80:363–370

Steel GG (2002) Basic clinical radiobiology. London/New York: Arnold/Oxford University Press

Strauss LG, Conti PS (1991) The applications of PET in clinical oncology. J Nucl Med 32:623–648

Su M, Miftena M, Whiddon C, Sun X, Light K, Marks L (2005) An artificial neural network for predicting the incidence of radiation pneumonitis. Med Phys 32:318–325

Thorwarth D, Eschmann S-M, Holzner F, Paulsen F, Alber M (2006) Combined uptake of [18F] FDG and [18F]FMISO correlates with radiation therapy outcome in head-and-neck cancer patients. Radiother Oncol 80:151–156

Thorwarth D, Eschmann S-M, Paulsen F, Alber M (2007) A model of reoxygenation dynamics of head-and-neck tumors based on serial 18F-fluoromisonidazole positron emission tomography investigations. Int J Radiat Oncol Biol Phys 68:515–521

Thorwarth D, Muller AC, Pfannenberg C, Beyer T (2013) Combined PET/MR imaging using (68) Ga-DOTATOC for radiotherapy treatment planning in meningioma patients. Recent Results Cancer Res 194:425–439

Tixier F, Hatt M, Le Rest CC, Le Pogam A, Corcos L, Visvikis D (2012) Reproducibility of tumor uptake heterogeneity characterization through textural feature analysis in 18F-FDG PET. J Nucl Med 53:693–700

Tofts PS (1997) Modeling tracer kinetics in dynamic Gd-DTPA MR imaging. J Magn Reson Imaging 7:91–101

Toloza EM, Harpole L, McCrory DC (2003) Noninvasive staging of non-small cell lung cancer: a review of the current evidence. Chest 123:137S–146S

Tomatis S, Rancati T, Fiorino C, Vavassori V, Fellin G, Cagna E, Mauro FA, Girelli G, Monti A, Baccolini M, Naldi G, Bianchi C, Menegotti L, Pasquino M, Stasi M, Valdagni R (2012) Late rectal bleeding after 3D–CRT for prostate cancer: development of a neural-network-based predictive model. Phys Med Biol 57:1399

Turkheimer FE, Aston JA, Asselin MC, Hinz R (2006) Multi-resolution Bayesian regression in PET dynamic studies using wavelets. NeuroImage 32:111–121

Vaidya M, Creach KM, Frye J, Dehdashti F, Bradley J D, El Naqa I (2012) Combined PET/CT image characteristics for radiotherapy tumor response in lung cancer. Radiothe Oncology J Eur Soc Therap Radiol Oncol 102:239–245

Vallieres M, Freeman CR, Skamene SR, El Naqa I (2015) A radiomics model from joint FDG-PET and MRI texture features for the prediction of lung metastases in soft-tissue sarcomas of the extremities. Phys Med Biol 60:5471–5496 van Rijswijk CSP, Geirnaerdt MJA, Hogendoorn PCW, Peterse JL, van Coevorden F, Taminiau AHM, Tollenaar RAEM, Kroon BBR, Bloem JL (2003) Dynamic contrast-enhanced MR imaging in monitoring response to isolated limb perfusion in high-grade soft tissue sarcoma: initial results. Eur Radiol 13:1849–1858

Vanel D, Bonvalot S, Guinebretière JM, Petrow P, Dromain C, Caillet H (2004) MR imaging in the evaluation of isolated limb perfusion: a prospective study of 18 cases. Skelet Radiol 33:150–156

Vapnik V (1998) Statistical learning theory. Wiley, New York

Verhagen AF, Bootsma GP, Tjan-Heijnen VC, van der Wilt GJ, Cox AL, Brouwer MH, Corstens FH, Oyen WJ (2004) FDG-PET in staging lung cancer: how does it change the algorithm? Lung Cancer 44:175–181

Watabe H, Ikoma Y, Kimura Y, Naganawa M, Shidahara M (2006) PET kinetic analysis – compartmental model. Ann Nucl Med 20:583–588

Webb S (2001) The physics of three-dimensional radiation therapy: conformal radiotherapy, radiosurgery, and treatment planning. Institute of Physics Pub, Bristol/Philadelphia

Willmann JK, van Bruggen N, Dinkelborg LM, Gambhir SS (2008) Molecular imaging in drug development. Nat Rev Drug Discov 7:591–607

Yang D-H, Min J-J, Jeong Y, Ahn J-S, Kim Y-K, Cho S-H, Chung I-J, Bom H-S, Kim H-J, Lee J-J (2009) The combined evaluation of interim contrast-enhanced computerized tomography (CT) and FDG-PET/CT predicts the clinical outcomes and may impact on the therapeutic plans in patients with aggressive non-Hodgkin's lymphoma. Ann Hematol 88:425–432

Zaidi H, Mawlawi O, Orton CG (2007) Point/counterpoint. Simultaneous PET/MR will replace PET/CT as the molecular multimodality imaging platform of choice. Med Phys 34:1525–1528

Zaidi H, Abdoli M, Fuentes CL, El Naqa IM (2012) Comparative methods for PET image segmentation in pharyngolaryngeal squamous cell carcinoma. Eur J Nucl Med Mol Imaging 39:881–891

Zhang J, Tan T (2002) Brief review of invariant texture analysis methods. Pattern Recogn 35:735–747

Index

H. Arimura (ed.), *Image-Based Computer-Assisted Radiation Therapy*,
DOI 10.1007/978-981-10-2945-5

Printed by Printforce, the Netherlands